CONTENTS

A Colour Handbook

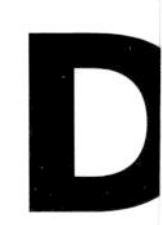

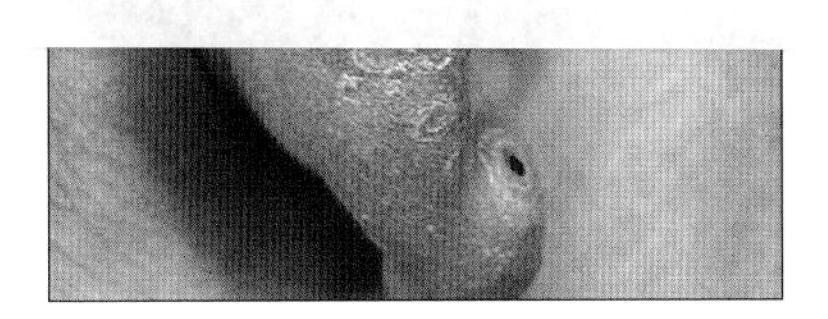

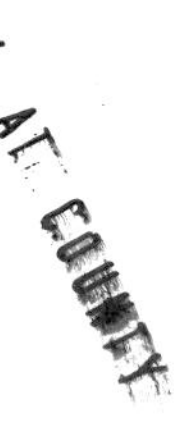

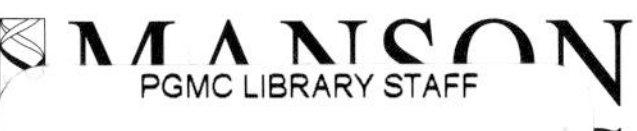

ISBN: 978-1-84076-110-8

A CIP catalogue record for this book is available from the British Library.

For full details of all Manson Publishing Ltd titles please write to:
Manson Publishing Ltd, 73 Corringham Road, London NW11 7DL, UK.
Tel: +44(0)20 8905 5150
Fax: +44(0)20 8201 9233
Email: manson@mansonpublishing.com
Website: www.mansonpublishing.com

Commissioning editor: Jill Northcott
Project manager: Ayala Kingsley
Copy editor: Ruth Maxwell
Cover and book design: Ayala Kingsley
Additional layout: DiacriTech, Chennai, India
Colour reproduction: Tenon & Polert Colour Scanning Ltd., Hong Kong
Printed by: New Era Printing Co Ltd., Hong Kong

PART 2
TUMOURS

Benign tumours arising from the epidermis

Benign tumours arising from the dermis

Benign tumours arising from skin appendages

Benign melanocytic lesions

Malignant neoplasms and their precursors

Cutaneous lymphoproliferative disorders

PART 3
INFECTIONS AND INFESTATIONS

Bacterial infections

Fungal diseases

Viral infections

Human immunodeficiency virus (HIV) infection

Infestations

Tropical infections

PREFACE TO THE SECOND EDITION

Stuart Robertson and I had hoped that, if we omitted treatment from this little book, then it would never need to be revised. We had underestimated the devotion of our readership to the cause of making patients better. Giving in eventually to the pleas of our publisher, our only stipulation was that we would need the help of a third editor. And who better, we thought, than Sarah Wakelin, already an experienced author in this field?

At the same time as this wholesale improvement, the opportunity was taken to correct deficiencies in the coverage of skin disorders, including HIV infection, while thoroughly revising the original text and illustrations. More than a hundred new illustrations have thus been incorporated, provided very largely by the indefatigable Stuart Robertson.

The result is an even more useful book than before, one that will be a dependable guide to those starting out on dermatological training, whether doctors or nurses, as well as to more experienced health professionals in other disciplines, including general practice and occupational health.

I thank both my fellow editors for working with me so attentively to breathe new life into the Colour Handbook.

RICHARD J G RYCROFT

History

Diagnosis in dermatology follows the standard approach of history taking and physical examination. Questions relating to the presenting dermatosis should answer the following: time and site of onset; ensuing course; provoking and relieving factors (sunlight, temperature, occupation, and so on.) and associated symptoms (itch, pain, and so on.). It is important to elicit a history of any previous general medical or surgical problems as well as details of past dermatological conditions. A past history of eczema or psoriasis is of particular relevance. Enquiry into the occurrence of the common inherited dermatoses (such as atopic eczema, psoriasis, or ichthyosis) in first-degree relatives is useful, as is a history of infectious illness in close personal contacts. Aspects of the patient's daily life are relevant to the diagnosis of many skin diseases: occupational or recreational contact with potentially sensitizing substances may be pertinent, as may a history of excess sun exposure. A detailed drug history is mandatory. A full list of medications taken for other conditions may reveal a possible culprit in iatrogenic skin disease, while knowledge of concomitant therapies may help to avoid drug interactions or polypharmacy. Current and past use of topical agents should be noted.

Examination

The diagnosis of skin disease is dependent on careful examination and the correct interpretation of cutaneous physical signs. In addition to an inspection of the area(s) of involvement, a dermatological examination should include visual assessment of the whole skin. Adequate illumination is imperative, while additional torch-light may be required to examine the oral cavity. At times, a light source positioned obliquely to the lesions can reveal important morphological information. Closer inspection of individual lesions is often helpful and is facilitated by the use of a hand lens. Palpation of the lesional skin should always be undertaken to provide information on temperature, consistency, and level of tissue involvement. Examination of the regional lymph nodes is sometimes necessary.

In order to extract the maximum amount of information for diagnostic purposes, four aspects of the lesion(s) under scrutiny need to be recorded:

- Morphology.
- Shape.
- Distribution.
- Colour.

Morphology

Most skin lesions have a characteristic morphology which, once defined, will narrow the differential diagnosis. The following list describes the features of the common primary lesions:

- Macule.
- Papule.
- Nodule.
- Plaque.
- Wheal.
- Vesicle.
- Bulla.
- Pustule.
- Erosion.
- Ulcer.
- Fissure.
- Telangiectasia.
- Comedone.

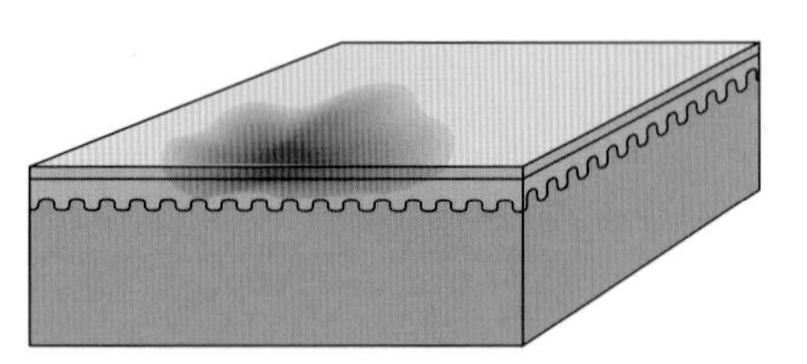

Macule – a flat, non-palpable lesion, distinguished from adjacent, normal skin by a change in colour.

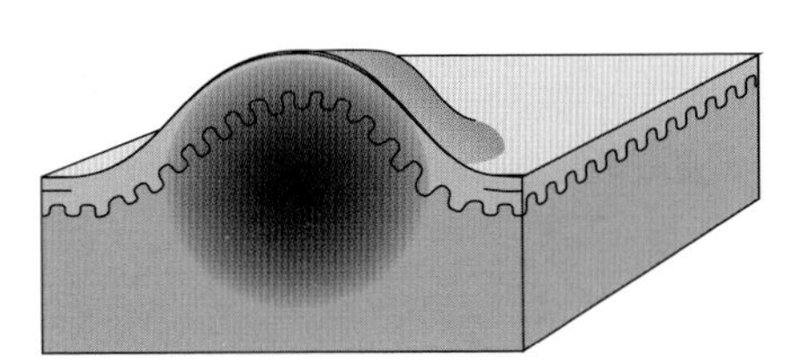

Papule – a small, solid and raised lesion less than 5 mm in diameter). A raised legion larger than 5 mm is a nodule.

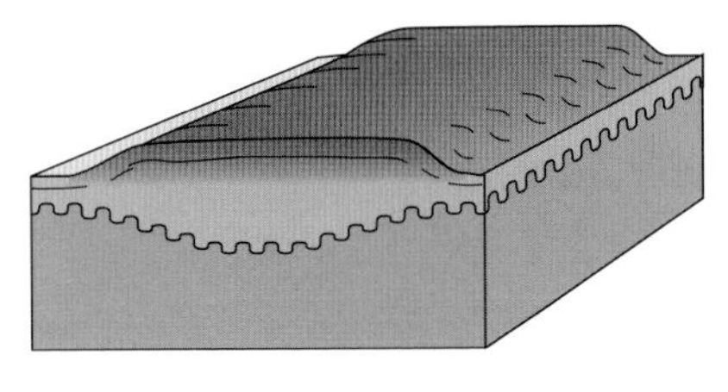

Plaque – a flat-topped lesion with a diameter considerably greater than its height.

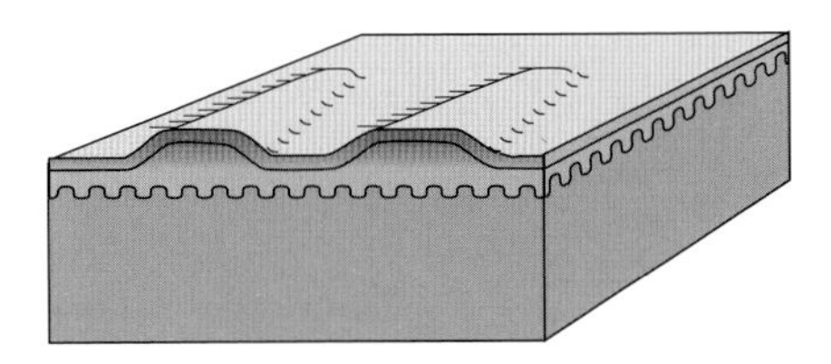

Wheal – a transient swelling of the skin of any size, often associated with surrounding, localized erythema (the flare).

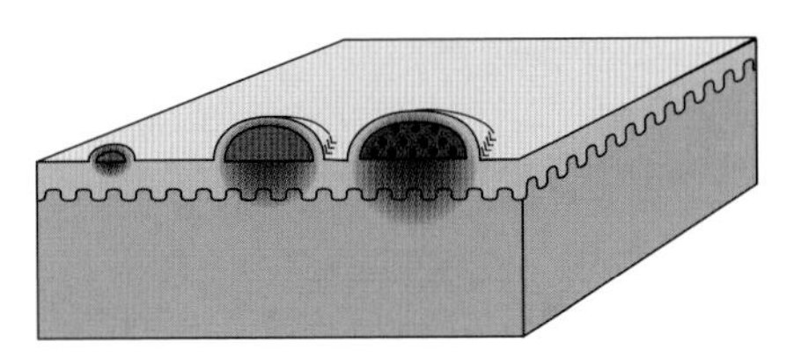

Vesicle – a blister less than 5 mm in diameter. A blister greater than 5 mm in diameter is a bulla.

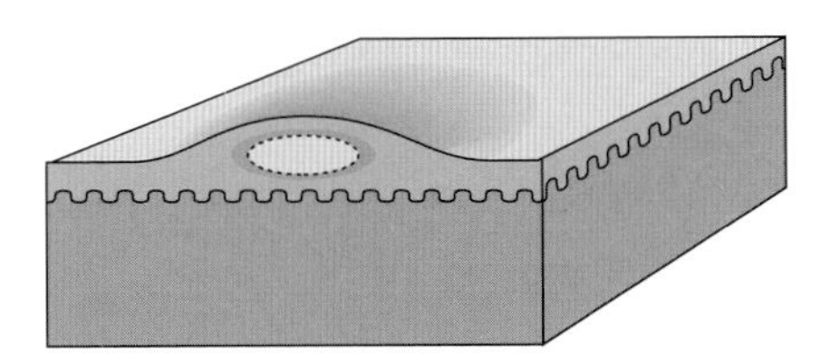

Pustule – a visible accumulation of pus, therefore white, yellow, or green in colour.

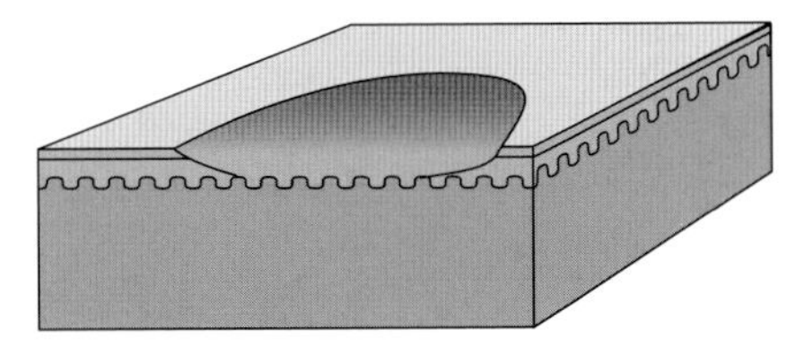

Erosion – an area of skin from which the epidermis alone has been lost.

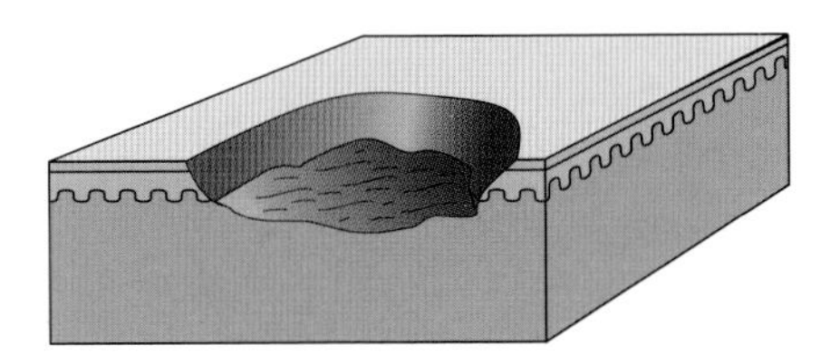

Ulcer – an area of skin from which the epidermis and part of the dermis has been lost.

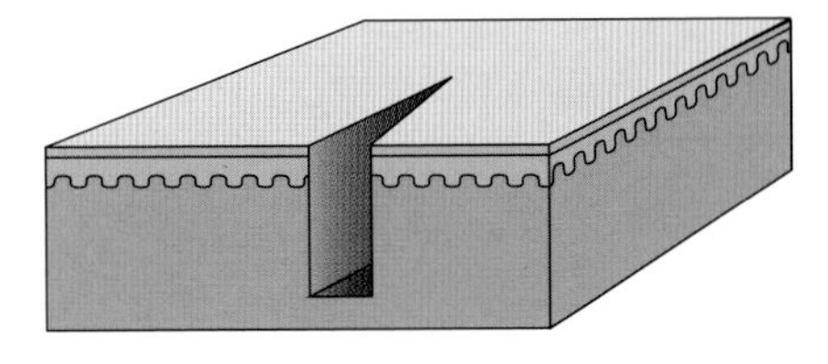

Fissure – a cleft-shaped ulcer.

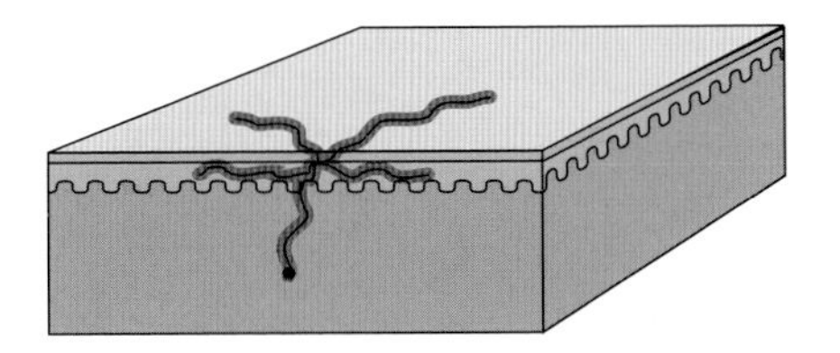

Telangiectasia – a visibly-dilated, small, dermal blood vessel.

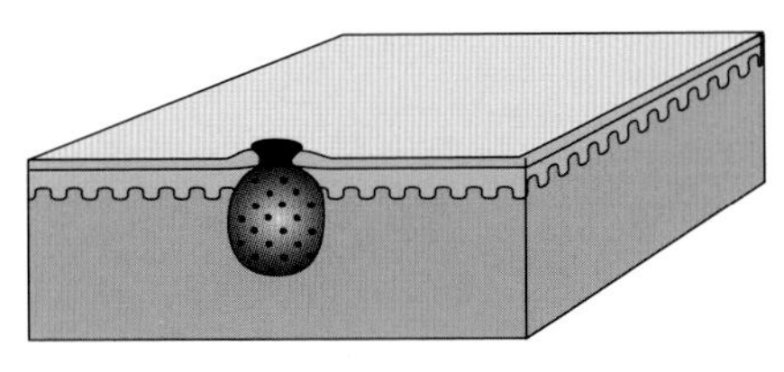

Comedone – accumulation of keratin and sebum lodged in dilated pilosebaceous orifice.

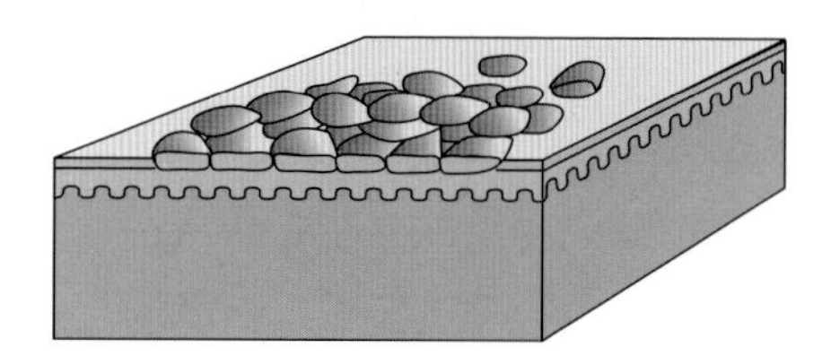

Scale – a flake of keratinized epidermal cells lying on the skin surface.

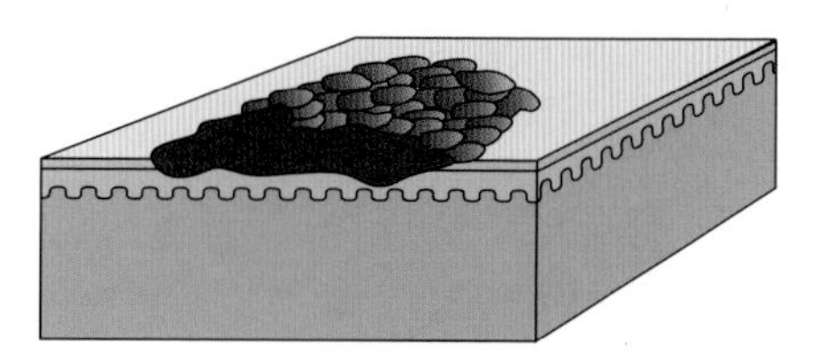

Crust – dried serous or sanguineous exudate.

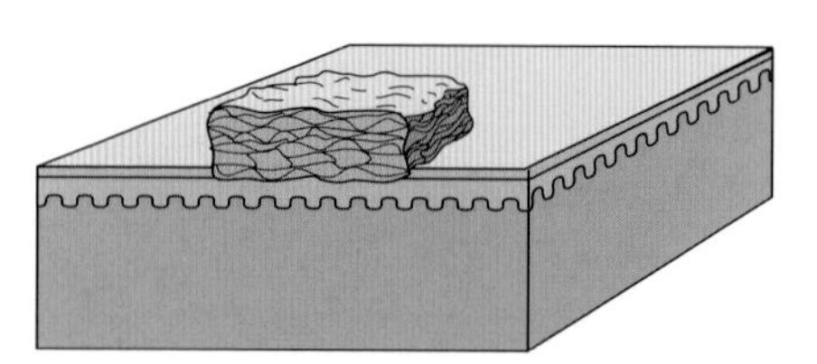

Hyperkeratosis – an area of thickened stratum corneum.

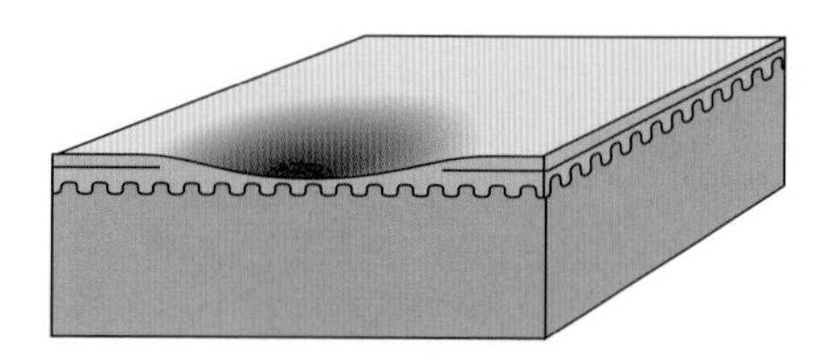

Atrophy – thinning of the skin due to the partial loss of one or more of the tissue layers of the skin (epidermis, dermis, sub-cutis).

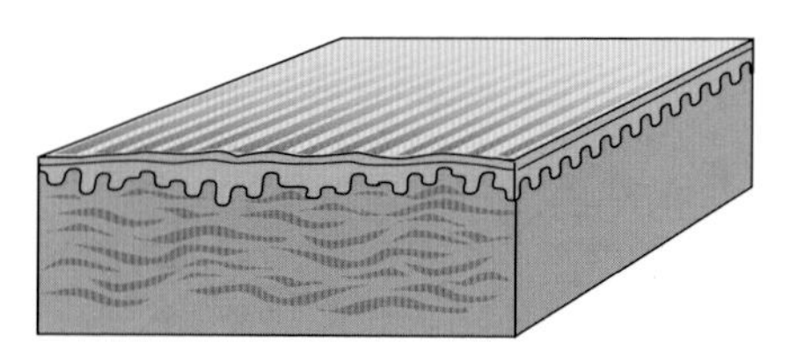

Sclerosis – hardening of the skin due to dermal pathological change (often an expansion of collagenous elements) characterized by induration.

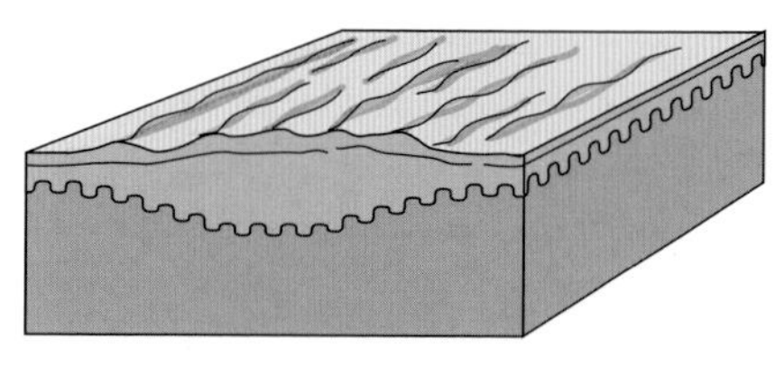

Lichenification – thickened skin with increased markings usually due to prolonged scratching.

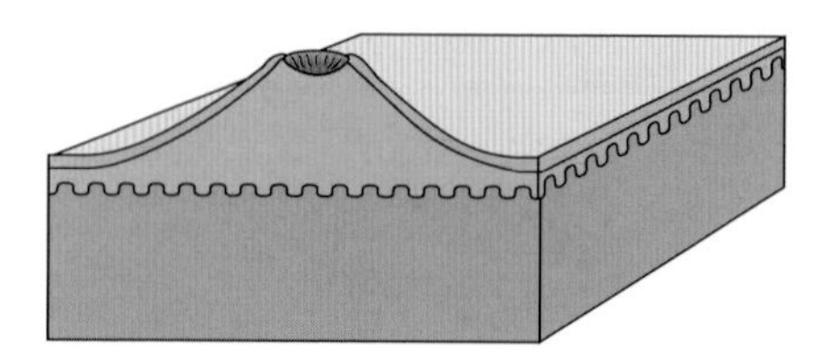

Umbilicated – shaped like the umbilicus .

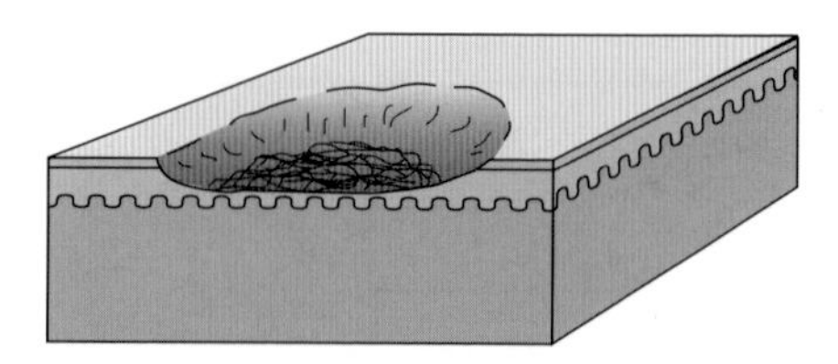

Exudate – material escaped from blood vessels with a high content of protein, cells, cellular debris, and so on.

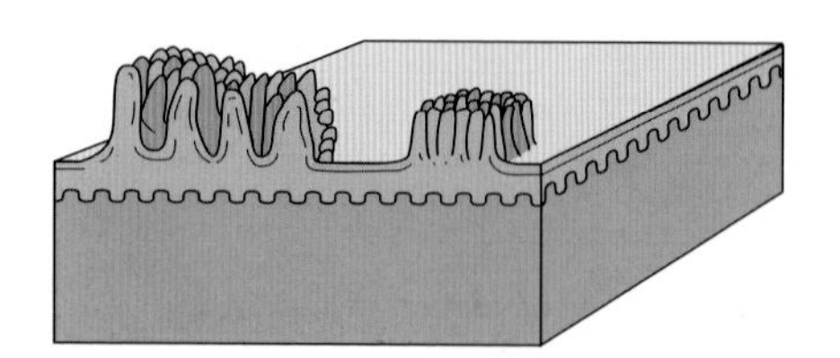

Warty – horny excrescence.

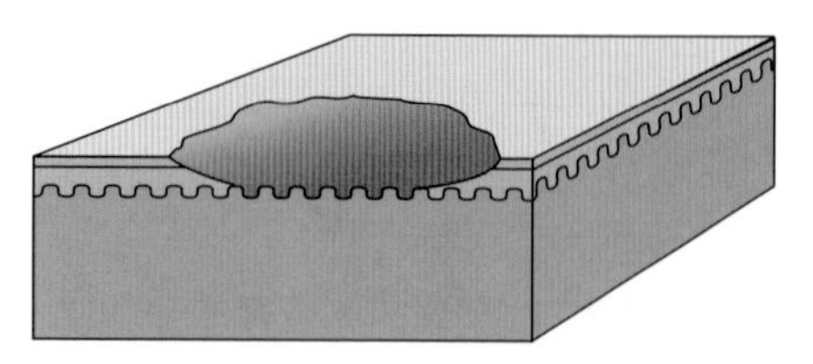

Excoriation – scratch or abrasion of the skin.

A primary lesion can be associated with additional, superimposed features:

- Scale.
- Crust.
- Hyperkeratosis.
- Atrophy.
- Sclerosis.
- Lichenification .
- Umbilicated.
- Exudate.
- Warty.
- Excoriation.

Shape

The shape of individual lesions has a clinical significance as certain dermatoses consist of lesions with a characteristic shape. Commonly observed shapes or patterns are as follows:

- Linear.
- Discoid refers to a coin-shaped lesion.
- Annular describes a ring-shaped lesion.
- Target describes a lesion consisting of concentric rings.
- Polycyclic describes a pattern of interlocking rings.
- Arcuate describes lesions that are arc shaped.
- Serpiginous describes a linear lesion which is wavy in shape.
- Whorled is used to describe lesions which follow the developmental lines of Blaschko and demonstrate a curved or spiral pattern.
- Digitate refers to lesions which are finger-like in shape.
- Zosteriform means resembling herpes zoster (see p. 231).

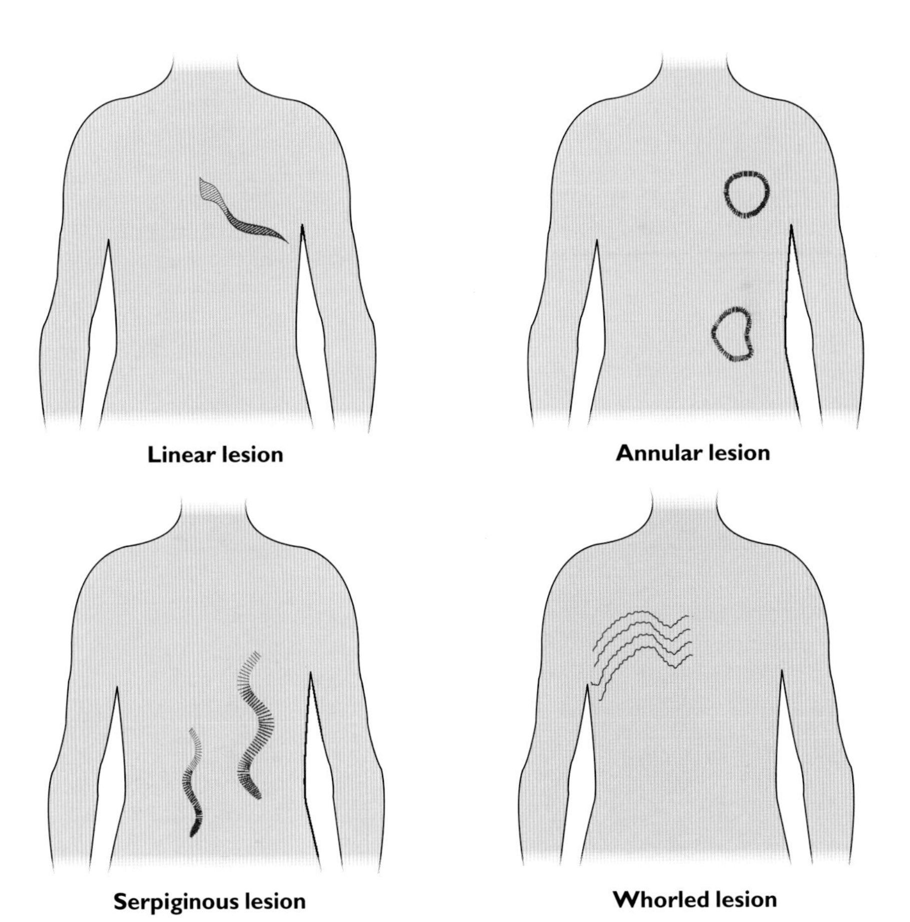

Distribution

The majority of skin diseases have a characteristic distribution or a predilection for certain sites. Other dermatoses vary in extent of involvement according to their severity. The recognition of particular configurations is important diagnostically, while defining the extent of involvement is useful for prognostic and therapeutic reasons. Discrete lesions occurring in a localized area are called *grouped*, while multiple lesions distributed over a wide area of skin are called *scattered*. There are terms which define widespread distributions more exactly:

- Exanthem refers to a predominantly truncal eruption consisting of multiple, symmetrical, erythematous, maculopapular lesions. Such dermatoses (called exanthematous) can be further described as being either morbilliform (meaning measles-like, comprised of blotchy, pink, slightly elevated lesions) or scarlatiniform (meaning scarlet fever-like, comprised of tiny erythematous papules).
- Confluent describes the appearance of a coalescence of individual lesions to form a large area of involvement.
- Erythroderma implies that a particular dermatosis involves more than 90% of the body surface area and that the involvement is confluent.

The distribution of lesions can also be described according to regional involvement, the recognition of which can help pinpoint a diagnosis:

- Centrifugal – mostly affecting the extremities, e.g. granuloma annulare.
- Centripetal – mostly affecting the trunk, e.g. pemphigus vulgaris.
- Centrifacial – mostly involving the forehead, nose, and chin, e.g. rosacea.
- Palmoplantar – affecting the palms and soles, e.g. palmoplantar pustulosis.
- Flexural – involving the flexural skin, e.g. erythrasma.
- Extensor – involving the extensor skin, e.g. plaque psoriasis.
- Dermatomal – affecting the skin of one or more dermatomes, e.g. shingles (herpes zoster).
- Periorbital – distributed around the eyes, e.g. syringomata.
- Perioral – distributed around the mouth, e.g. perioral dermatitis.
- Light-exposed – involving the skin routinely exposed to sunlight, e.g. chronic actinic dermatitis.

Colour

Cutaneous lesions can be flesh-coloured, demonstrate a change in pigmentation (hyper- or hypopigmentation), or be characterized by redness. Erythema is redness due to microvascular dilatation which can be blanched by pressure. Purpura is a darker cutaneous redness due to erythrocyte extravasation; purpura cannot be blanched by pressure.

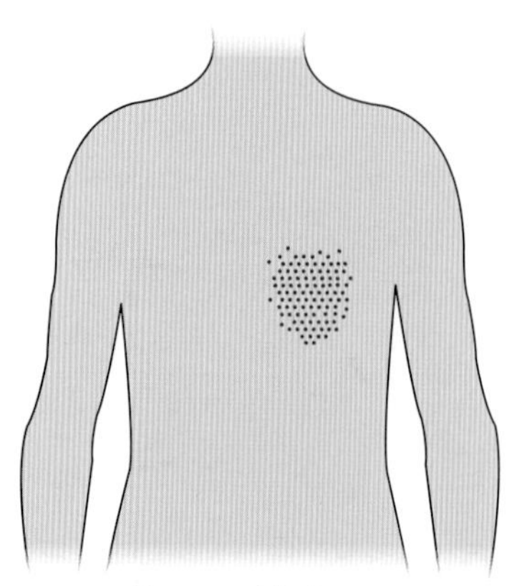

Grouped lesions

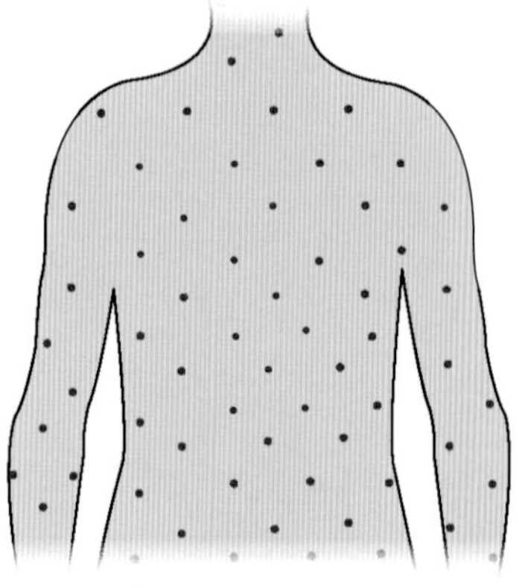

Scattered lesions

PART 1

Dermatoses

- **Eczema/dermatitis**
- **Non-dermatitic occupational dermatoses**
- **Urticaria**
- **Papulosquamous eruptions**
- **Blistering diseases**
- **Disorders of keratinization**
- **Disorders of the sebaceous and apocrine glands**
- **Genital and perianal dermatoses**
- **Hair disorders**
- **Pigmentation disorders**
- **Photosensitivity disorders**
- **Disorders of the blood vessels**
- **Skin manifestations of systemic disease**
- **Drug eruptions**

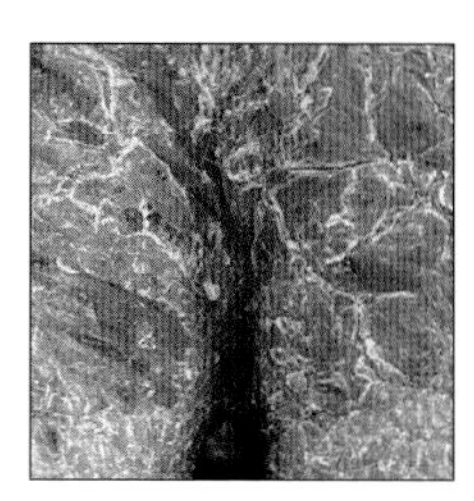
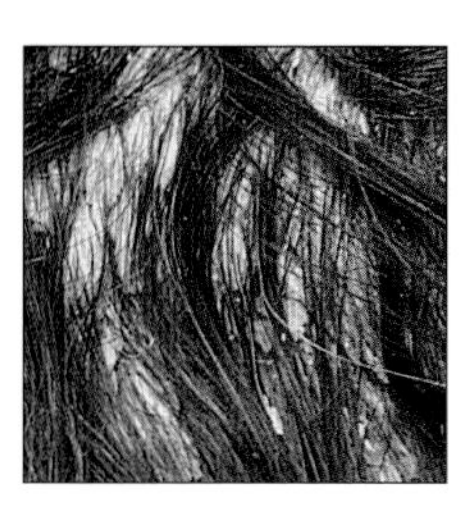
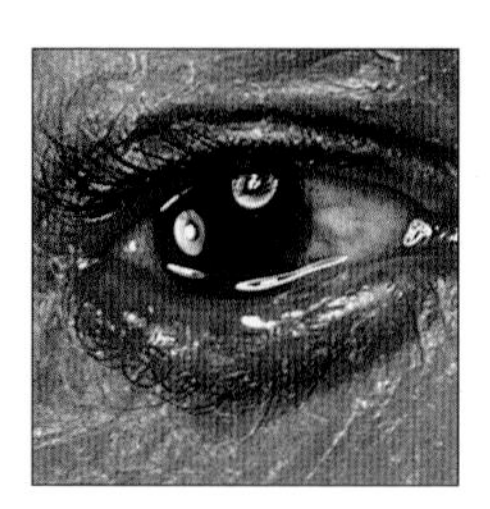
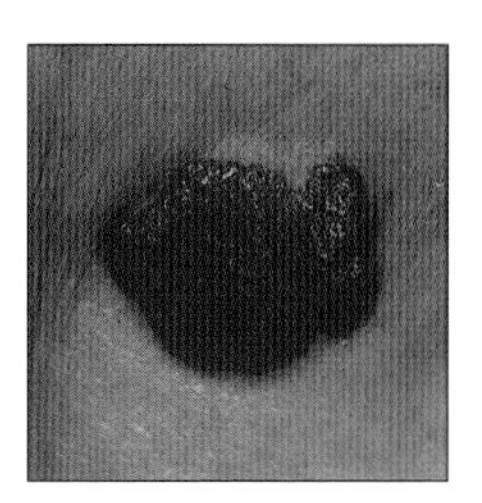

ECZEMA/DERMATITIS

Endogenous or constitutional eczemas are a group of dermatoses where a primary external cause is not established. Like anaemia, the word eczema is not a diagnosis in itself and should prompt further enquiry to identify the subtype of eczema or a treatable cause.

Atopic eczema
(atopic dermatitis)

DEFINITION AND CLINICAL FEATURES

A chronic, pruritic condition which affects the skin flexures and usually starts in the first 2 years of life. The prevalence of atopic eczema in developed countries has increased in recent decades and approximately 20% of children are affected at some time. There is often a family history of atopy and sufferers are at increased risk of having food allergies and developing asthma and hay fever. It is thought that environmental factors such as a reduction in early exposure to infections and increased exposure to household allergens are responsible for the rise in prevalence of atopic diseases.

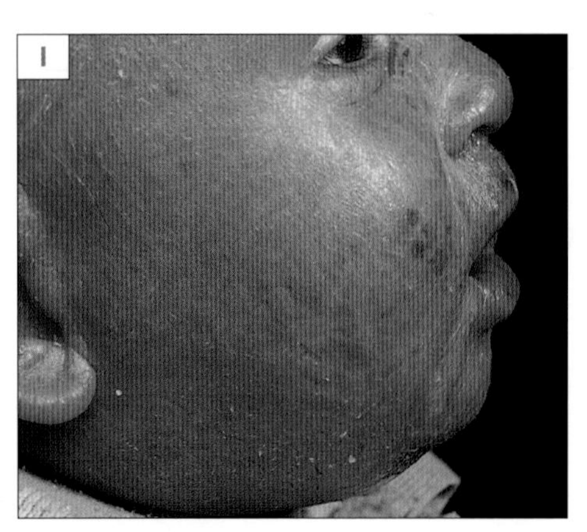

1 Infantile eczema.

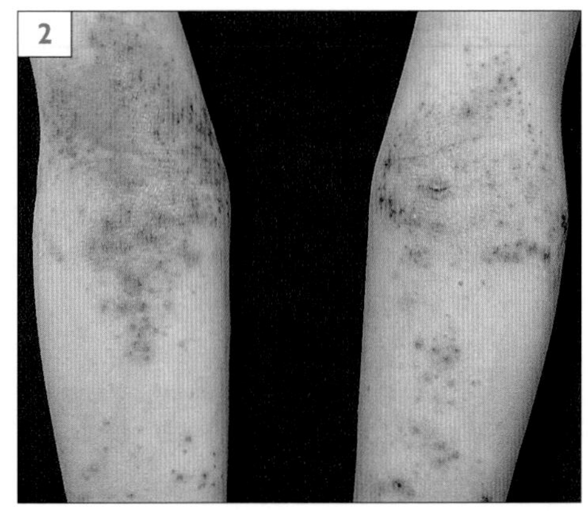

2 Flexural eczema.

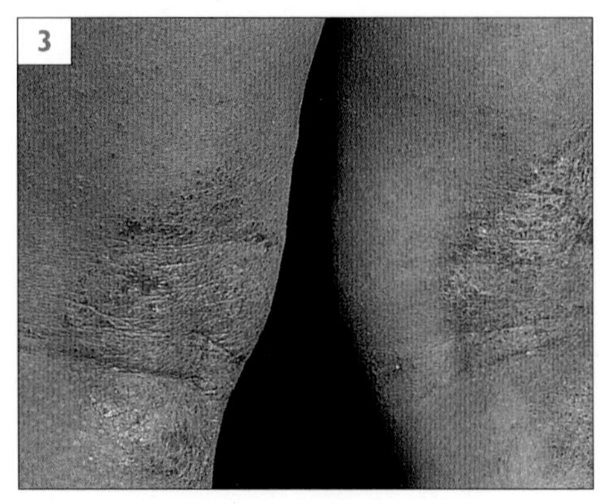

3 Flexural eczema.

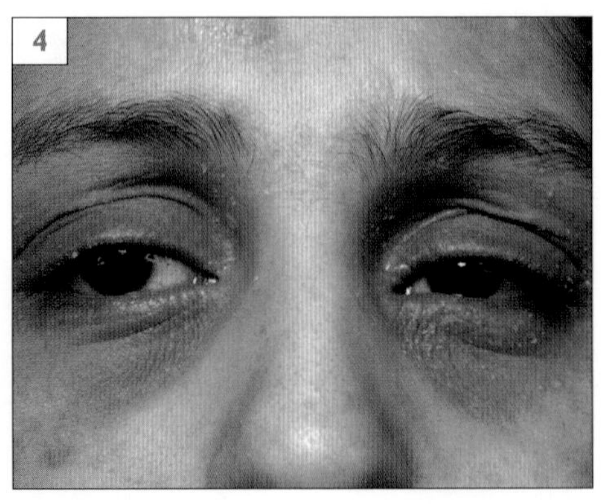

4 Orbital eczema.

Eczematous lesions often present on exposed areas such as the cheeks (**1**) or outer aspects of the forearms or legs. The lesions are red, poorly defined, and surface changes such as scaling, erosions, papules, or vesicles are present. In the older child, eczema usually affects flexural sites such as the antecubital (**2**) and popliteal fossae (**3**), and the neck and face (**4**).

Children are often upset by intractable itching which disturbs their sleep and disrupts family life. Repeated rubbing and scratching leads to lichenification (**5**). Follicular eczema may occur, especially in black skin (**6**). A generally dry skin (xerosis) is almost always present even in the absence of active eczema. Two-thirds of children with atopic eczema are clear by the age of 16, but the condition may recur as hand eczema in adulthood (**7**).

DIFFERENTIAL DIAGNOSIS

Scabies (see p.244) must be excluded in any widespread pruritic eruption of recent onset. Contact dermatitis is not usually flexural except in the case of clothing, wood dust dermatitis, or autosensitization eczema.

INVESTIGATIONS

These are not usually necessary but a raised serum IgE level and positive skin prick tests to aeroallergens support the diagnosis. Skin swabs should be taken when secondary bacterial infection is suspected to determine microbial sensitivities. Patch testing may be helpful to exclude a coexistent allergic contact dermatitis.

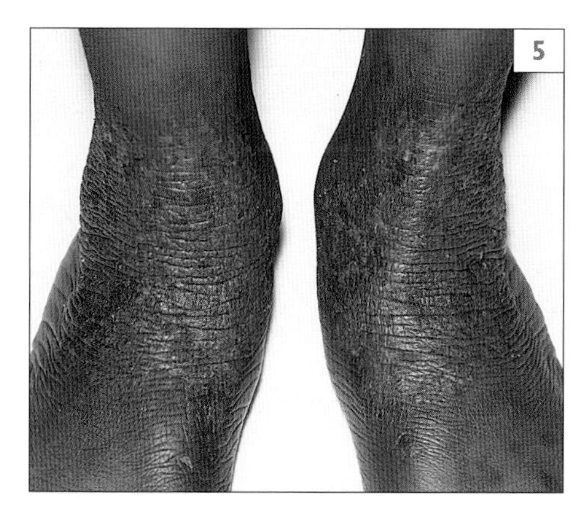

5 Lichenified eczema on the ankles.

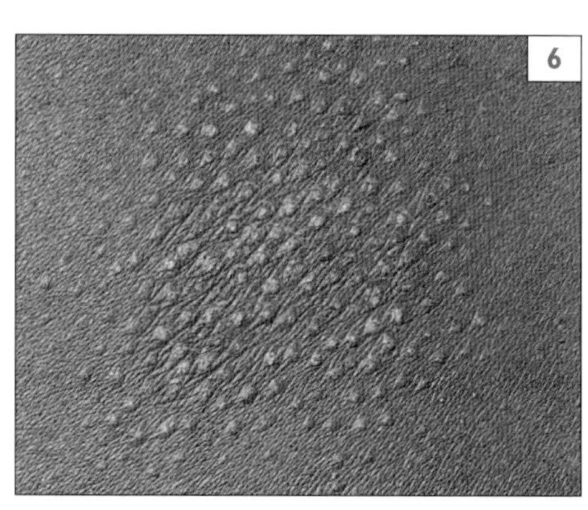

6 Follicular eczema.

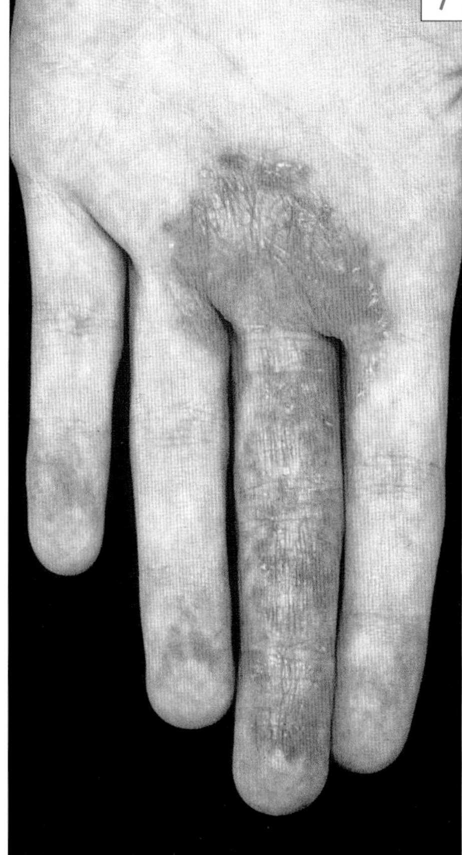

7 Hand eczema.

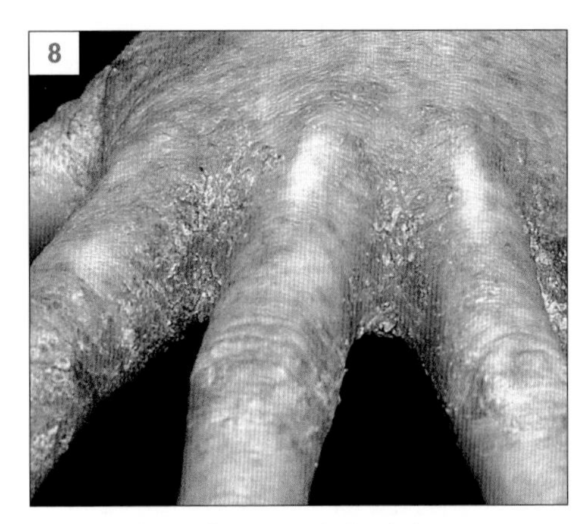

8 Secondary infection with *Staphylococcus aureus*.

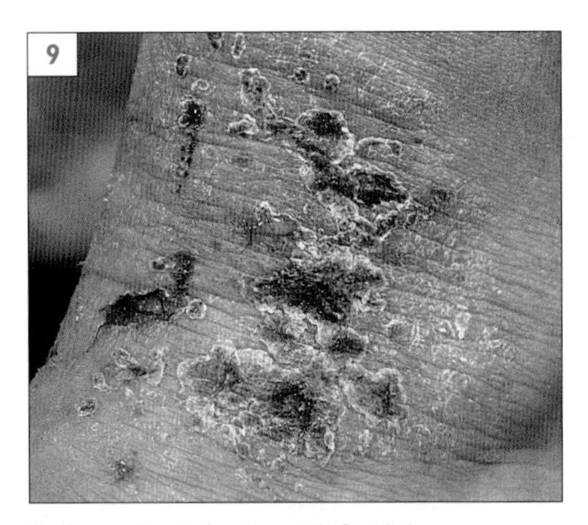

9 Secondary infection with *Staphylococcus aureus*.

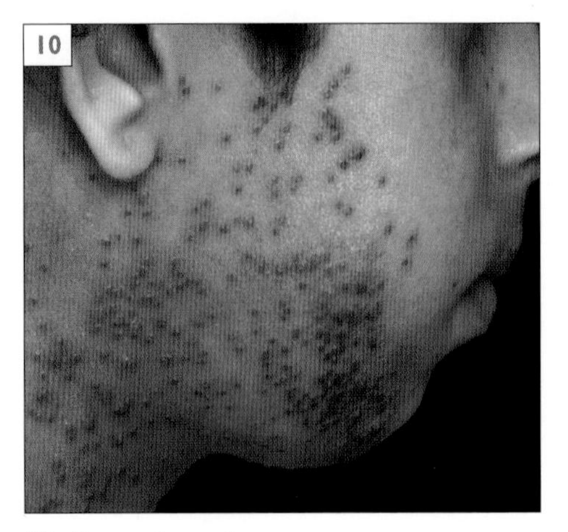

10 Eczema herpeticum.

SPECIAL POINTS

Secondary infection with *Staphylococcus aureus* is common where soreness, crusting, and pustules may be present (**8**, **9**). Occasionally *Herpes simplex* virus infection spreads widely on areas of atopic eczema (eczema herpeticum) (**10**). This requires urgent systemic antiviral therapy.

TREATMENT

First-line therapies include liberal use of emollients and soap substitutes to help restore the impaired skin barrier. Topical corticosteroids reduce the inflammation and itch of eczema and are available in different formulations (creams, ointments, and lotions) and potencies. Milder potency corticosteroids should be used to treat facial or flexural eczema to minimize the risk of skin atrophy. More potent corticosteroids are usually required to control disease on palmoplantar skin. Topical calcineurin inhibitors may be useful to manage facial eczema because they do not cause atrophy. Other second-line therapies include UVB phototherapy, ciclosporin, and azathioprine.

Venous eczema
(gravitational, varicose, or stasis eczema)

DEFINITION AND CLINICAL FEATURES
Eczema secondary to venous hypertension. Venous eczema occurs on the lower legs (**11**). The inner aspect of the lower leg is the first area to be affected. There are often accompanying changes such as pigmentation from haemosiderin deposition, small white areas of atrophy (atrophie blanche), oedema, purpura, and venous varicosities. Trivial injury can often lead to the development of a venous ulcer (**12**). The exact mechanism of venous eczema is still unknown, but venous hypertension secondary to a previous deep vein thrombosis is the most common cause. The condition is commonest in middle and old age, and females outnumber males.

DIFFERENTIAL DIAGNOSIS
Contact dermatitis secondary to rubber hosiery or impregnated bandages usually involves the whole of the lower leg and shows a sharp cut-off point. Cellulitis usually develops acutely and the patient feels unwell with a fever. The affected skin is tender and inflamed.

INVESTIGATIONS
Colour flow Doppler studies identify incompetent veins which may be amenable to surgery and assesses the adequacy of the peripheral arterial circulation. Swabs may be indicated if secondary infection is suspected. Patch testing is indicated in unresponsive cases to exclude medicament allergy.

SPECIAL POINTS
Contact dermatitis from medicaments is a common problem at this site, so treatment should be kept as simple as possible.

TREATMENT
Bland emollients and moderate or potent topical corticosteroids are usually effective in controlling this condition. Ointment formulations are preferable as they contain fewer potential allergens such as preservatives.

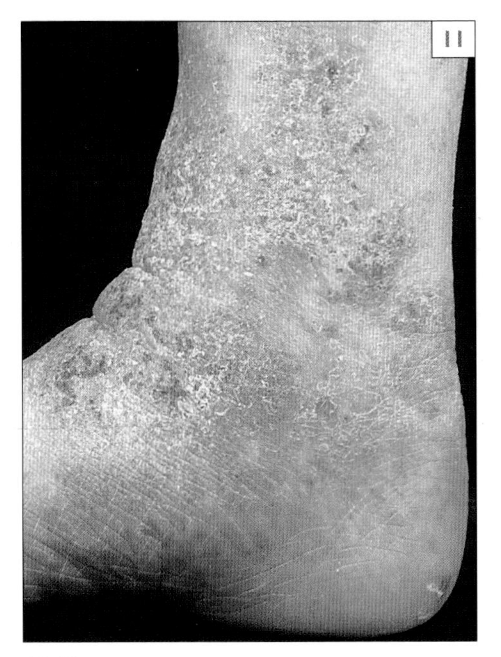

11 Venous eczema..

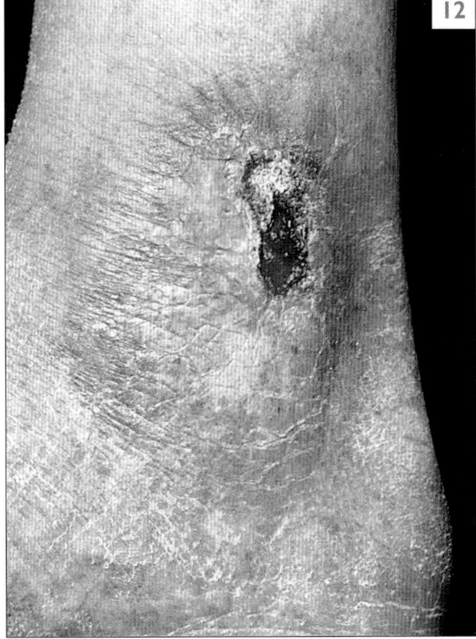

12 Venous ulcer.

Seborrhoeic eczema
(seborrhoeic dermatitis)

DEFINITION AND CLINICAL FEATURES

A relapsing eczema affecting seborrhoeic areas of the scalp, face, and upper trunk. Patients usually complain of the cosmetic effects of scaling and redness rather than itching. Lesions of seborrhoeic eczema have fine scaling and are often quite well demarcated. The scalp may be diffusely involved or lesions may be localized to the scalp margins. On the face, the paranasal areas (**13**), eyebrows, and external ears are typically affected. Elsewhere the presternal area (**14**), interscapular area (**15**), axillae, and groins may be involved.

Although the exact aetiology is unknown, there is strong evidence to link seborrhoeic eczema with the presence of the lipophilic yeast *Pityrosporum ovale*. A variant of seborrhoeic eczema may occur in infants (**16**), but its precise relationship to adult seborrhoeic eczema is unclear. Seborrhoeic eczema may affect adults of all ages and is commoner in men.

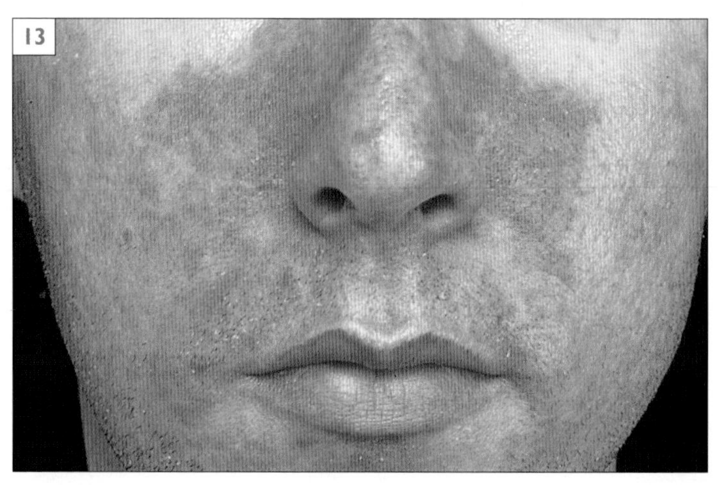

13 Seborrhoeic eczema.

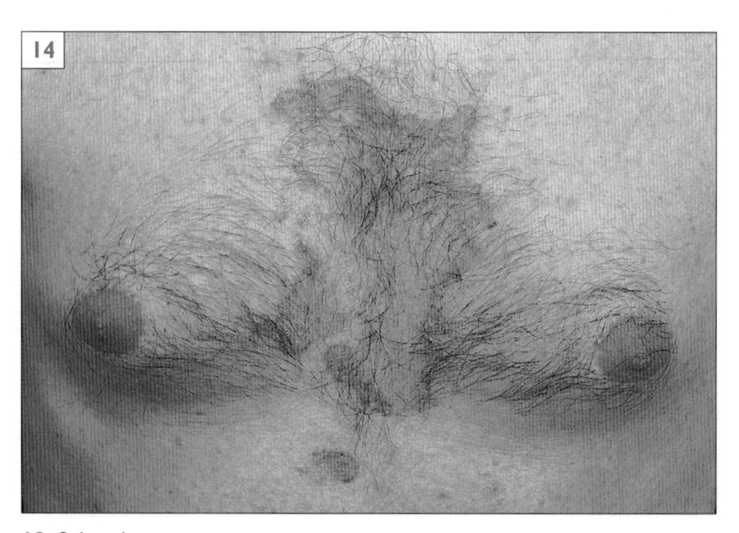

13 Seborrhoeic eczema.

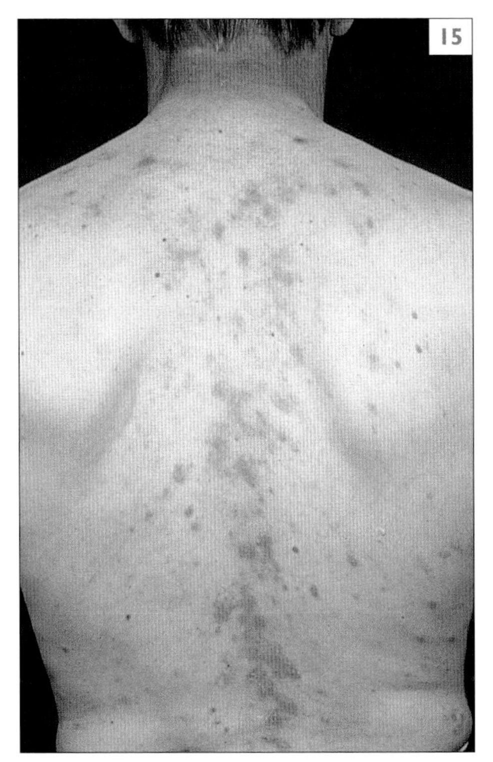

15 Seborrhoeic eczema.

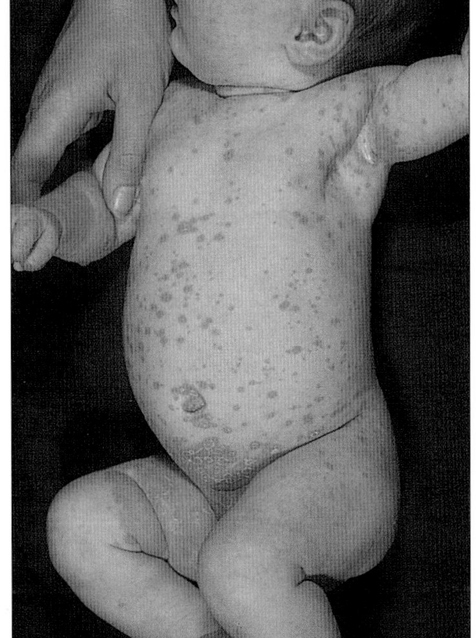

16 Seborrhoeic eczema of infancy.

DIFFERENTIAL DIAGNOSIS

Mild facial and scalp psoriasis can be difficult to distinguish from seborrhoeic eczema. However, the lesions of the latter are usually less well demarcated and less scaly than those of psoriasis. Systemic lupus erythematosus usually affects the malar as opposed to the paranasal areas, and is associated with systemic symptoms such as malaise and arthralgia.

INVESTIGATIONS

None are usually necessary. Patch testing should be considered in any facial dermatitis which does not fit the above description to exclude contact allergies.

SPECIAL POINTS

While most seborrhoeic eczema occurs in healthy adults, the sudden appearance of widespread involvement should raise the possibility of underlying HIV infection.

TREATMENT

Mild potency topical corticosteroids and topical antiyeast agents are usually effective in controlling seborrhoeic eczema, but relapses are common if treatment is discontinued. Scalp disease should be treated with an antiyeast shampoo and this can be continued prophylactically.

Discoid eczema
(nummular eczema)

DEFINITION AND CLINICAL FEATURES

This is an eczema of unknown cause characterized by discrete round lesions on the limbs and trunk. It is very pruritic and consists of multiple, well demarcated, coin-shaped lesions measuring 2–6 cm in diameter (**17**, **18**). Lesions show oozing, crusting, and scaling (**19**) and vesicles may be present. The hands may also be affected.

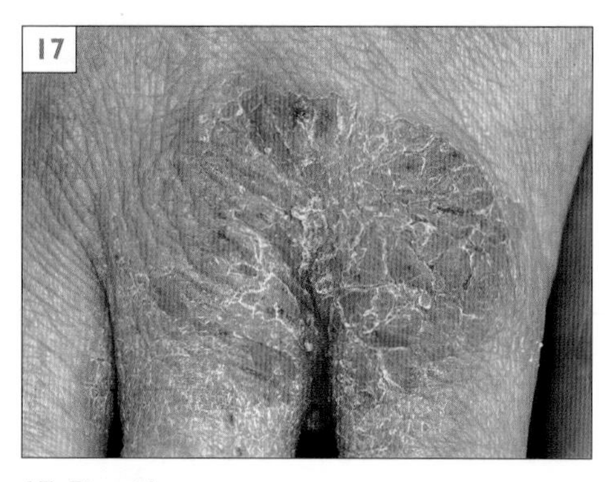

17 Discoid eczema.

Discoid eczema may be seen at any age but is most common in middle-aged adults. Its precise relationship to atopic eczema is unknown. Emotional stress, excessive drying of the skin, and secondary infection may be important factors in the dissemination of lesions.

DIFFERENTIAL DIAGNOSIS

The lesions of guttate psoriasis are usually smaller (1–2 cm) than in discoid eczema and are not intensely pruritic. Tinea corporis lesions are annular with a distinct scaly margin. Bowen's disease may be difficult to distinguish especially on the lower legs, but is usually not pruritic.

INVESTIGATIONS

None are usually required. Swabs for microbial culture may reveal secondary infection. Skin scrapings should be taken from solitary lesions to exclude tinea infection.

TREATMENT

Potent topical corticosteroids are usually needed for disease control and preparations with added antibiotics may be useful. Emollients and soap substitutes are also indicated.

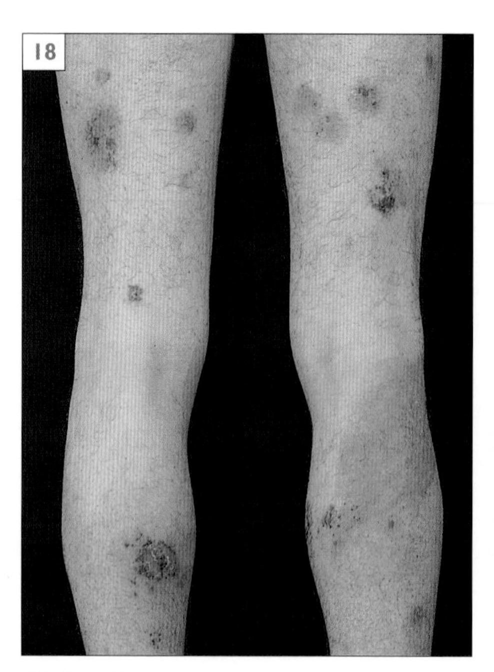

18 Discoid eczema.

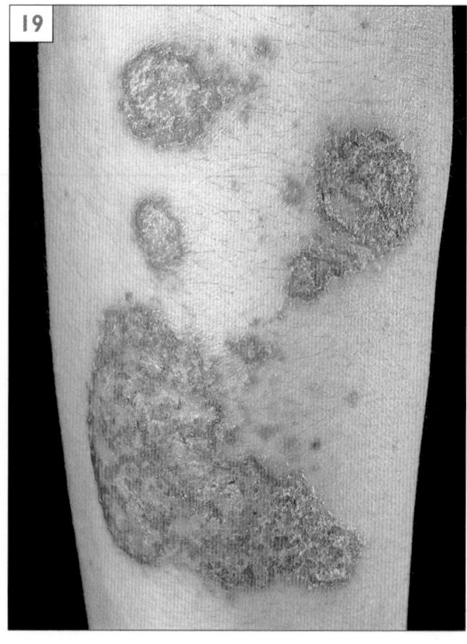

19 Discoid eczema.

Asteatotic eczema

DEFINITION AND CLINICAL FEATURES

Eczema caused by the excessive loss of skin lipids. The elderly are particularly prone with the lower limbs most commonly affected. The exact prevalence of this condition is unknown but it is one of the commonest reasons for a dermatologist to be called to see a hospital inpatient. Lesions develop because natural skin lipid production diminishes with age and can no longer compensate for its removal by frequent washing with soaps. High ambient temperatures and low humidity also play a role. The skin is generally dry (**20**) and in some areas cracks appear which become red (eczéma craquelé) (**21**). A generalized eczema or discoid pattern may eventually develop.

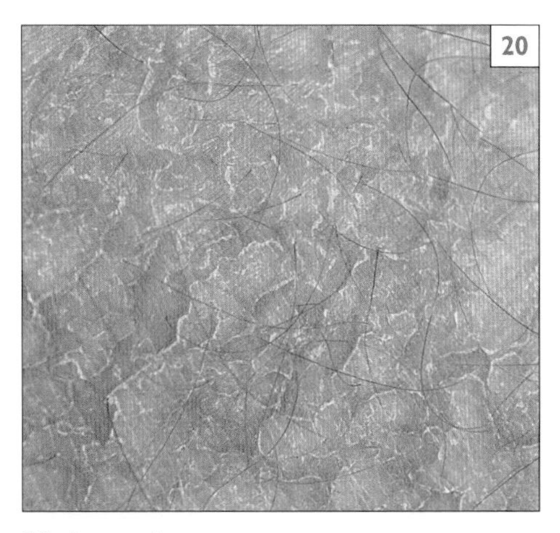

20 Asteatotic eczema.

DIFFERENTIAL DIAGNOSIS

Drug eruptions are usually more proximal and symmetrical, inflamed cracks in the skin surface being unusual. Congenital ichthyosis, as the name implies, is present from birth. Lymphoma or treatment with clofazimine may occasionally give rise to a generalized dryness of the skin.

INVESTIGATIONS

No investigations are usually necessary.

TREATMENT

Soaps and detergents should be strictly avoided. Liberal use of soap substitutes and emollients is usually all that is required to treat and prevent this condition.

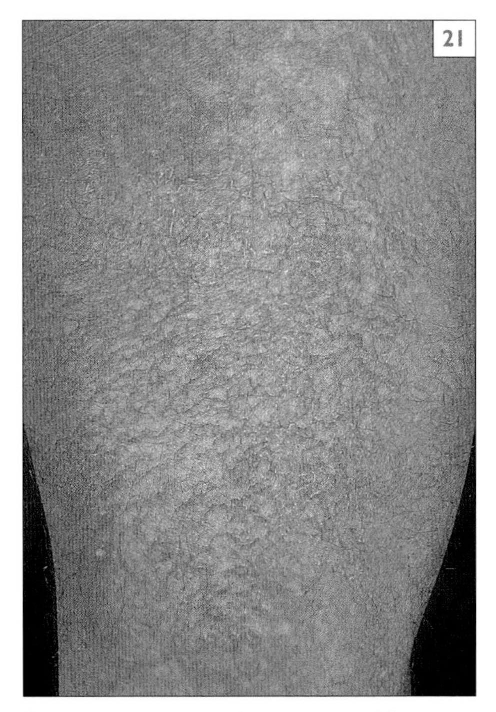

21 Asteatotic eczema (eczéma craquelé).

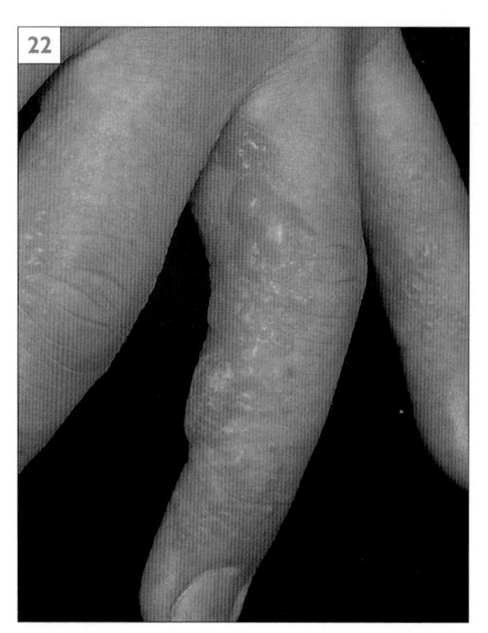

22 Pompholyx.

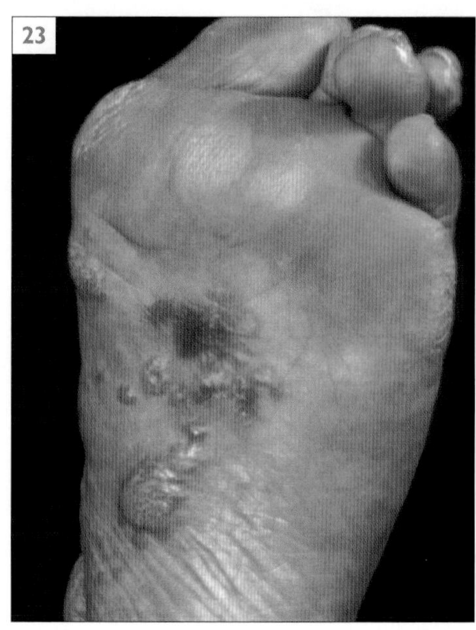

23 Pompholyx.

Vesicular hand and foot eczema (Pompholyx)

DEFINITION AND CLINICAL FEATURES

A severe form of eczema of the palms and/or soles in which there are numerous small blisters or vesicles. These often affect the lateral aspects of the fingers and can appear acutely in crops. They may become confluent producing large bullae (**22**, **23**). Itching is usually intense. Secondary bacterial infection may complicate the condition. Pompholyx may occur at any age but its onset is usually between the ages of 10 and 40 years. Recurrence is often over long periods, especially in the summer when sweating increases.

DIFFERENTIAL DIAGNOSIS

Vesicular changes may occur in acute irritant or allergic contact dermatitis. Pustular psoriasis has characteristic yellow pustules which turn brown and scaly and is usually less pruritic. A vesicular eruption may also occur in tinea of the hands and feet. Bullous pemphigoid may rarely present with palmoplantar blistering.

INVESTIGATIONS

Mycological and/or bacterial examination, as well as patch testing, may be indicated.

TREATMENT

Moderate to potent topical corticosteroids should be applied twice daily. Cream formulations are preferable for exudative lesions. Daily soaking of affected areas in an aqueous solution of potassium permanganate (1 in 10,000) helps to dry the blisters. Large blisters can be lanced and drained, leaving the roof intact. In severe cases, short tapering courses of systemic corticosteroids may be needed, and hand–foot psoralen with UVA (PUVA) can provide longer term disease control.

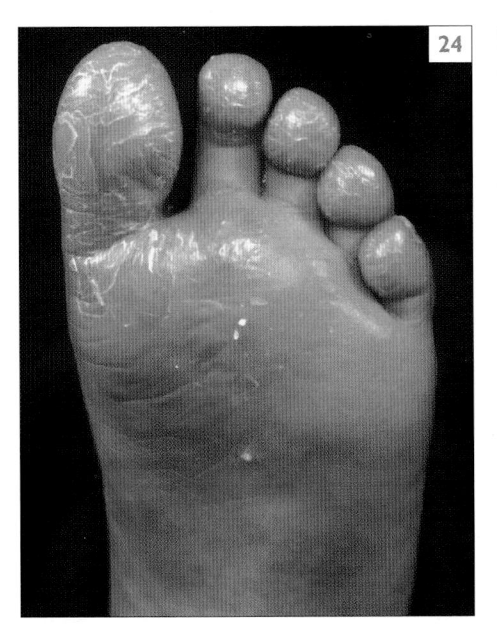

24 Juvenile plantar dermatosis.

Juvenile plantar dermatosis

DEFINITION AND CLINICAL FEATURES

This distinctive form of eczema is characterized by glazed, fissured erythematous skin on the pressure bearing areas of the soles of the forefeet (**24**). It typically affects young boys and is thought to occur due to prolonged wearing of occlusive footwear, especially trainers.

DIFFERENTIAL DIAGNOSIS

The toe webs are normal, which helps to differentiate this complaint from tinea pedis.

INVESTIGATIONS

None are routinely needed, but patch testing may be helpful in excluding a footwear allergy if there is diagnostic doubt.

TREATMENT

Changing footwear to absorbent, natural fabrics may help. Most cases clear spontaneously in adolescence.

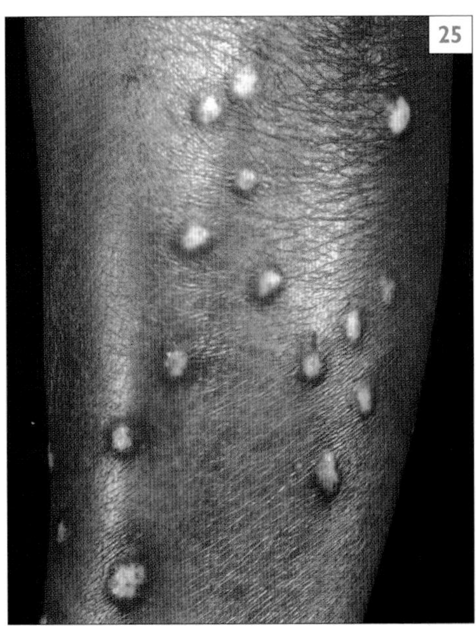

25 Nodular prurigo.

Nodular prurigo

DEFINITION AND CLINICAL FEATURES

This condition is usually seen in association with chronic eczema and is characterized by intensely itchy nodules, usually on the distal limbs. Lesions are repeatedly excoriated (**25**) and may become secondarily infected. Some regress to leave scars. The cause is unknown, but abnormalities in cutaneous neuropeptides have been identified.

DIFFERENTIAL DIAGNOSIS

The appearance and disturbing itch is usually characteristic. Bullous pemphigoid may rarely present with nodular rather than blistered lesions.

INVESTIGATIONS

Histology shows marked hyperkeratosis and acanthosis. Direct IMF to exclude immunobullous disorders.

TREATMENT

Superpotent or intralesional corticosteroids may be used as a first line therapy with a sedating antihistamine at night and topical antipruritic. Other options include PUVA, immunosuppressants, and thalidomide.

Lichen simplex

DEFINITION AND CLINICAL FEATURES

An intensely itchy localized form of eczema where there is no known predisposing skin disorder. The condition usually runs a chronic course, and repeated scratching and rubbing leads to well circumscribed lichenified patches and papules with peripheral hyperpigmentation. The peak incidence is between the ages of 30 and 50, but it may be seen at any time after puberty. Common sites are the nape (**26**) of the neck, outer calves and ankles (**27**), pubis, vulva, perianal area, and scrotum. Scratching is usually worse at night.

DIFFERENTIAL DIAGNOSIS

Lichen planus, tinea, and allergic contact dermatitis (e.g. nail varnish or hair dye).

INVESTIGATIONS

None usually necessary, but in atypical cases a skin biopsy, mycological examination, or patch testing may be required.

SPECIAL POINTS

There is often underlying emotional distress and patients may benefit from learning stress management techniques such as relaxation therapy.

TREATMENT

Patients should be advised that habitual rubbing and scratching perpetuates lichen simplex. Potent topical corticosteroids can be effective in relieving pruritus and helping to break the itch–scratch cycle. They may be used under occlusion for a limited period, with close supervision to monitor for signs of skin atrophy. A topical formulation of 2% menthol in aqueous cream can be applied as needed for immediate itch relief.

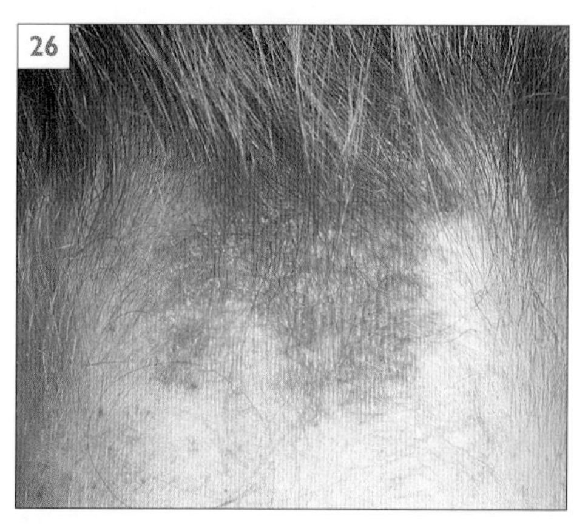

26 Lichen simplex.

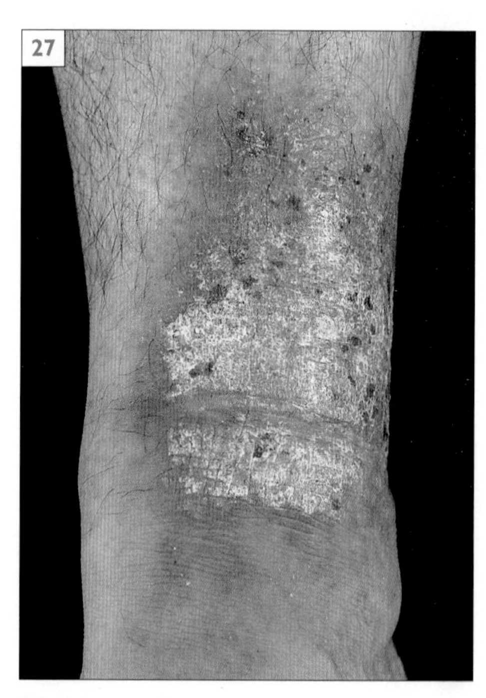

27 Lichen simplex.

Contact dermatitis

DEFINITION AND CLINICAL FEATURES

This is a dermatitis (i.e. an eczema) caused by contact with external substances (contact factors). It may be allergic (immunological) or irritant (non-immunological)

Irritant contact dermatitis/eczema is more common than allergic, and most cases nowadays occur because of repeated exposure to weak irritants such as detergents. This complaint mainly affects adults of working age, and its prevalence is higher in certain occupations such as hairdressing, catering, and heavy industry; this form of eczema almost invariably affects the hands. Typical features include dryness and chapping in the finger webs (**28**) and dorsal hands, or palmar aspects of the fingers (**29**). This may evolve to a more inflammatory pattern of eczema which is clinically indistinguishable from an endogenous eczema.

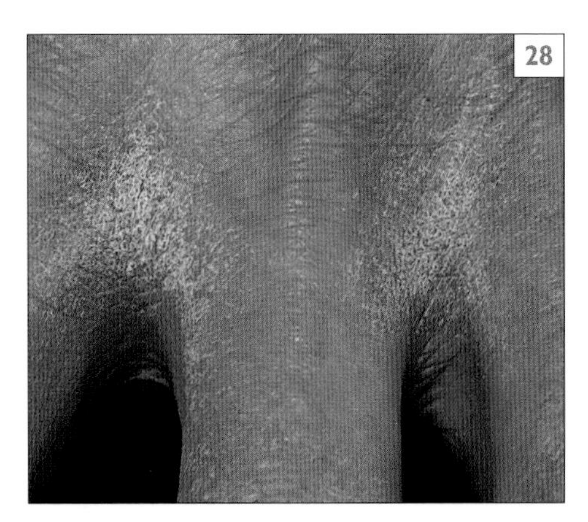

28 Irritant contact dermatitis.

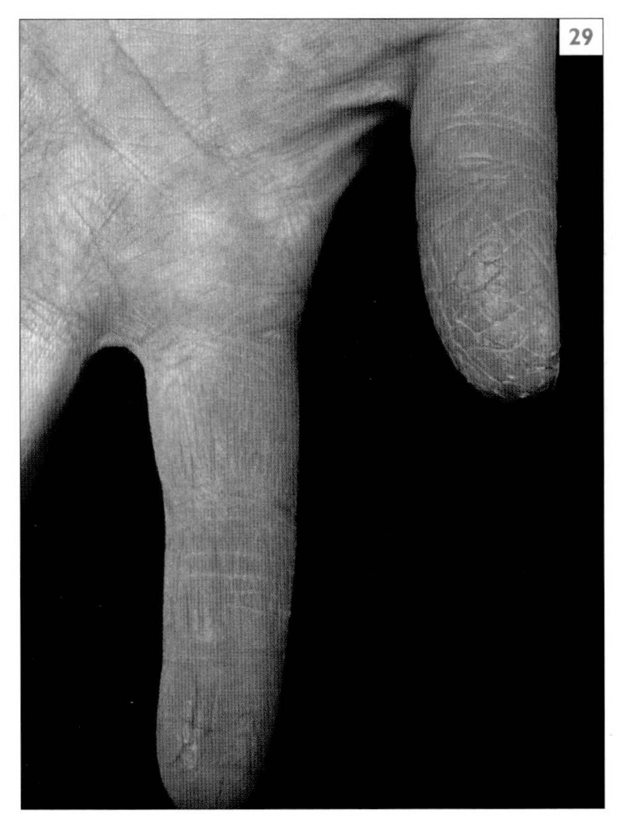

29 Irritant contact dermatitis.

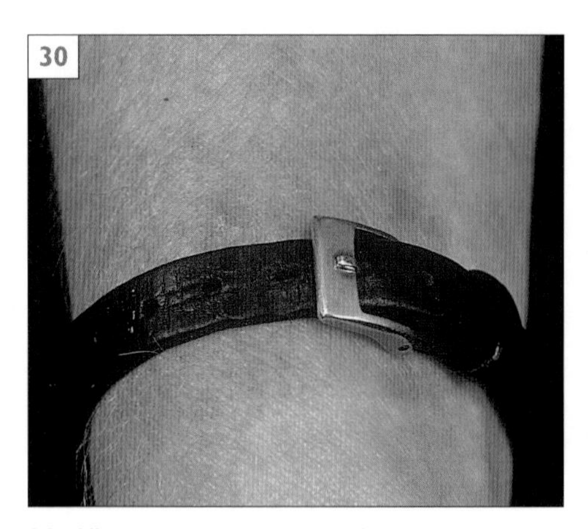

30 Allergic contact dermatitis from nickel.

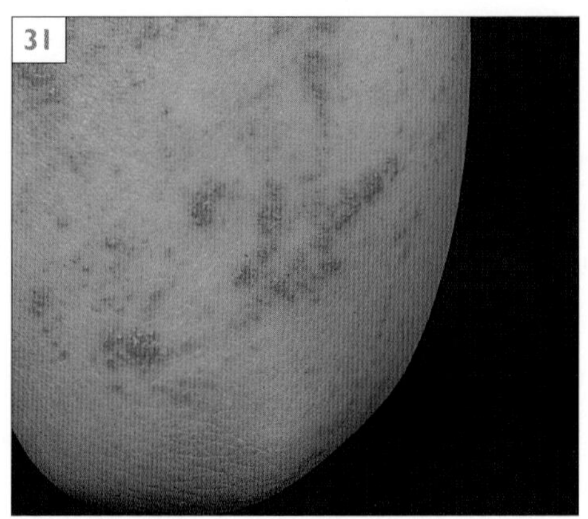

31 Allergic contact dermatitis from primula.

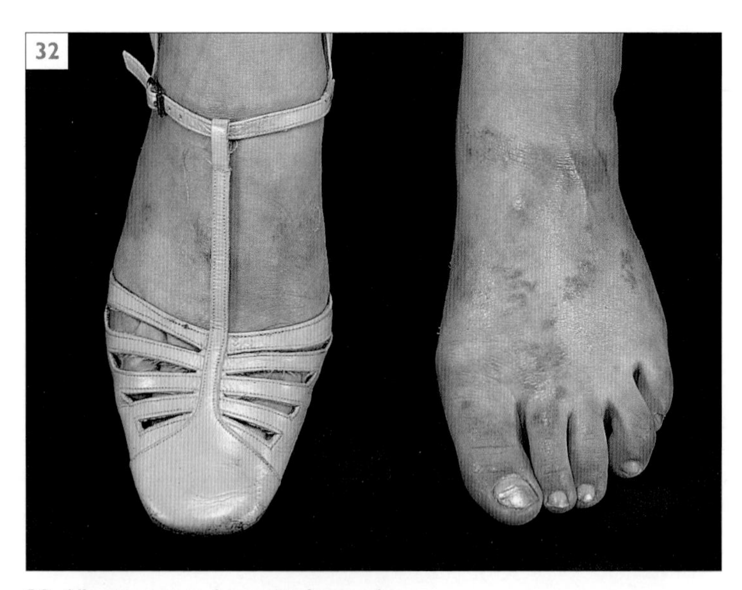

32 Allergic contact dermatitis from a shoe.

Allergic contact dermatitis can affect all ages, although it is rare in infants. It may arise after years of trouble-free exposure to a particular allergen, but once established, such allergies are usually lifelong. Many cases are morphologically indistinguishable from endogenous eczema (see above). Certain patterns are characteristic of some contact allergens, e.g. nickel (**30**), primula (**31**), shoe dermatitis (**32**), and fragrances (**33**).

DIFFERENTIAL DIAGNOSIS

As the clinical features may be identical with endogenous eczema a high level of suspicion is required, particularly in chronic eczema, eczema subject to rapid and recurrent relapse, eczema of an unusual clinical pattern (**34**), and hand eczema (**35**). Psoriasis and tinea are the main non-eczematous causes of confusion, particularly on the hands.

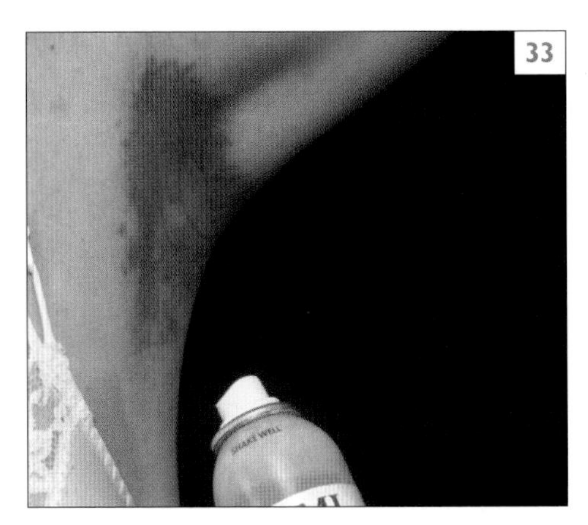

33 Allergic contact dermatitis from fragrance.

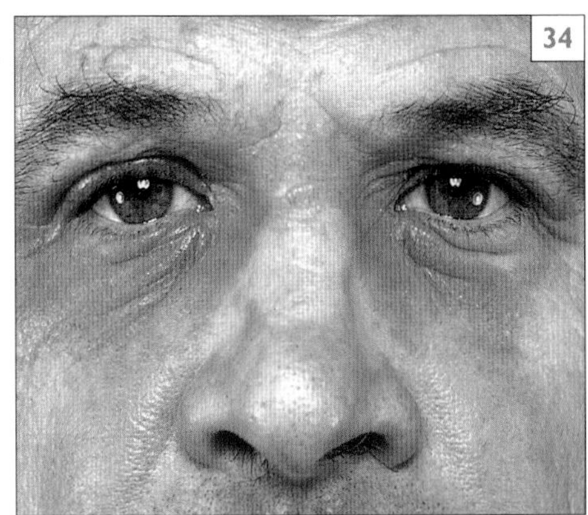

34 Occupational allergic contact dermatitis from airborne epoxy resin.

INVESTIGATIONS

Patch testing is essential in order to identify or exclude allergic contact dermatitis.

SPECIAL POINTS

Occupational contact dermatitis is among the commonest of all occupational diseases.

TREATMENT

The mainstay of managing irritant contact dermatitis is to reduce exposure to the irritant substance(s). This may include use of personal protective equipment especially gloves in the workplace, as well as active treatment of the dermatitis with emollients, soap substitutes, and topical corticosteroids. Allergic contact dermatitis management involves careful avoidance of the allergen(s). In some situations, e.g. a medicament allergy, another agent which the patient is not allergic to can easily be chosen, but in an occupational setting, this may involve a change of job.

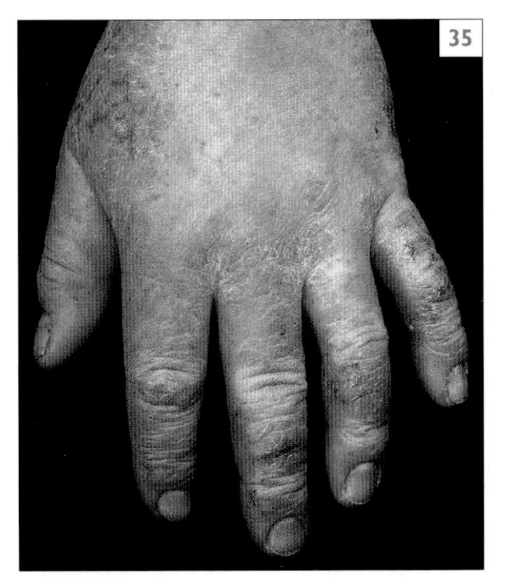

35 Occupational allergic contact dermatitis from chromate in wet cement.

Dermatitis artefacta

DEFINITION AND CLINICAL FEATURES

Dermatitis artefacta is the result of self-inflicted skin damage. This form of deliberate self-harm is most common in young women. Lesions may be variable according to the nature of the skin damage, but are often linear with sharp edges and are in accessible sites (**36**, **37**). The sufferer may appear remarkably indifferent to the problem and needs to be approached with sympathy and tact in order to explore the underlying psychological problems.

INVESTIGATIONS

Other possible causes of skin lesions need to be excluded. A skin biopsy can help identify features consistent with physical trauma.

TREATMENT

Directly confronting the patient with this diagnosis usually has a negative effect and their care should ideally be shared with a psychiatrist. Skin lesions may be treated with bland emollients, antiseptics, and occlusion.

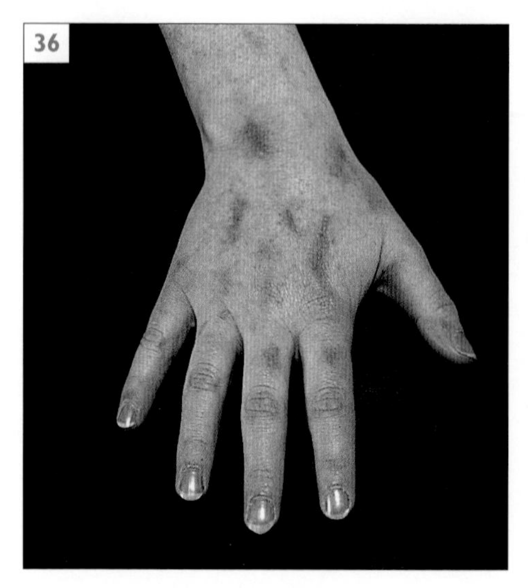

36 Excoriated dermatitis artefacta.

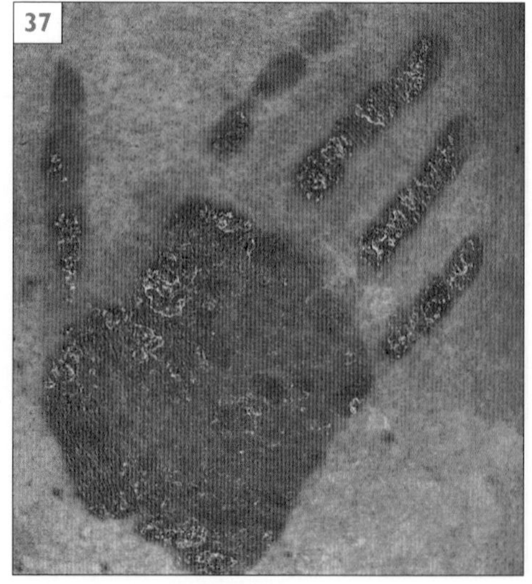

37 Dermatitis artefacta on the thigh from a chemical applied on a glove.

NON-DERMATITIC OCCUPATIONAL DERMATOSES

Chloracne

DEFINITION AND CLINICAL FEATURES

A refractory follicular dermatosis caused by occupational or environmental exposure to halogenated aromatic compounds of a specific molecular shape (e.g. dioxins) which may be accompanied by systemic toxicity. Epidemics have occurred from accidental ingestion or inhalation as well as from external skin contact in chemical plants (and surrounding populations after plant explosions) and chemical waste disposal plants. All ages are susceptible.

Open comedones (blackheads) (**38**) with small, pale-yellow cysts (**39**) predominate in milder cases. In more severe cases, inflammatory pustules and even cold abscesses develop. The skin just below and to the outer side of the eye and behind the ear (**39**) is the most sensitive, next the cheeks, forehead (but not the nose), and male genitalia, followed in severe cases by the shoulders, chest, and back (**38**), buttocks, and abdomen. Lesions may continue to appear after exposure ceases and tend to persist in spite of treatment.

DIFFERENTIAL DIAGNOSIS

Acne vulgaris in younger patients, senile comedones in older patients, cystic acne in severe cases.

INVESTIGATIONS

Occupational or community clustering of similar cases and appropriate exposure should be enquired for. Biopsy shows characteristic keratinous cysts replacing sebaceous glands. The patient's weight, peripheral nervous system, lung function, liver function, blood lipids, and urinary porphyrins should be checked.

SPECIAL POINTS

Chloracne is generally the most sensitive indicator of toxic exposure to such chemicals. Mild cases are easily missed.

TREATMENT

Conventional antiacne therapy may be given but the response is typically poor and chronicity is usual.

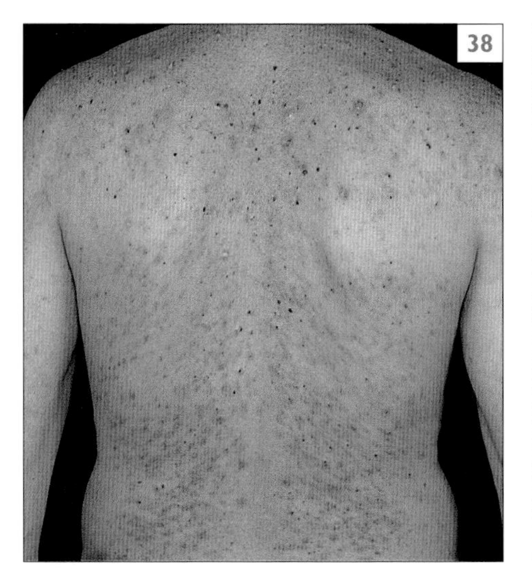

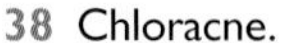

38 Chloracne.

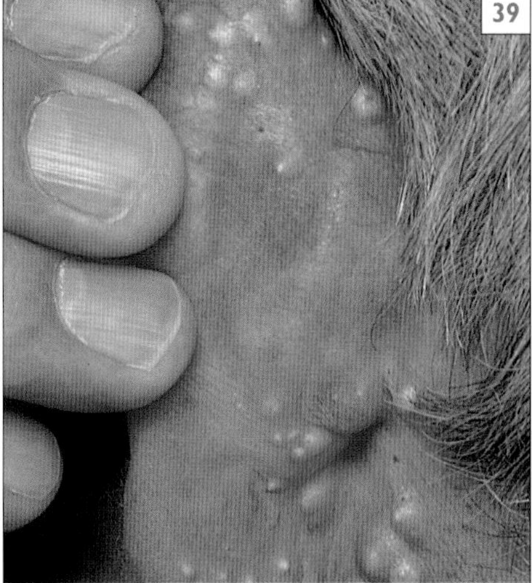

39 Chloracne cysts.

Other occupational dermatoses

These non-dermatitic conditions are primarily caused by the patient's work and account for 10% or less of occupational dermatoses. A wide variation exists, e.g. glass-fibre dermatitis (**40**), contact urticaria, oil acne (**41**), chrome ulceration (**42**), cement burns (**43**), leukoderma, scleroderma-like disease (see p. 101), squamous cell carcinoma (**44**), and koilonychia (**45**).

DIFFERENTIAL DIAGNOSIS

Non-occupational forms of, for example, contact urticaria and epithelioma, and idiopathic forms of such conditions as leukoderma, scleroderma, and koilonychia.

INVESTIGATIONS

These are indicated by the condition in question, e.g. prick testing in contact urticaria.

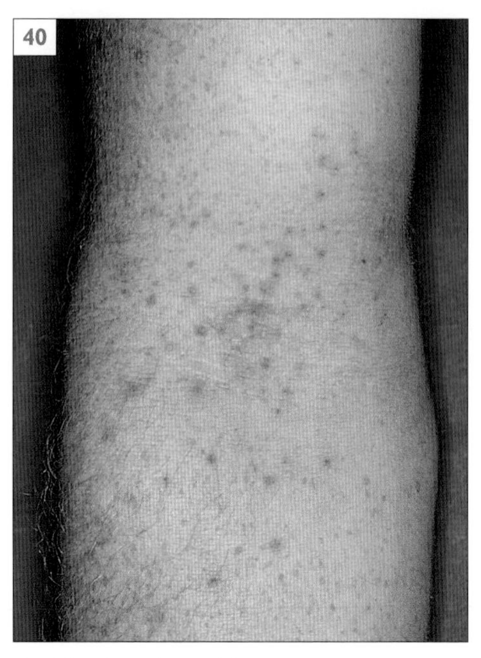

40 Glass-fibre dermatitis.

41 Oil acne.

TREATMENT

Management of these conditions may include use of personal protective equipment or redeployment in the workplace.

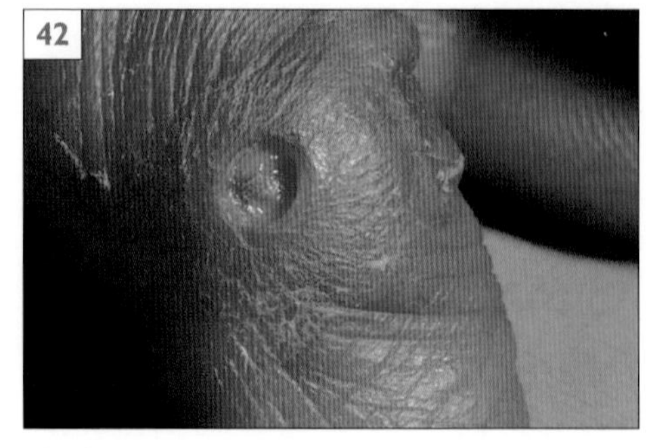

42 Chrome ulceration.

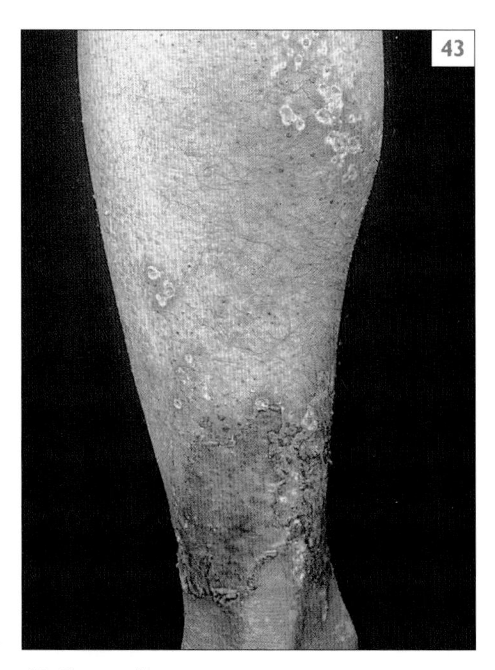

43 Cement burns.

Hyperhidrosis

Hyperhidrosis is the result of excessive production of eccrine sweat. Most cases are idiopathic and affect the hands, feet, and axillae. Generalized hyperhidrosis may occur with metabolic or endocrine diseases, while localized hyperhidrosis may result from injury to the central or peripheral nervous systems, and these must be distinguished by thorough history taking and examination.

People with palmar hyperhidrosis may cause ferrous material to rust if repeatedly handled, for example in engineering (**46**). They are colloquially known as 'rusters'. Problems arise especially when this occurs to finished metal products in transit to the customer.

TREATMENT

Adequate control of the hyperhidrosis may be achieved by use of topical aluminium chloride hexahydrate solution, tap water iontophoresis or, in severe cases, endoscopic transthoracic sympathectomy.

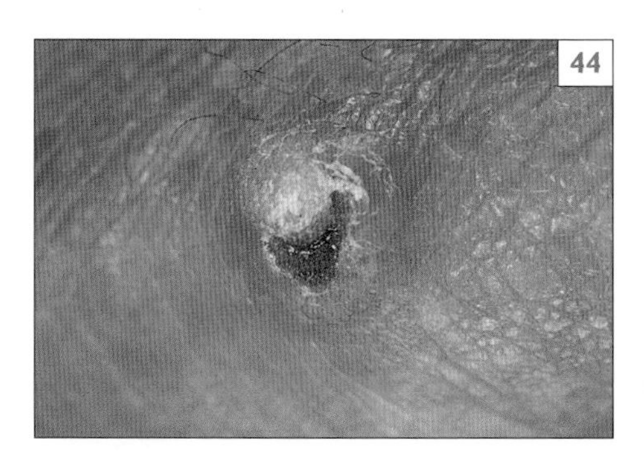

44 Squamous cell carcinoma.

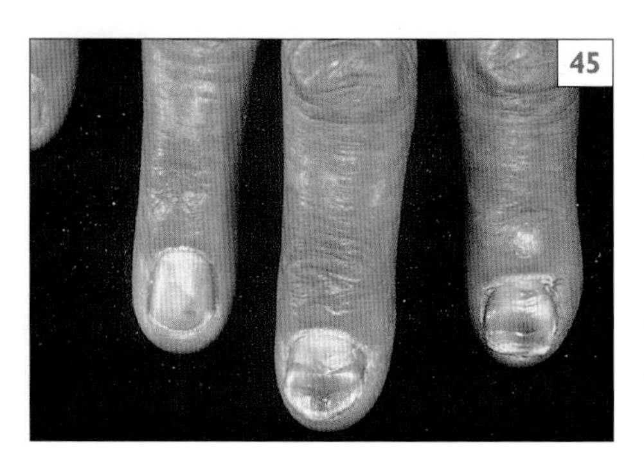

45 Koilonychia.

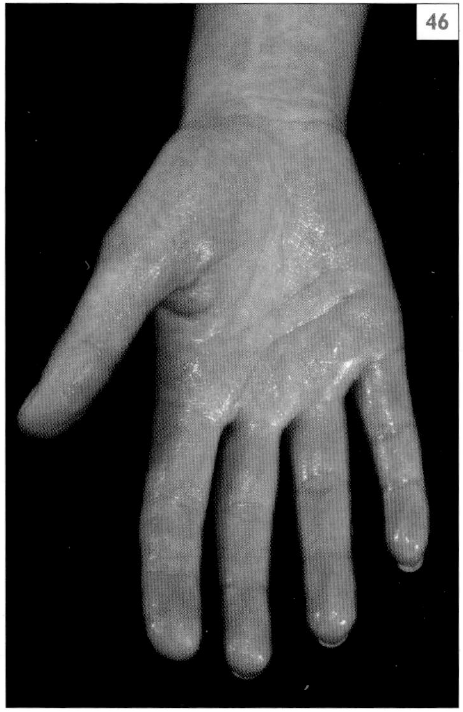

46 Palmar hyperhidrosis in a 'ruster'.

URTICARIA

The urticarias are a group of dermatoses commonly known as hives. They consist of transient pruritic areas of erythema and dermal oedema which occur due to plasma leakage and resolve within hours without leaving residual cutaneous signs such as scaling or dryness. Lesions may take the form of focal papules, plaques, or annular areas of palpable dermal oedema with or without erythema (**47**). The time course, distribution, and morphology of the lesions is influenced by the precipitating cause.

Contact urticaria

DEFINITION AND CLINICAL FEATURES

Contact urticaria is a localized wheal-and-flare reaction to contact with external substances; it may be immunological or non-immunological. The morphology of individual lesions resembles other forms of urticaria but the history and localized site are characteristic. Lesions usually develop within minutes of contact with the urticant and resolve within an hour or so without any residual signs of skin damage. Immunological contact urticaria may be associated with severe, systemic allergic symptoms.

The prevalence of non-immunological contact urticaria is unknown, as mild reactions are easily overlooked. Natural rubber latex allergy has evolved as one of the most important causes of immunologic contact urticaria in recent decades. The incidence peaked in the 1990s due to a surge in the use of poor quality rubber gloves with high residual levels of latex protein and glove powder (**48**). This condition is important to diagnose because of the risk of anaphylaxis from invasive medical interventions with natural rubber latex containing devices.

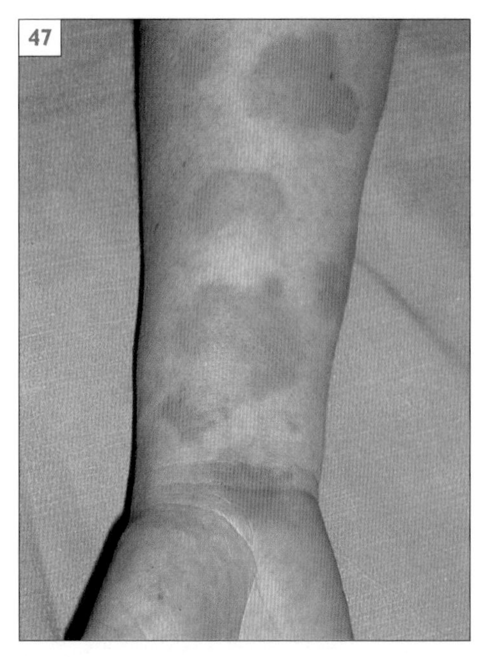

47 Urticaria.

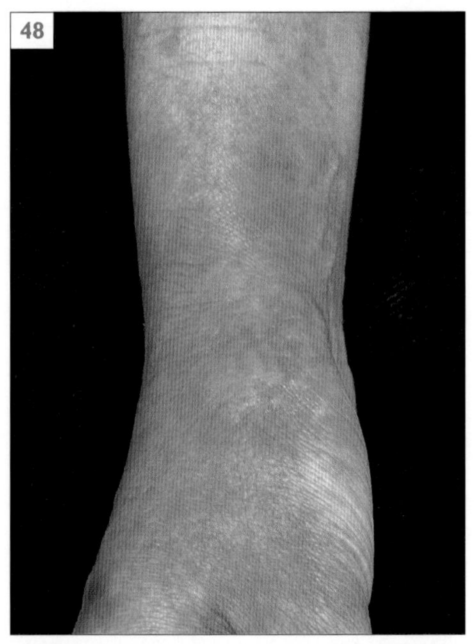

48 Immunological contact urticaria from rubber latex glove.

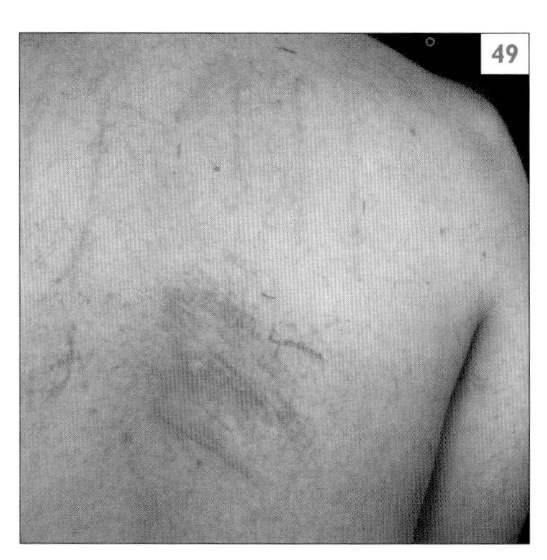

49 Dermographism.

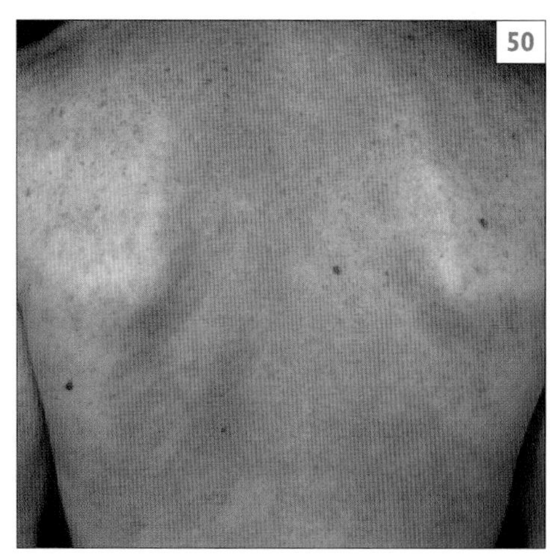

50 Cholinergic urticaria.

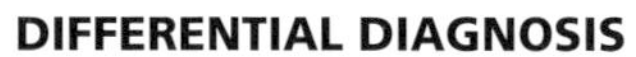

DIFFERENTIAL DIAGNOSIS

Idiopathic urticaria is usually more widespread and wheals are longer lasting. Contact dermatitis evolves over several days and is associated with skin surface changes.

INVESTIGATIONS

Non-immunological contact urticaria is not routinely investigated. Skin prick tests or measurement of allergen specific IgE (RAST) may be helpful to confirm a diagnosis of immunological contact urticaria.

TREATMENT

Treatment is not usually required because of the short lived nature of contact urticaria. Medical therapy is indicated for more generalized urticarial reactions and those associated with systemic symptoms.

Physical urticaria

DEFINITION AND CLINICAL FEATURES

This is a subgroup of urticaria where a specific physical stimulus induces wheals. These are typically short lived, so the skin often appears normal when examined. Dermographism, the most common physical urticaria, consists of urticated wheals developing at sites where the skin is firmly stroked (**49**).

Other forms of physical urticaria include pressure, vibration, cold, heat, sunlight, and water. Cholinergic urticaria is triggered by sweating which usually occurs with stress, exercise, or heat (**50**). It is a common complaint and usually affects fit young people. It presents with pruritic small papules and wheals on the upper body. The wheals of delayed pressure urticaria are more persistent and develop several hours after sustained pressure. They are often painful as well as pruritic, and may occur in patients with chronic ordinary urticaria.

INVESTIGATIONS

None are routinely necessary. The diagnosis may be confirmed by a provocation test such as an ice cube test for cold urticaria.

TREATMENT

Reassurance may be all that is needed, but prophylactic treatment with non-sedating oral antihistamines may be used when symptoms are troublesome.

Ordinary urticaria

DEFINITION AND CLINICAL FEATURES

Ordinary urticaria is a term used when other forms of urticaria have been excluded. It is a common complaint and most cases are mild. Many cases are self-limiting and resolve within days or weeks; these are classified as acute urticaria. Chronic urticaria is defined by daily wheals for 6 or more weeks. Some patients also suffer from angioedema and this is associated with a longer disease course. Chronic urticaria is seldom due to an underlying allergy and an underlying autoimmune cause has been identified in about 40% of patients. They may suffer from other autoimmune diseases, particularly those affecting the thyroid. In some patients there are precipitating factors including drugs such as salicylates, opiates, and antibiotics. These are more likely to be found in acute urticaria than chronic urticaria. Food allergy may cause acute urticaria but the diagnosis is usually clear from the history.

DIFFERENTIAL DIAGNOSIS

The diagnosis of urticaria is rarely a problem, although urticarial vasculitis should be considered in patients with lesions that persist for longer than 24 hours or that resolve leaving postinflammatory changes (see p.103).

INVESTIGATIONS

Acute urticaria, especially when episodic, may require investigation for suspected allergies as indicated by the history. In patients with chronic urticaria, investigations can be limited to a full blood count and ESR. Thyroid function tests and thyroid autoantibodies may also be tested. Food allergy testing is not indicated in chronic urticaria.

TREATMENT

Non-sedating H1 antihistamines are the first line of therapy and help symptom control in most cases. Sedating antihistamines may be useful at night. In patients who fail to respond, combination of H1 and H2 antihistamines can be used. Strict pseudoallergen-free diets have been found to help some patients with chronic idiopathic urticaria. Oral corticosteroids are effective in treating various forms of urticaria, especially acute severe urticaria, but they should not be used as for long-term treatment because of their side-effects. Ciclosporin is an alternative in refractory cases.

Urticarial vasculitis

DEFINITION AND CLINICAL FEATURES

Urticarial vasculitis is an uncommon variant of urticaria in which the individual lesions persist for more than 24 hours and resolve with bruising or staining of the skin (**51**). This may simply represent the more severe end of the spectrum of common urticaria, but may be the presenting feature of an underlying connective tissue disease, particularly systemic lupus erythematosus (SLE). Such patients more frequently have arthralgia and reduced complement C2 and C4.

DIFFERENTIAL DIAGNOSIS

Urticarial vasculitis needs to be distinguished from a reactive erythema or exanthem, as well as from simple urticaria.

INVESTIGATIONS

A general physical examination of patients with urticarial vasculitis is important. Urine must be tested for proteinuria or haematuria and, if either is present, sent for microscopy and culture. Full blood count, ESR, urea and electrolytes, creatinine, liver function tests, C2, C4, and ANF should be done as baseline investigations, as well

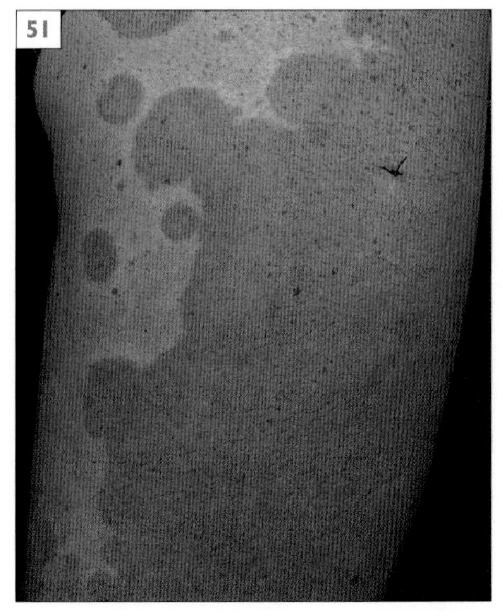

51 Urticarial vasculitis.

as a skin biopsy for routine histology. Infective triggers, such as recent streptococcal infection or mycoplasma, should also be considered.

TREATMENT

There is usually a limited response to oral antihistamines, and systemic corticosteroids are indicated for initial disease control. Other second-line drugs including dapsone may be substituted for long-term management.

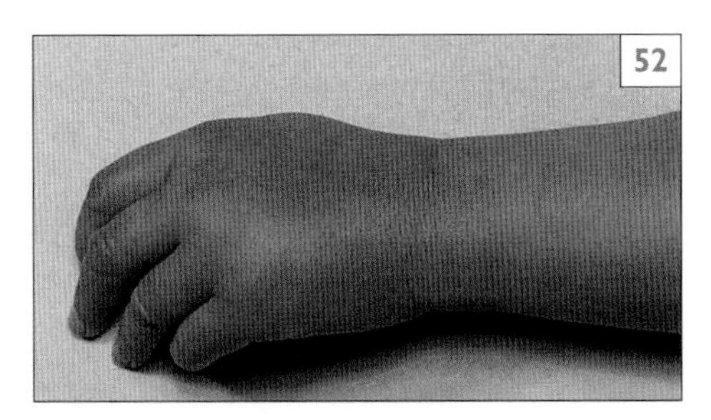

52 Angio-oedema.

Angio-oedema

DEFINITION AND CLINICAL FEATURES

Angio-oedema consists of transient episodes of focal subcutaneous and dermal oedema (**52**) which may affect any body site but which are most commonly seen in a perioral or periorbital distribution. Glottal (**53**) and laryngeal angio-oedema are of particular concern because, in rare instances, sudden severe episodes may cause obstruction of the airway. Lesions are usually non-pruritic and frequently last for 24–48 hours (**54**).

Angioedema associated with urticaria is usually idiopathic. In patients with an underlying allergy, for example to food or venomous insects, this diagnosis is usually evident on taking a careful history. Hereditary angio-oedema is a rare autosomal dominant disorder in which there is a deficiency or inactivity of complement C1-esterase inhibitor. Patients suffer from symptoms related to subcutaneous and gastrointestinal angio-oedema. These patients are at risk of sudden death due to laryngeal oedema. C1-esterase inhibitor deficiency may also arise as an acquired disorder in association with B-cell lymphoma and SLE.

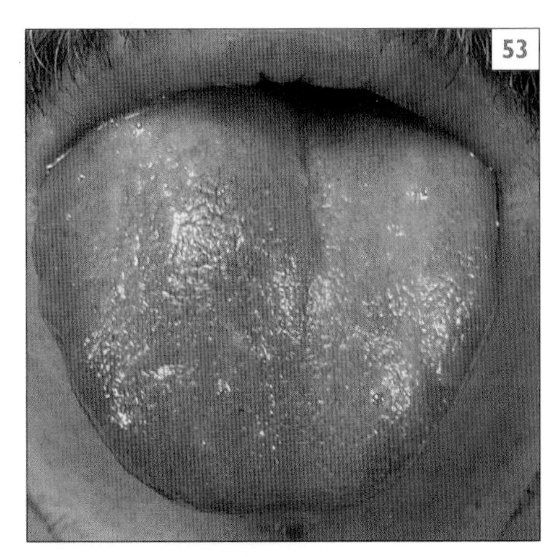

53 Glottal angio-oedema.

DIFFERENTIAL DIAGNOSIS

Acute facial allergic contact dermatitis, especially from hair dye, may present with gross periorbital swelling resembling angio-oedema, but resolves over several days to leave eczematous changes.

INVESTIGATIONS

Routine blood tests including a full blood count, ESR, and ANF and complement C2 and C4 levels should be measured. If complement levels are reduced, C1-esterase inhibitor levels and functional assays should be performed.

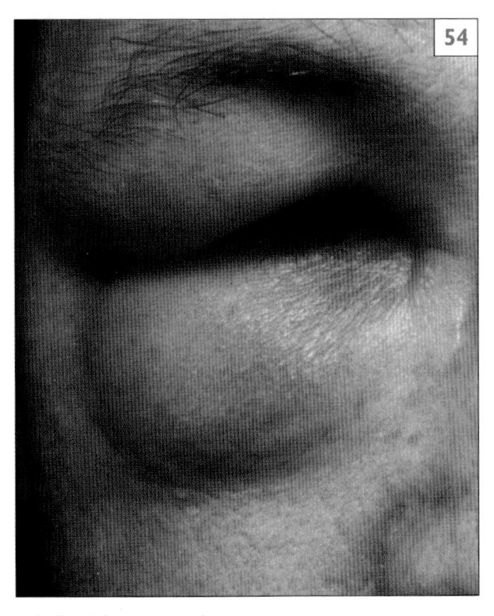

54 Eyelid angio-oedema.

SPECIAL POINTS

Angiotensin-converting enzyme inhibitors may be overlooked as the cause of acquired angio-oedema because the onset can be delayed for several months after starting medication.

TREATMENT

Treatment of idiopathic angio-oedema is essentially the same as for chronic urticaria. Hereditary angio-oedema requires prophylactic treatment with attenuated androgens (danazol and stanazolol). C1-inhibitor concentrate is the first-line therapy for an acute attack. An intramuscular adrenaline autoinjector is indicated for allergic angio-oedema.

Mastocytosis and urticaria pigmentosa

DEFINITION AND CLINICAL FEATURES

Mastocytosis is a rare condition characterized by an excessive number of normal mast cells in the skin, bone marrow, and gut. Urticaria pigmentosa is the commonest cutaneous form, and may develop in early infancy or adulthood.

Childhood (paediatric) urticaria pigmentosa usually presents with a number of brownish dermal papules and plaques widely distributed over the body (**55**). When rubbed, these plaques become urticated (Darier's sign). Solitary lesions (mastocytomas) can also occur, and tend to

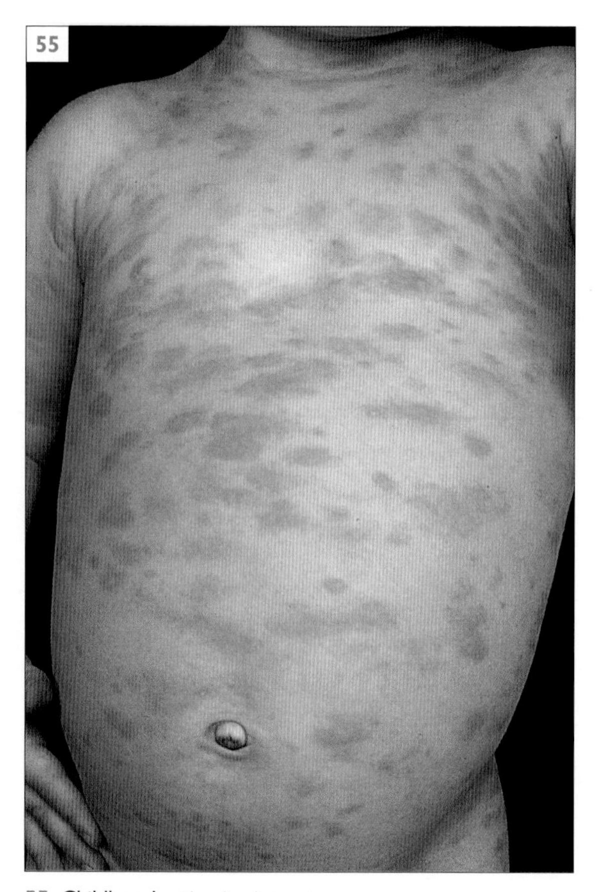

55 Childhood urticaria pigmentosa.

blister with friction (**56**). Patients suffer from pruritus due to the release of mast cell mediators and, in severe cases with extensive involvement, may have systemic symptoms including wheezing, diarrhoea, and syncope. Mast cell mediator release may be triggered by physical stimuli such as temperature extremes, towelling, alcohol, and medication, particularly non-steroidal anti-inflammatory drugs and opiates. Clinical evidence of systemic involvement is uncommon in children and spontaneous resolution of the cutaneous manifestations is the rule.

Adult urticaria pigmentosa presents with an insidious onset of monomorphic pigmented reddish-brown maculopapular lesions, sometimes with prominent telangiectasia on the trunk and limbs (**57**, **58**). Involvement of the bone marrow may be asymptomatic, but symptoms include diarrhoea, nausea and vomiting, palpitations, headache, and fatigue. Bone cysts, osteoporosis, and spontaneous fracture may occur.

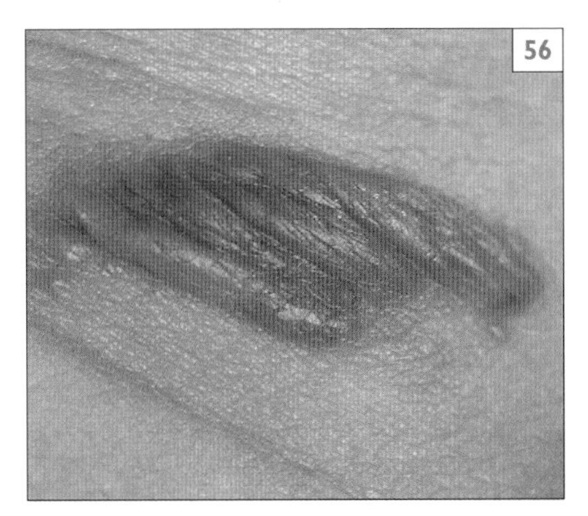

56 Bullous lesions in urticaria pigmentosa.

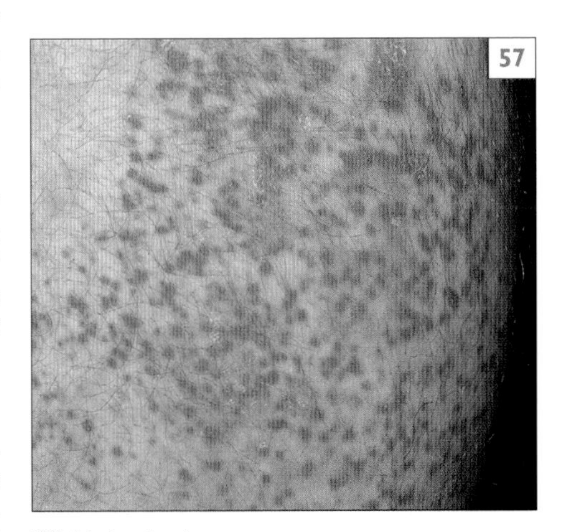

57 Urticaria pigmentosa.

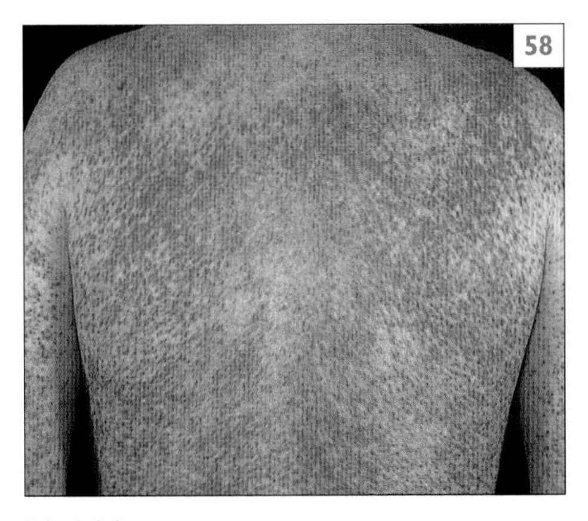

58 Adult urticaria pigmentosa.

DIFFERENTIAL DIAGNOSIS

Paediatric urticaria pigmentosa is usually confirmed by the presence of Darier's sign but other infiltrative processes, such as Langerhans' cell histiocytosis and sarcoidosis, need to be considered. The differential diagnosis is similar for adult urticaria pigmentosa.

INVESTIGATIONS

A skin biopsy is desirable to confirm the diagnosis, although this may be deferred in younger children. Symptoms suggesting systemic involvement should be investigated. A full blood count should be performed at presentation to exclude significant bone marrow involvement; other symptoms should be investigated on merit.

SPECIAL POINTS

It is important to advise the pathologist of the possible diagnosis of urticaria pigmentosa actively as skin biopsies may not be diagnostic unless special stains for mast cells are performed.

TREATMENT

There is no specific treatment, but management includes avoidance of triggers for mast cell degranulation, antihistamines for symptomatic relief, and monitoring for significant systemic disease. UVB phototherapy and oral PUVA may temporarily improve symptoms and appearance of adult disease.

PAPULOSQUAMOUS ERUPTIONS

Psoriasis

DEFINITION AND CLINICAL FEATURES

Psoriasis is a common chronic inflammatory papulosquamous eruption with a prediliction for the extensor aspects of limbs and scalp. Both sexes are equally affected and there is a bimodal distribution of the age of onset which peaks in adolescence and middle age. The severity of disease may vary with time and a range of clinical patterns are recognized. Family studies indicate a strong genetic component, and precipitating or exacerbating factors include trauma (Köbner phenomenon) (**59**), streptococcal infection, various drugs (e.g. lithium, beta-blocking agents, antimalarials), stress, alcohol, and smoking.

Chronic plaque psoriasis (psoriasis vulgaris), the commonest form, is characterized by well-demarcated, thickened, deep-red plaques, surmounted by silvery scale (**60**). They may be distributed anywhere, although characteristically occur on the extensor aspects of limbs, particularly the knees (**61**) and elbows, sacrum, scalp (along the hairline) (**62**) and ears. The plaques vary in size from small (1–2 cm) to very large (e.g. covering the entire extensor aspect of a limb). The disease may be localized to one or two areas only, or cover most of the body (**63**).

Rupioid psoriasis is a term given to grossly hyperkeratotic limpet-like plaques (**64**).

Guttate psoriasis classically occurs following a streptococcal throat infection in children and young adults: showers of red, oval or round, scaly plaques up to 1 cm in diameter rapidly appear on the trunk and proximal limbs (**65**).

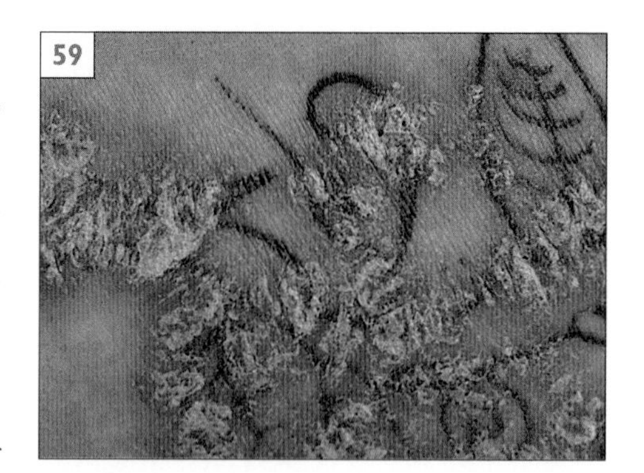

59 Köbner phenomenon.

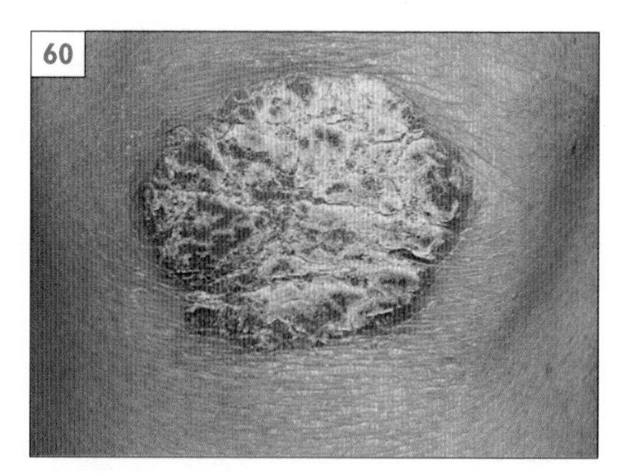

60 Psoriatic plaque.

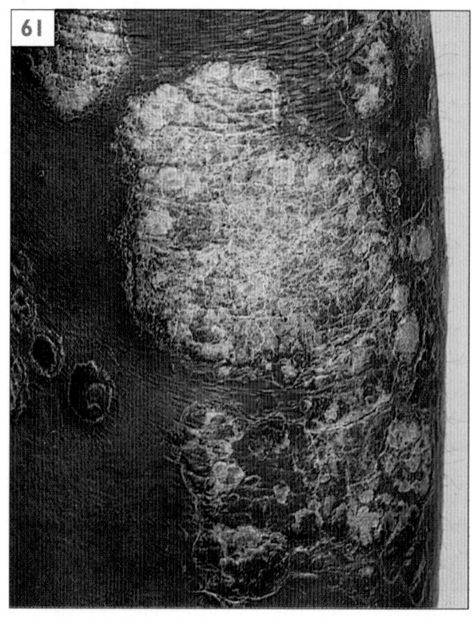

61 Psoriatic knee.

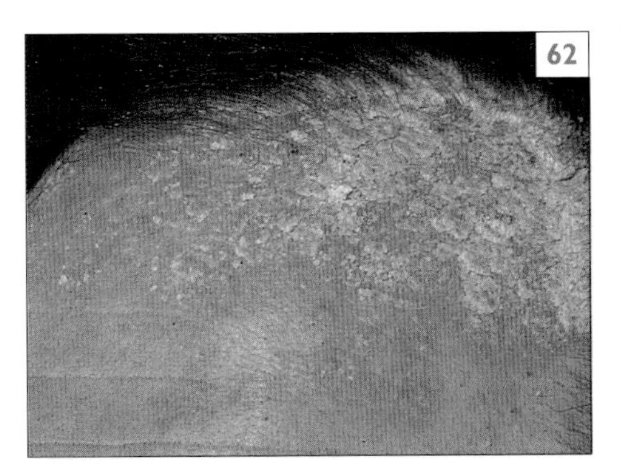

62 Psoriatic scalp.

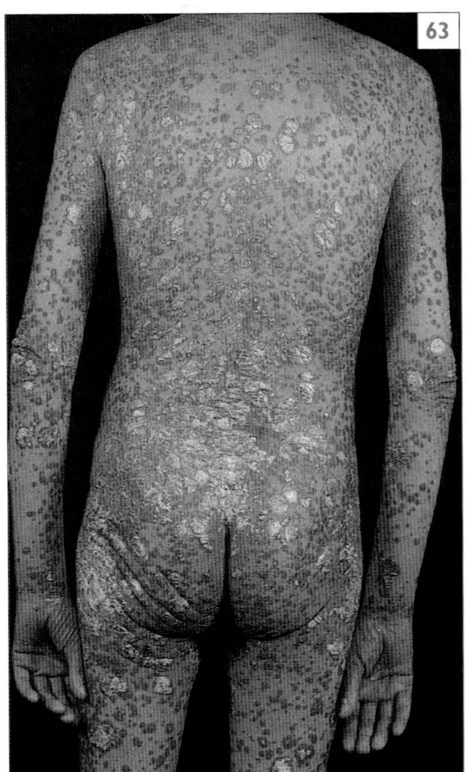

63 Widespread psoriasis.

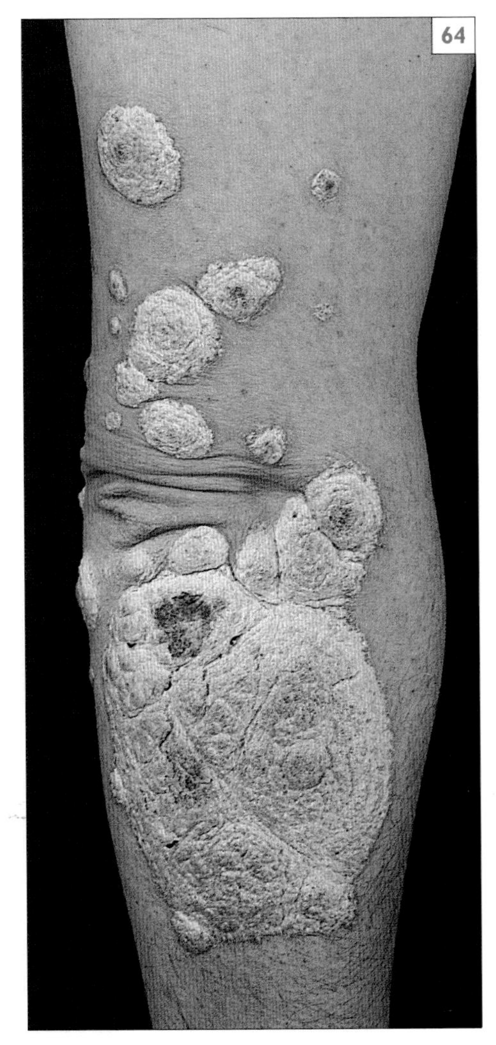

64 Rupioid psoriasis.

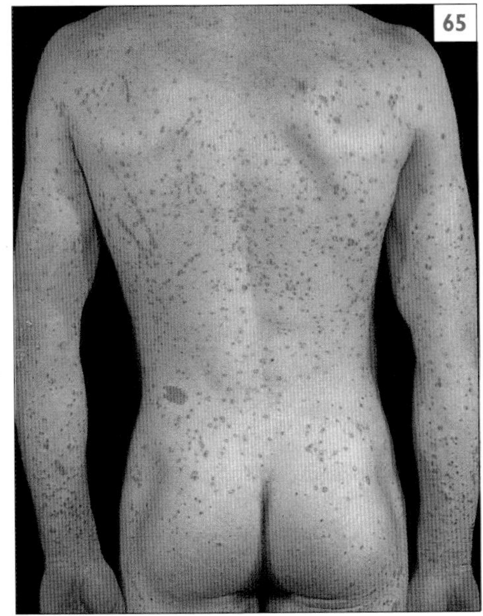

65 Guttate psoriasis.

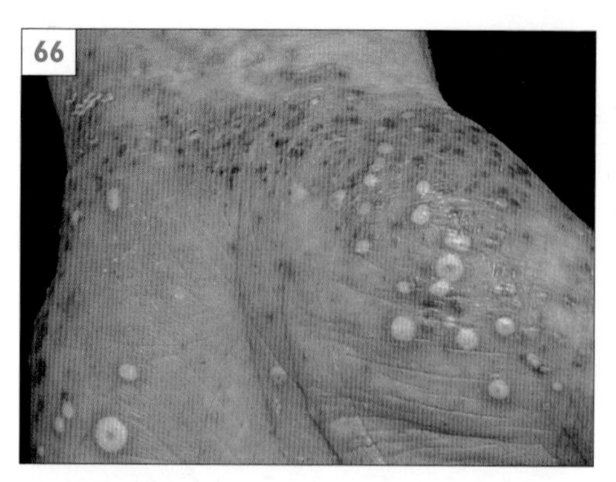

66 Pustular psoriasis.

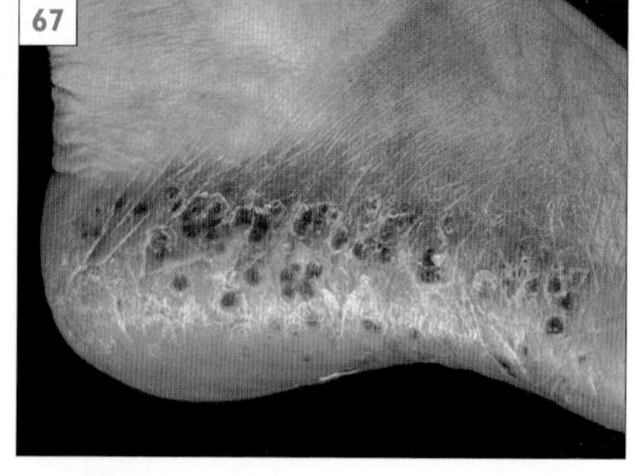

67 Pustular psoriasis.

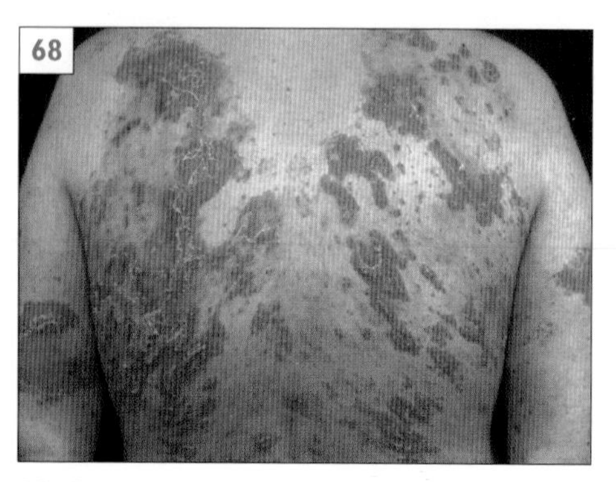

68 Generalized pustular psoriasis.

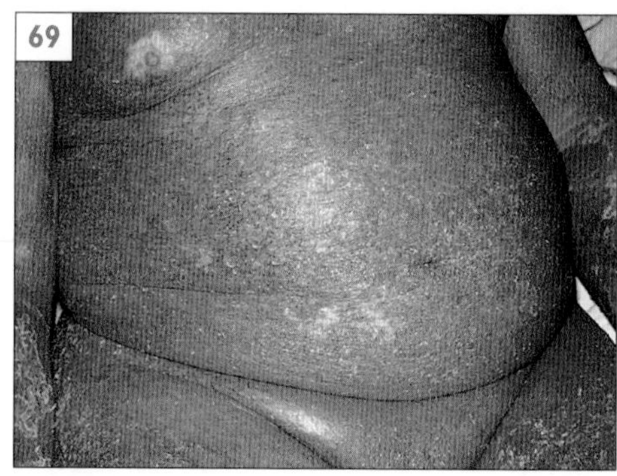

69 Erythrodermic psoriasis.

Pustular psoriasis may be localized or generalized. Chronic, localized pustular psoriasis (also called palmoplantar pustulosis) occurs predominantly in adults and manifests as recurrent crops of sterile yellow pustules, 0.1–0.5 cm in diameter, on the palms and soles (**66**, **67**). The pustules involute to leave red-brown macules with scaling. Generalized pustular psoriasis is an unstable, severe form of psoriasis. Erythematous plaques studded with pustules rapidly appear at any site and may become confluent (**68**). Fever and malaise are common. Erythrodermic psoriasis is a widespread severe variant with generalized erythema, and scaling. It is associated with systemic symptoms, and if untreated, carries a significant mortality (**69**). It may evolve from pustular psoriasis or be triggered by infection, over-treatment with tar, dithranol, or the sudden withdrawal of corticosteroids. Patients are at risk of fluid and protein loss, poor temperature control, and infection.

The clinical features of psoriasis may be modified by site. Involvement of flexures leads to loss of scale, with erythema and maceration only (**70**). Scalp psoriasis, particularly in children and young adults, may be associated with thick, white scale adhering to the scalp and hair shaft (pityriasis amiantacea) (**71**). Nail changes are common, especially in association with arthropathy, and manifest as pitting, onycholysis, yellow-brown areas of discolouration (salmon patches or oil-drop sign) (**72**), and subungual hyperkeratosis (**73**).

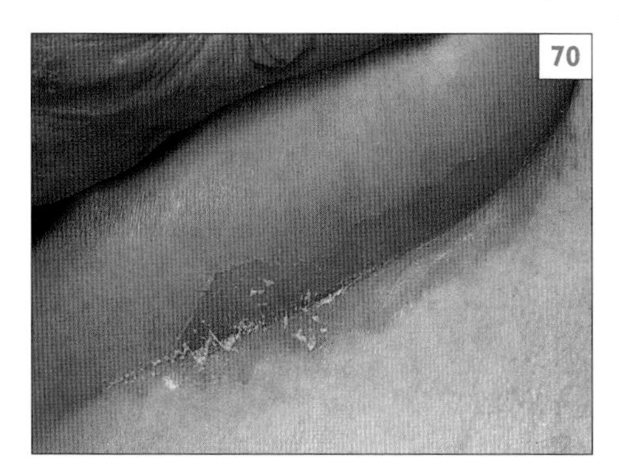

70 Flexural psoriasis.

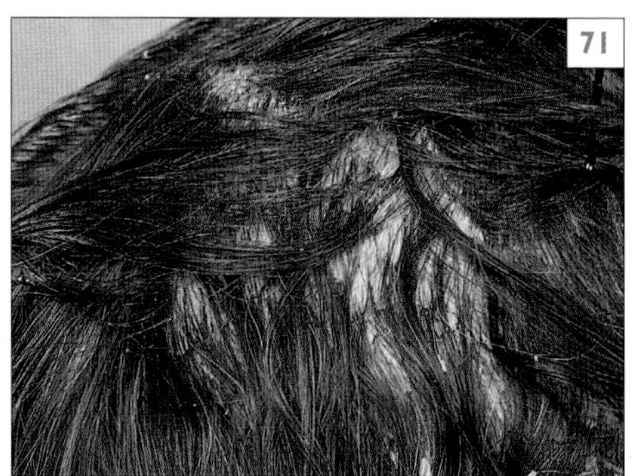

71 Pityriasis amiantacea.

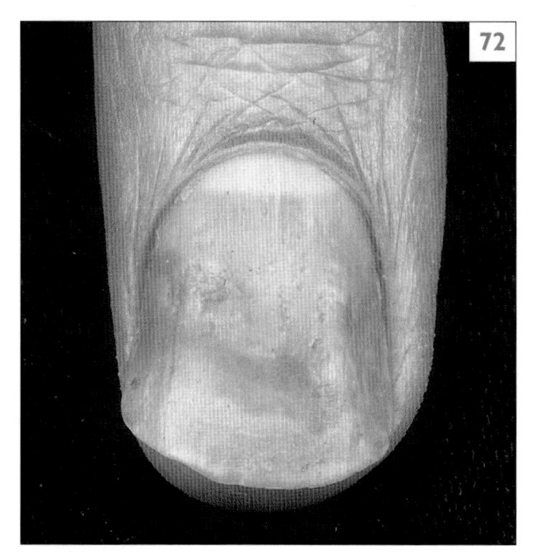

72 Psoriatic pitting, onycholysis, and salmon patch.

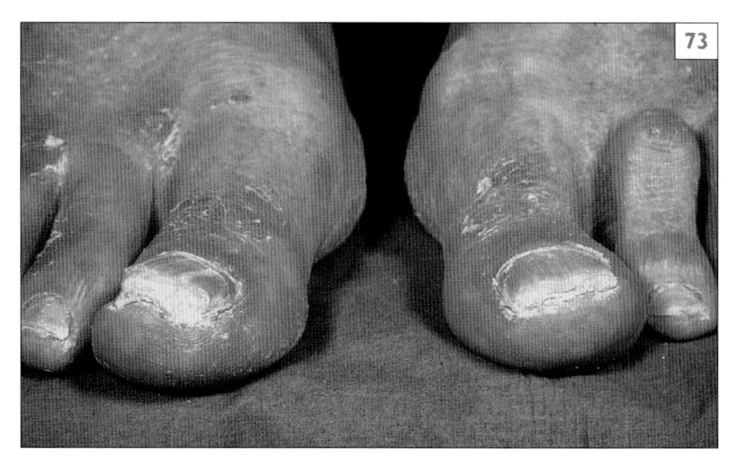

73 Subungual hyperkeratosis.

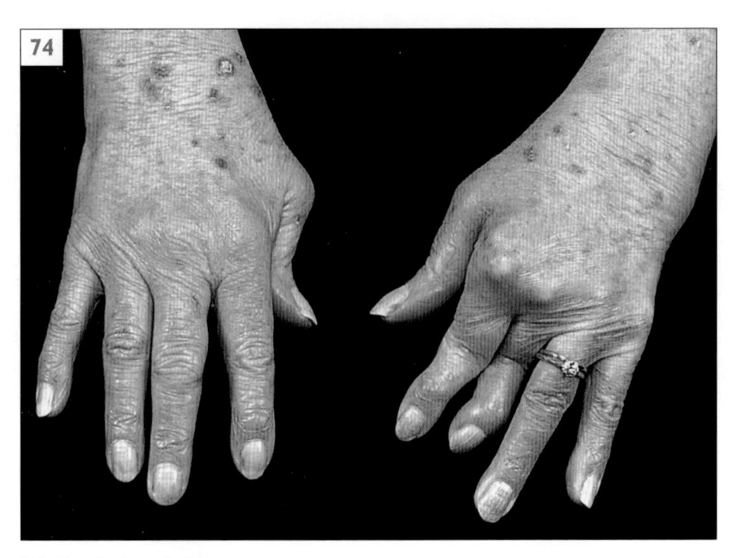

74 Psoriatic arthritis.

Psoriatic arthritis (**74**) is an inflammatory arthritis associated with psoriasis of the skin or nails, in the absence of circulating rheumatoid factor. The prevalence amongst psoriasis patients is uncertain, but it appears more common in those with severe skin disease. Different clinical patterns are recognized including an asymmetrical oligoarthritis, erosive deforming disease, and an ankylosing spondylitis-like variant.

DIFFERENTIAL DIAGNOSIS

The diagnosis of psoriasis is usually made clinically. Chronic plaque psoriasis confined to the palms or soles may closely resemble chronic eczema or tinea. Facial psoriasis may share features and be difficult to distinguish from seborrhoeic eczema (see **14–16**). Guttate psoriasis can simulate pityriasis rosea, pityriasis lichenoides, and secondary syphilis. Flexural psoriasis is often misdiagnosed as chronic intertrigo, but is characteristically well demarcated. Erythrodermic psoriasis may be indistinguishable from other causes of erythroderma, particularly pityriasis rubra pilaris.

INVESTIGATIONS

No investigations are routinely necessary unless the diagnosis is unclear in which case a skin biopsy may be helpful. Patch testing or mycology of skin scrapings should be considered in hand and foot disease where there is diagnostic doubt to exclude allergic contact dermatitis and tinea.

TREATMENT

Although psoriasis is incurable, the majority of patients with mild disease can benefit from topical treatments including corticosteroids, vitamin D analogues, coal tar, and dithranol. UVB and PUVA phototherapy are indicated for more widespread involvement, and a range of systemic drugs are indicated for more severe disease. These include methotrexate, retinoids, ciclosporin and, more recently, biologics. Their efficacy in terms of disease control and improvement in quality of life needs to be balanced against long-term safety and side-effect profiles.

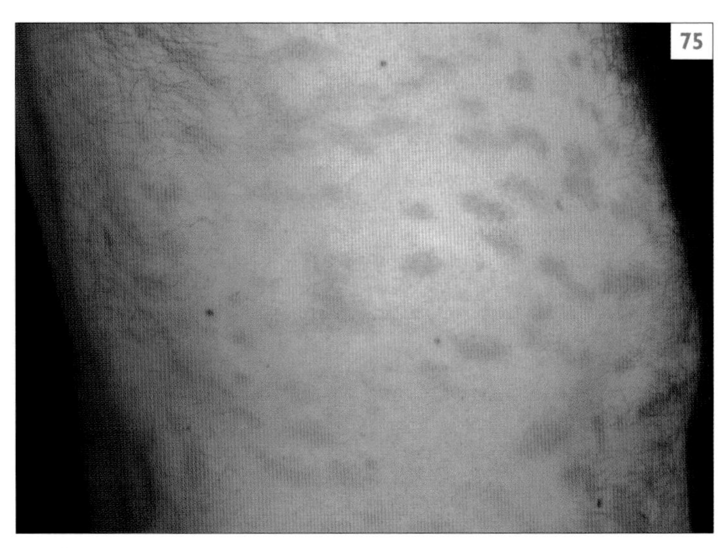

75 Chronic superficial scaly dermatitis.

Small plaque parapsoriasis

DEFINITION AND CLINICAL FEATURES

Also known as chronic superficial scaly dermatitis, and digitate dermatosis, this is a chronic asymptomatic condition that typically affects middle aged adults. The rash is characterized by small, thumb-print-like superficial, pink plaques with fine surface scaling on the trunk and limbs (**75**). Lesions may show signs of atrophy. The cause is unknown, and the condition is usually asymptomatic with a tendency to improve on sun exposure. Emollients and mild topical corticosteroids can be used if there is any associated pruritus. The classification of this condition is confusing as it was once grouped amongst the so-called pre-mycotic eruptions which have a tendency to evolve into mycosis fungoides. However, small plaque parapsoriasis is now considered to be a benign entity that does not progress to a cutaneous lymphoma.

DIFFERENTIAL DIAGNOSIS

Other eczematous disorders and psoriasis. Lesions of early mycosis fungoides are usually larger, and show evolving histological features of lymphoma.

OTHER INVESTIGATIONS

Histology shows mild eczematous features and lacks epidermotropism, or lymphocyte atypia. There is no change in the histological features with time, which helps to differentiate this condition from early mycosis fungoides. In cases of doubt, follow-up skin biopsies should be performed.

Pityriasis rosea

DEFINITION AND CLINICAL FEATURES

This is an acute, self-limiting, rash, probably of infectious origin, which mainly affects young adults. The first lesion to appear, or 'herald patch' (**76**) is larger than the subsequent oval pink scaly patches that appear several days later in crops over subsequent weeks. These mainly affect the trunk and proximal limbs in a Christmas tree pattern (77). There may be mild pruritus. Spontaneous resolution usually occurs within 6 weeks and recurrences are rare.

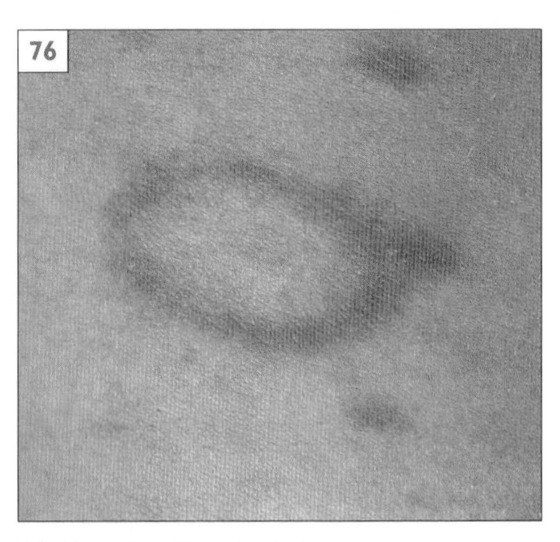

76 Herald patch in pityriasis rosea.

DIFFERENTIAL DIAGNOSIS

Seborrhoeic dermatitis, guttate psoriasis, lichen planus, pityriasis lichenoides, tinea corporis, drug reactions, and secondary syphilis.

INVESTIGATIONS

None are routinely necessary. In atypical cases, skin scrapings should be taken for mycology and serological tests for secondary syphilis considered.

TREATMENT

An emollient and moderate potency topical corticosteroid may be prescribed if pruritis is troublesome.

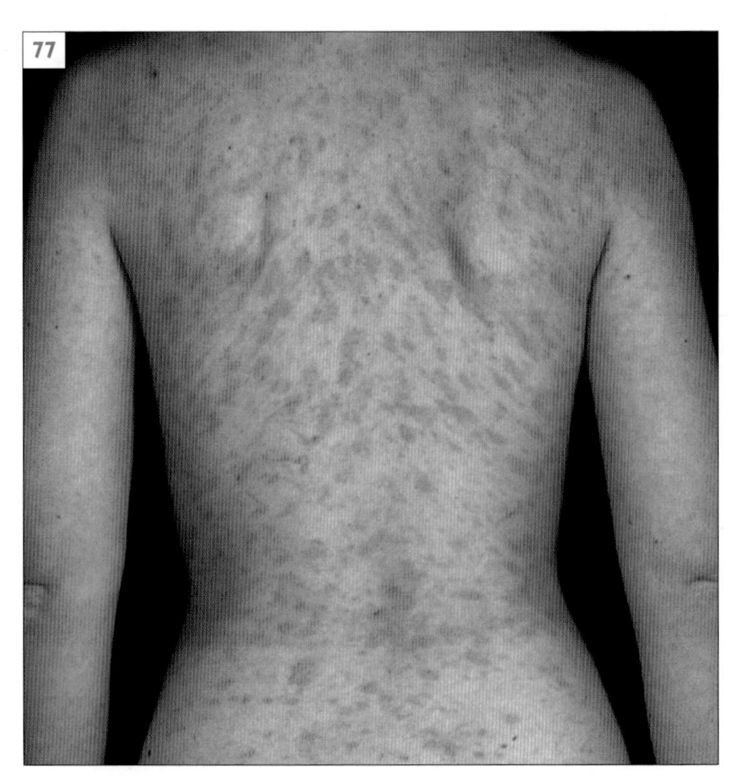

77 Christmas tree pattern in pityriasis rosea.

Pityriasis rubra pilaris

DEFINITION AND CLINICAL FEATURES

Pityriasis rubra pilaris (PRP) is a rare, acquired group of inflammatory disorders of keratinization of unknown cause. Griffiths' classification has identified five subtypes:

- Type 1 or classical adult PRP.
- Type 2 or atypical adult form.
- Type 3 or classical juvenile form.
- Type 4 or circumscribed juvenile PRP.
- Type 5 or atypical juvenile PRP.

Their common features are follicular hyperkeratosis, branny scale on a background of orange-red erythema (**78**). This typically spreads from the head downwards over a period of weeks or months. The extensor proximal digits are often affected producing a nutmeg-grater effect. Palmoplantar keratoderma and a nail dystrophy consisting of thickened nail plates may develop (**79**, **80**) and, later in the course, an erythroderma with islands of spared normal skin may result. Mild pruritus is common. Many cases, especially Type 3, improve spontaneously but the disease can persist for years and may progress to erythroderma.

DIFFERENTIAL DIAGNOSIS

Psoriasis, erythrokeratoderma, and extensive seborrhoeic eczema. In the early and late stages of disease a confident diagnosis may be difficult.

INVESTIGATIONS

Histology of a typical lesion may support the diagnosis, but features can be non-specific.

TREATMENT

Bland emollients are used to reduce scaling. Systemic retinoids or methotrexate may be of benefit in widespread disease, but their effectiveness in PRP is less predictable than in the treatment of psoriasis.

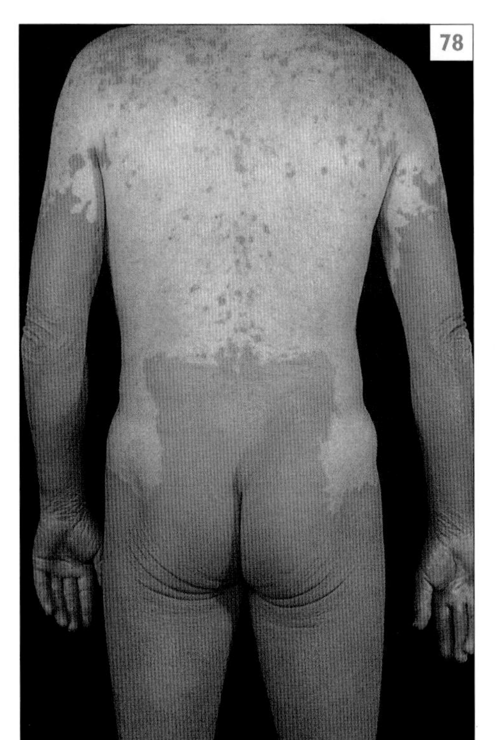

78 Pityriasis rubra pilaris.

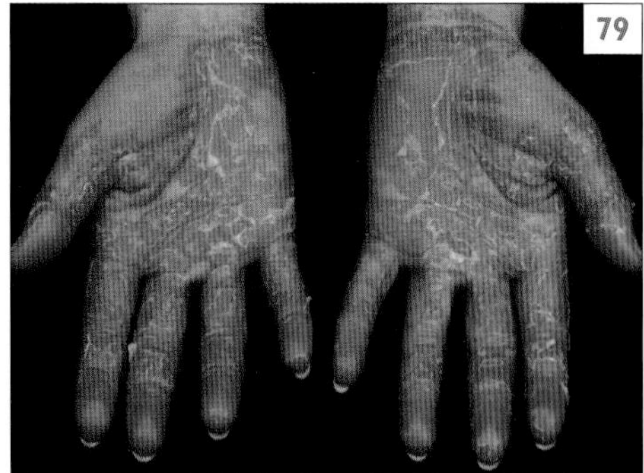

79 Palmoplantar keratoderma.

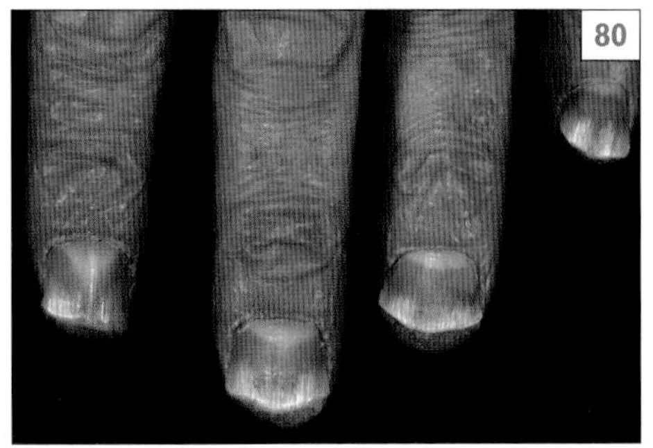

80 Nail dystrophy.

Pityriasis lichenoides

DEFINITION AND CLINICAL FEATURES

Pityriasis lichenoides is a dermatosis of unknown aetiology characterized by multiple papules and plaques which develop in crops on the trunk and limbs. The chronic form, pityriasis lichenoides chronica, is more common and mainly affects young adults with a 2:1 male predominance. It is characterized by small reddish-brown papules with an adherent mica-like scale (**81**) and scarring is unusual. The more acute form, pityriasis lichenoides acuta et varioliformis (pleva or Mucha–Habermann disease), mainly affects children, with an equal sex incidence. Lesions evolve from erythematous papules into haemorrhagic vesicles and necrotic ulcers, and heal with chickenpox-like scars (**82**). Systemic upset with fever and malaise may occur rarely (febrile ulceronecrotic variant). Both acute and chronic forms may follow a relapsing course over several months or years. Cases have been reported in association with a variety of infections, and one hypothesis is that pityriasis lichenoides represents a vascular injury response following hypersensitivity to an infective organism.

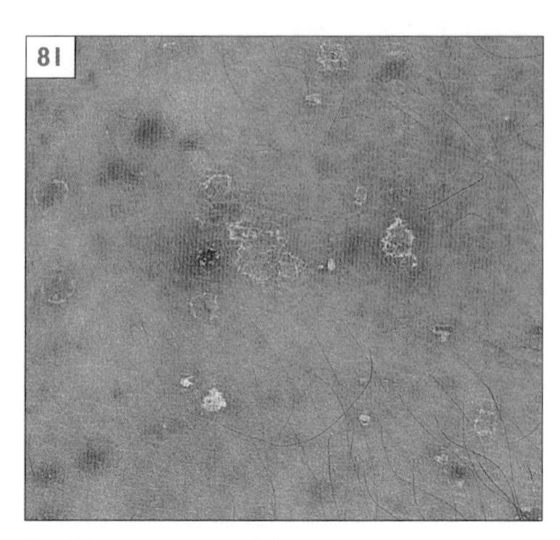

81 Chronic pityriasis lichenoides.

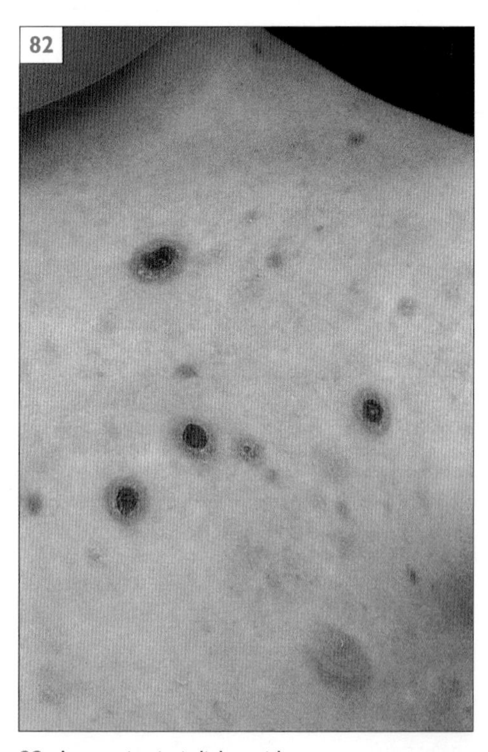

82 Acute pityriasis lichenoides.

DIFFERENTIAL DIAGNOSIS

The acute form is usually distinctive, but may resemble other vesicobullous disorders, including viral eruptions and insect bites and, in severe cases, may be difficult to differentiate from lymphomatoid papulosis. The chronic form should be differentiated from other papulosquamous disorders, including psoriasis, lichen planus, and secondary syphilis.

INVESTIGATIONS

Histology usually helps support the diagnosis, with features varying according to the stage of the lesion and severity. Early lesions show a dense lymphocytic infiltrate with dilated superficial blood vessels and erythrocyte extravasation, while chronic lesions show epidermal changes such as spongiosis, acanthosis, and parakeratosis.

TREATMENT

Success has been reported with long-term erythromycin or tetracycline treatment or phototherapy.

Lichen planus

DEFINITION AND CLINICALFEATURES

Lichen planus (LP) is an intensely pruritic eruption of purple-tinted, polygonal flat-topped papules (**83**). On clearing, these characteristically leave post-inflammatory hyperpigmentation (**84**). All races and ages are susceptible, although the greatest incidence is from 20 to 50 years of age. The cause is unknown though an immunological basis is suggested. Some drugs can induce LP-like eruptions (e.g. antimalarials, heavy metals, antituberculous therapy). An association with hepatitis C infection has also been reported in some countries.

LP can affect any part of the body but is most commonly seen symmetrically on the flexor surfaces of the wrists, forearms, ankles, and lower back. White streaks (Wickham's striae) (**85**) overlie the lesions and are frequently observed on the buccal mucosa where they form a lacy pattern (**86**). Unlike candidiasis, these cannot be removed by gentle wiping with a swab. Lesions on the lower legs and palmoplantar surfaces

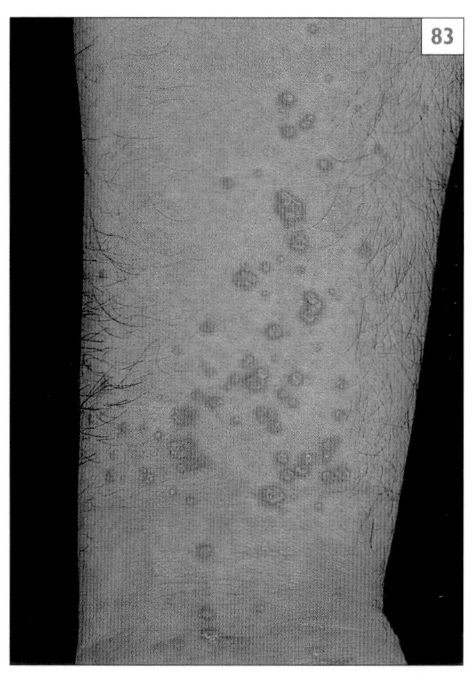

83 Flat-topped papules.

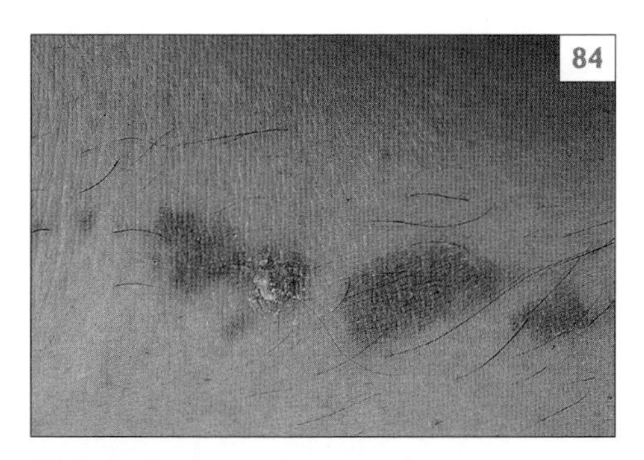

84 Lichen planus hyperpigmentation.

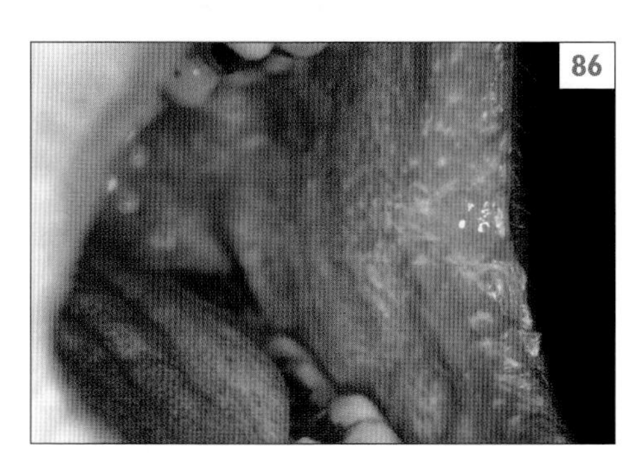

86 Oral lichen planus.

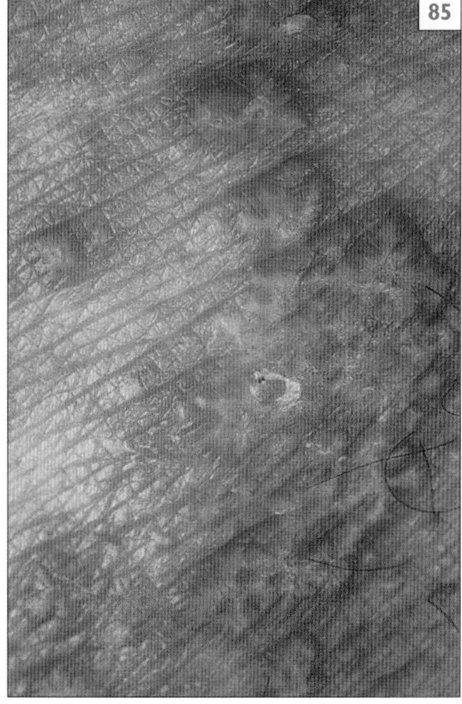

85 Wickham's striae.

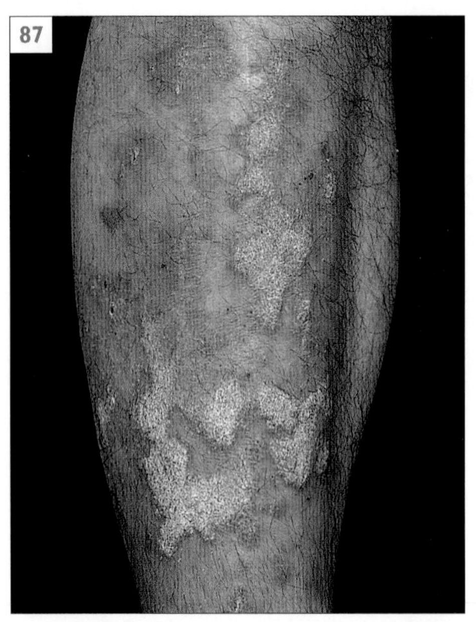

87 Hyperkeratotic lichen planus.

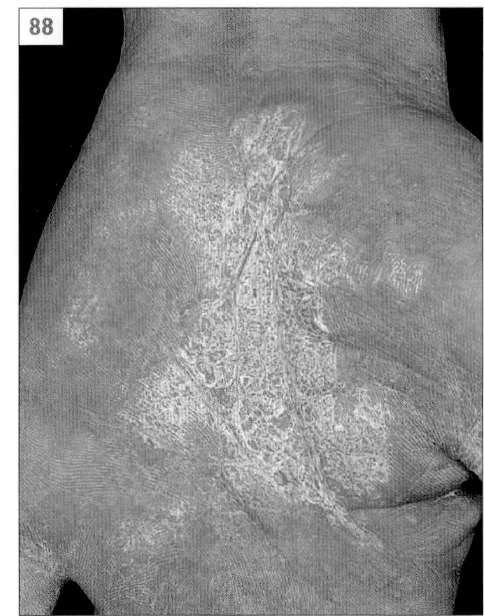

88 Palmar lichen planus.

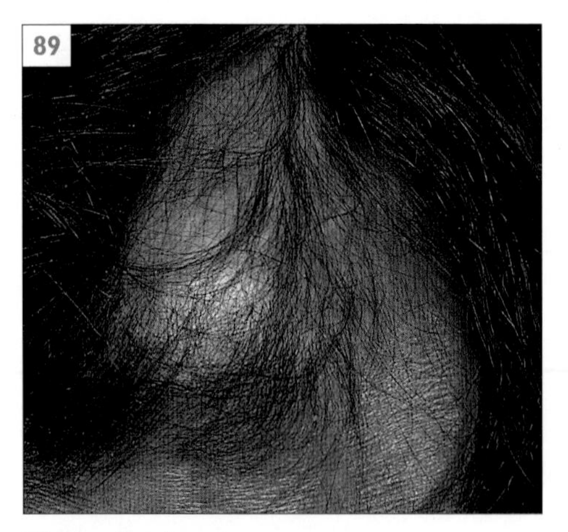

89 Scarring alopecia.

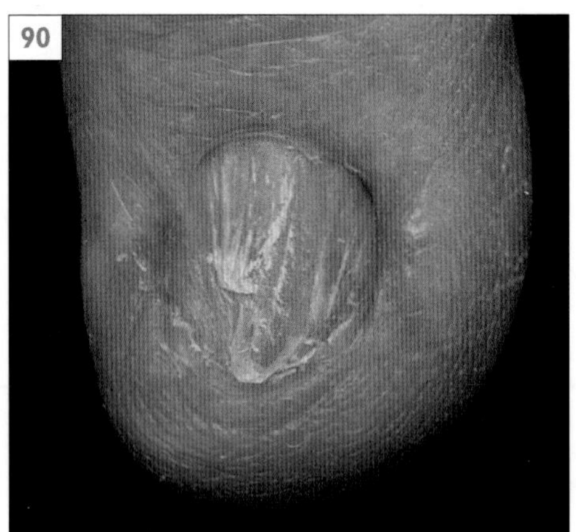

90 Pterygium.

are frequently hyperkeratotic (**87**) and share features with chronic lichenified eczema (**88**) and scalp involvement produces scarring alopecia (**89**). Nail involvement causes longitudinal ridges, variable atrophy, and permanent scarring (pterygium) (**90**). Lesions occur at sites of trauma (Köbner phenomenon) (**91**). Annular lesions may occur, especially on the penis (**92**). Spontaneous recovery is usual within 9 months, but hypertrophic lesions can persist for many years, especially on the lower legs. An uncommon variant affecting the oro-genital mucosa typically runs a recalcitrant course (see p.86). Lichen nitidus is an uncommon variant of LP which presents with multiple minute grouped papules (**93**) that typically affect the forearms, penis, torso, and buttock. It affects children and young adults.

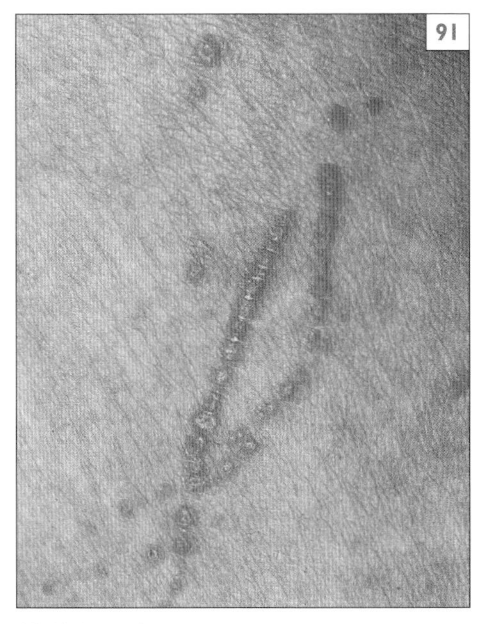

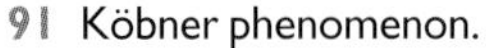

91 Köbner phenomenon.

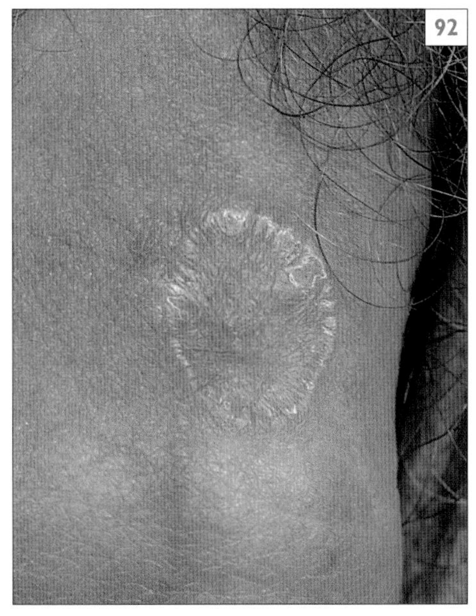

92 Annular lichen planus.

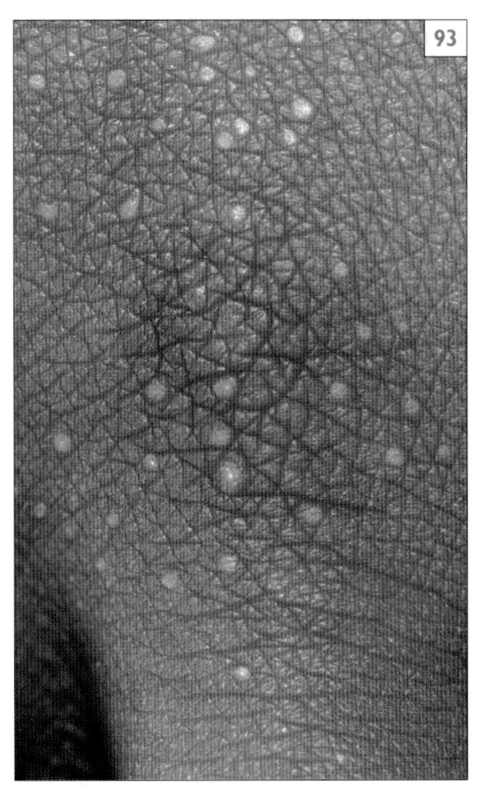

93 Lichen nitidus.

DIFFERENTIAL DIAGNOSIS

Oral lesions may be confused with candidiasis and frictional hyperkeratosis. Hyperkeratotic lesions on the palmo-plantar skin and legs may resemble chronic eczema.

INVESTIGATIONS

Histology of active lesions shows lichenoid inflammation and supports the diagnosis.

SPECIAL POINTS

A drug history is important in patients with atypical lichenoid eruptions to exclude drug-induced disease.

TREATMENT

Potent topical, intralesional, or occasionally systemic corticosteroids are helpful in reducing pruritus. Hypertrophic lesions may benefit from occlusive dressings. Widespread acute LP may occasionally require a reducing course of oral corticosteroids. Other second-line treatments which are used for severe cutaneous or mucosal LP include acitretin, phototherapy, and ciclosporin.

BLISTERING DISEASES

Blistering may be a feature of a wide range of skin diseases. The morphology of the blister depends on the level of the split within the skin (**94**). Subcorneal (beneath the stratum corneum) and intraepidermal blisters (within the prickle cell layer) rupture easily, whereas subepidermal blisters (between the dermis and epidermis) are less fragile.

The autoimmune blistering disorders are a rare acquired group of diseases characterized by blistering and erosions of the skin and/or mucous membranes. Immunofluorescence (IF) techniques are the mainstay of diagnosis and classification of this group of diseases. In pemphigus, pemphigoid, dermatitis herpetiformis, and linear IgA bullous dermatosis the findings are specific for the particular disease (*Table 1*). Direct IF of the skin or mucosal surface demonstrates where immunoglobulins, components of complement 3 (C3), and fibrinogen have been deposited. Indirect IF of the serum detects circulating autoantibodies. Split skin techniques, which artificially cleave the lamina lucida of the basement membrane zone (BMZ), improve the sensitivity of indirect IF and aid diagnosis of subepidermal bullous diseases.

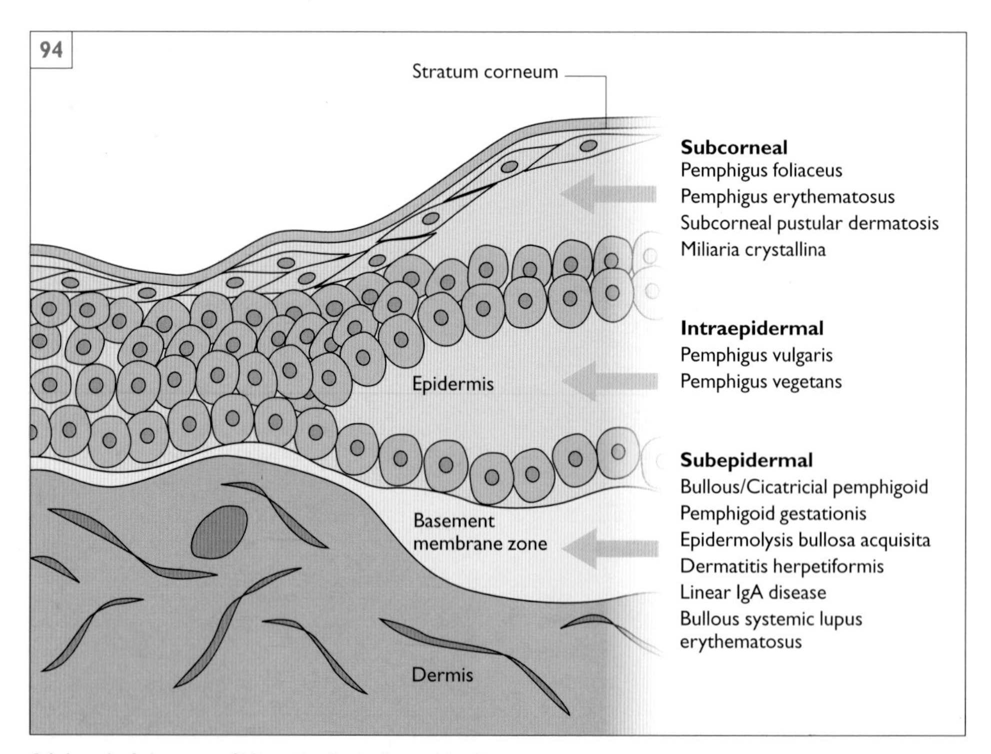

94 Level of cleavage of blister in the bullous skin diseases.

Table 1
Immunofluorescence findings

Disease	Direct	Indirect
Pemphigus foliaceus vulgaris	Intercellular IgG When disease is active, C3 is present	Intercellular IgG
vegetans erythematosus	Mixed IF pattern with intercellular IgG/C3 associated with granular BMZ	Intercellular IgG
Pemphigoid bullous cicatricial	Linear BMZ IgG/C3	Anti-BMZ IgG. The binding on split skin is to the roof
Pemphigoid gestationis	Linear BMZ C3	Complement binding and anti-BMZ IgG. The binding on split skin is to the roof
Epidermolysis bullosa acquisita	Linear BMZ IgG	Anti-BMZ IgG. The binding on split skin is to the base
Linear IgA bullous dermatosis (LAD and CBDC)	Linear BMZ IgA	Anti-BMZ IgA. The binding on split skin is usually to the roof
Dermatitis herpetiformis	Granular deposits of IgA in the dermal papillae	No circulating antibodies to BMZ or dermal papillae components. IgA endomysial antibodies*
Discoid lupus erythematosus	Granular BMZ IgM band (lupus band) in lesional skin; uninvolved skin is negative	
Systemic lupus erythematosus	Granular BMZ IgM band (lupus band) in both lesional and uninvolved skin	

* This is a specific marker for the presence of underlying gluten-sensitive enteropathy

Subcorneal blisters

Miliaria crystallina

DEFINITION AND CLINICAL FEATURES

Miliaria crystallina follows the superficial obstruction of sweat ducts, leading to the development of subcorneal vesicles. They are often seen in febrile illnesses in association with profuse sweating or after heavy exertion. The proposed mechanism is that sweat accumulates under the stratum corneum leading to the appearance of vesicles without underlying erythema. Clear thin-walled vesicles about 1–2 mm in diameter develop on non-inflamed skin (**95**). Lesions occur in crops, especially on the trunk, and are asymptomatic. The vesicles rupture easily and are followed by a superficial brawny desquamation. Lesions may become secondarily infected with bacteria.

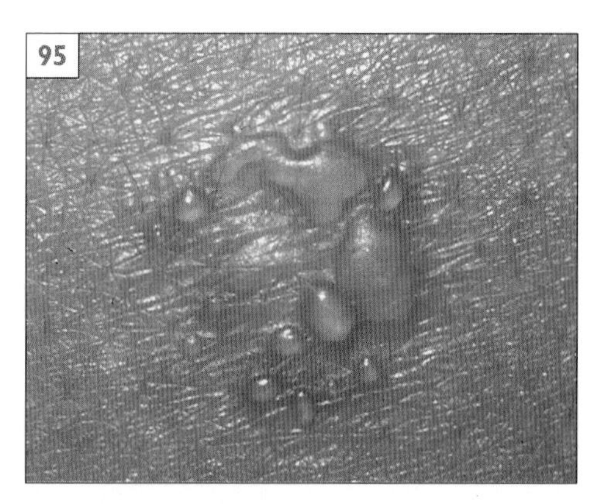

95 Miliaria crystallina.

DIFFERENTIAL DIAGNOSIS

Folliculitis.

INVESTIGATIONS

None routinely necessary.

TREATMENT

Avoidance of sweating, proper cooling and ventilation of the skin are all that is necessary to treat this self-limiting process.

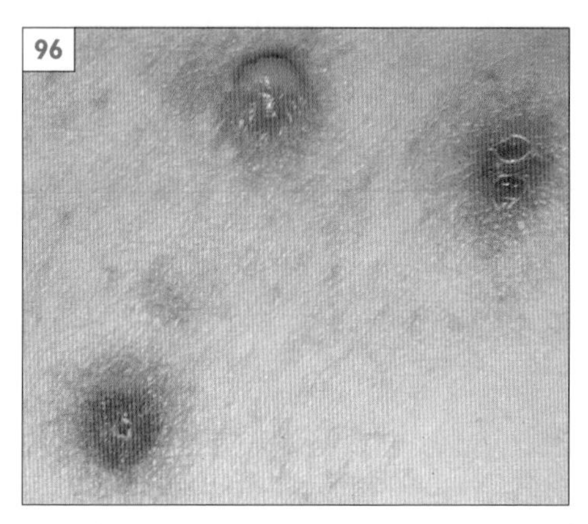

96 Subcorneal pustular dermatosis.

Subcorneal pustular dermatosis

DEFINITION AND CLINICAL FEATURES

Subcorneal pustular dermatosis (Sneddon–Wilkinson disease) is a chronic, benign, relapsing, pustular eruption which has a distinctive histology with subcorneal blisters containing neutrophils. It mainly affects women over the age of 40. Pea-sized oval-shaped pustules develop on normal or erythematous skin and these may rupture easily or coalesce (**96**). Some may demonstrate a level of pus with clear fluid above. Pustules dry up within a few days resulting in impetigo-like crusting and scaling. The eruption occurs mainly in the large flexures and spares the face and mucous membranes.

DIFFERENTIAL DIAGNOSIS

Impetigo, pemphigus foliaceus, dermatitis herpetiformis, chronic bullous disease of childhood, eosinophilic spongiosis, erythema multiforme, and pustular psoriasis must all be considered. IgA pemphigus may present with very similar clinical features, but shows intercellular IgA in the upper epidermis on direct IF.

INVESTIGATIONS

Histology shows numerous neutrophils in a subcorneal blister. Immunofluorescence is negative.

TREATMENT

Dapsone is the treatment of choice. Sulphapyridine and sulphamethoxypyridazine may be used as alternatives.

Intraepidermal blisters

Hailey–Hailey disease
(benign familial chronic pemphigus)

DEFINITION AND CLINICAL FEATURES
Hailey–Hailey disease is a rare autosomal dominant genodermatosis, characterized by defective keratinocyte adhesion. It is caused by mutations in a gene that controls a calcium pump, and is similar to the defect that underlies Darier's disease. Small blisters develop in the intertriginous areas, such as the axillae, groin, and submammary regions. The neck may also be involved. The blisters easily rupture resulting in erythematous eroded areas on which crusts form. A typical feature is small linear fissures in the affected skin (**97**). The disease usually presents in early or middle adult life and may be exacerbated by cutaneous yeast or bacterial infection. *Herpes simplex* virus can cause a widespread vesicular flare.

DIFFERENTIAL DIAGNOSIS
Seborrhoeic eczema, psoriasis, fungal and especially candidal infections.

INVESTIGATIONS
Skin biopsy shows separation of suprabasal keratinocytes (acantholysis) leading to splits, lacunae, and blisters. Direct and indirect IF are negative.

TREATMENT
Simple measures to reduce sweating with loose absorbent clothing helps to keep flexures dry and prevent bacterial overgrowth. Moderate to potent topical corticosteroids and topical or oral antibiotics and antiseptics can be of benefit.

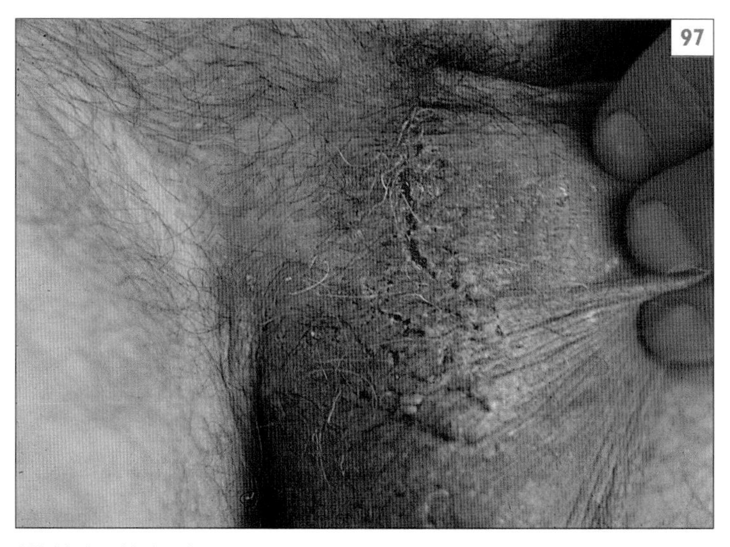

97 Hailey–Hailey disease.

Pemphigus

DEFINITION AND CLINICAL FEATURES

Pemphigus is an uncommon autoimmune bullous dermatosis caused by a circulating IgG autoantibodies directed against epidermal antigens. There are several forms of pemphigus, which differ in their geographical distribution, clinical presentation, histology, and target antigens. Pemphigus vulgaris and pemphigus foliaceus are the two main forms, and the rarer variants include pemphigus vegetans, pemphigus erythematosus, and pemphigus herpetiformis. Pemphigus mediated by IgA antibodies has also been described (IgA pemphigus).

The disease affects the skin and mucous membranes. Widespread flaccid blisters develop and rapidly rupture forming generalized erosions and crusts, often with secondary bacterial infection. The blisters are not haemorrhagic. Shearing stresses on normal skin may cause a new lesion to form (Nikolsky's sign). The oral cavity is the commonest mucous membrane affected, and in one-third of cases the mouth is affected prior to the skin (**98**). Pemphigus vulgaris is the commonest type, in which blisters and erosions predominate (**99**). In pemphigus foliaceus, widespread very superficial blisters rupture, leaving predominantly erosions and crusts (**100**).

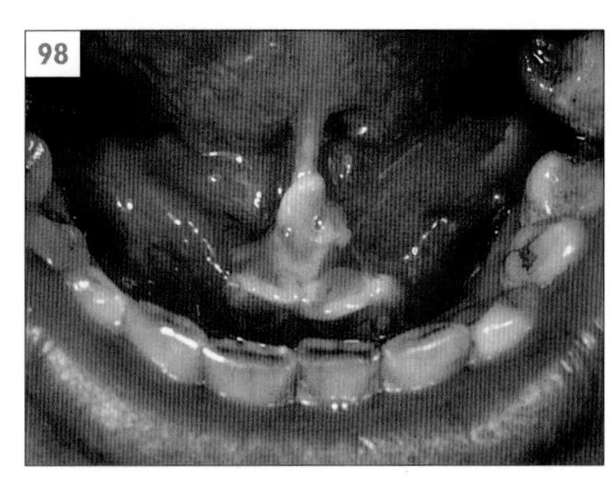

98 Oral pemphigus vulgaris.

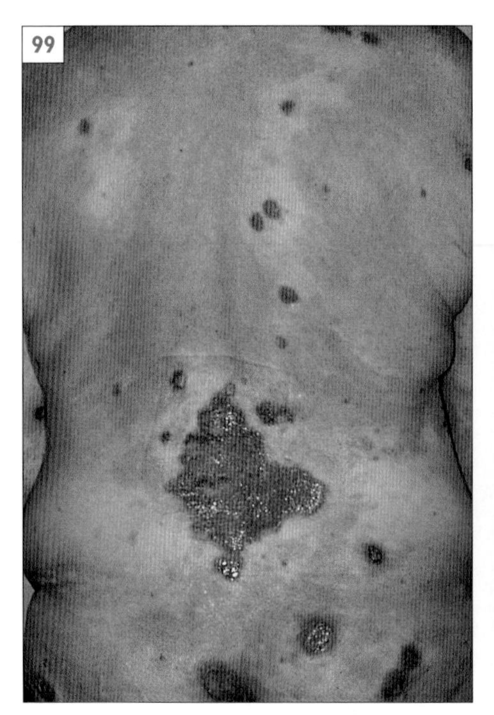

99 Pemphigus vulgaris.

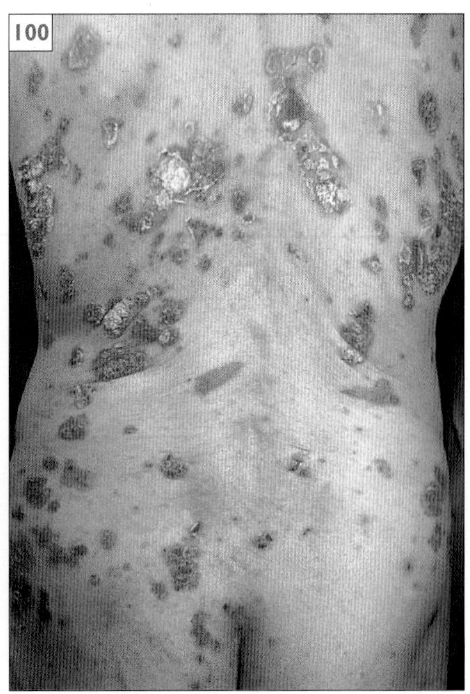

100 Pemphigus foliaceus.

There is no mucosal involvement. Pemphigus vegetans is a more localized form in which heaped-up or cauliflower-like lesions are present, especially in flexural sites such as the groins and axillae (**101**). Pemphigus erythematosus (also called Senear– Usher disease) probably represents coexistence of pemphigus and lupus erythematosus. Paraneoplastic pemphigus has been described in patients with underlying malignancy and is characterized by severe mucosal erosions and polymorphic skin lesions which overlap with erythema multiforme and lichen planus.

Pemphigus may affect all ages and shows marked racial and geographical variation. Pemphigus vulgaris tends to be common in people of Jewish or Indian origin. Pemphigus foliaceus is endemic in Brazil, where it is thought to be initiated by an insect-borne trigger. Drug-induced cases may also occur. Transient neonatal disease may occur in the offspring of mothers with pemphigus, due to transplacental transfer of IgG autoantibodies.

DIFFERENTIAL DIAGNOSIS

Other immunobullous disorders, impetigo, and seborrhoeic eczema (pemphigus foliaceus).

INVESTIGATIONS

Lesional skin shows intraepidermal blistering and acantholysis of the epidermal cells. Direct IF of perilesional skin shows characteristic intercellular epidermal deposits of IgG and C3. Approximately 90% of patients also have circulating autoantibodies and the titre of circulating autoantibody often correlates with disease activity.

TREATMENT

High-dose systemic corticosteroids are usually started to initiate disease control followed by the introduction of a steroid-sparing drug. A number of immunosuppressants have been used including azathioprine, cyclophosphamide, and mycophenolate mofetil. Intravenous immunoglobulin, plasmapheresis, and rituximab have been used in resistant cases.

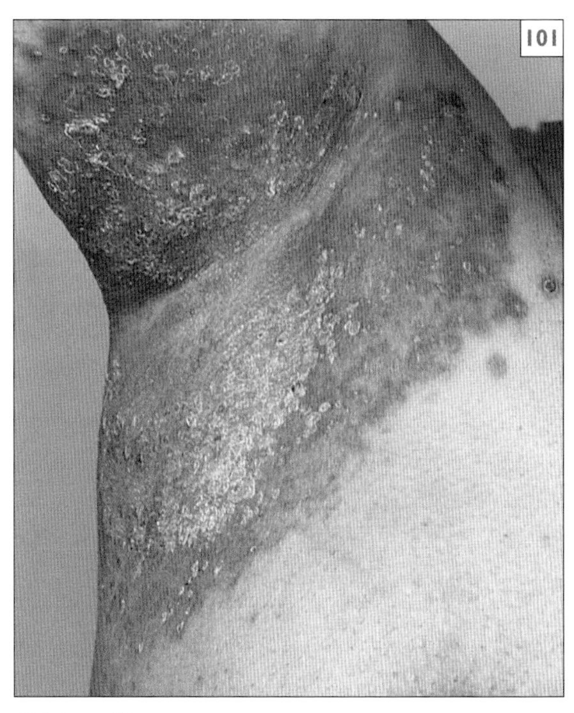

101 Pemphigus vegetans.

Subepidermal blisters

Bullous pemphigoid

DEFINITION AND CLINICAL FEATURES

Bullous pemphigoid is a chronic autoimmune condition in which subepidermal blisters develop due to a circulating IgG autoantibody directed against antigens in the dermo–epidermal junction. Bullous pemphigoid is predominantly a disease of the elderly. Tense blisters develop on erythematous urticarial areas, especially on the flexural aspects of the limbs (**102**). The lesions may be very itchy and the blisters may become large and remain intact for days, sometimes becoming haemorrhagic. The face and scalp are not usually affected, but the oral mucosal may develop small blisters. Nikolsky's sign is negative (see under Pemphigus).

DIFFERENTIAL DIAGNOSIS

Other immunobullous diseases, bullous systemic lupus erythematosus, and erythema multiforme. Drugs may induce or trigger pemphigoid.

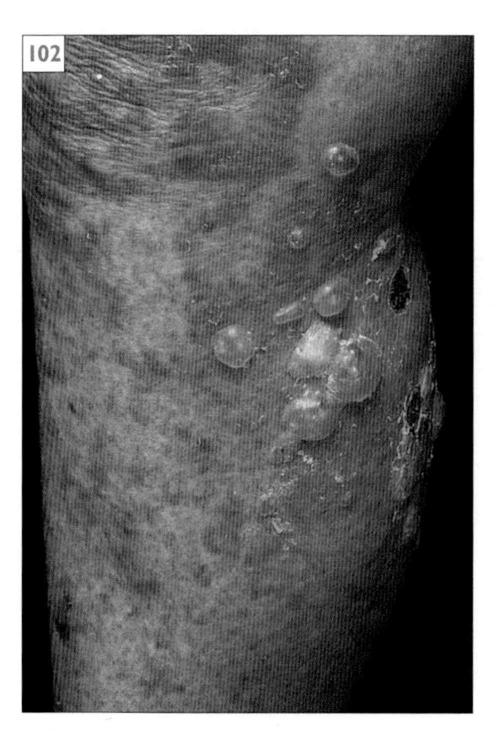

102 Bullous pemphigoid.

INVESTIGATIONS

Biopsy shows subepidermal blisters often with an infiltrate of eosinophils. Direct IF of perilesional skin demonstrates linear deposition of IgG and C3 along the BMZ. Indirect IF demonstrates circulating autoantibodies, which bind to the roof of salt-split skin.

TREATMENT

Localized disease may respond to superpotent topical corticosteroids. More widespread disease usually requires systemic corticosteroid treatment for adequate control of blistering. Dapsone or tetracycline and nicotinamide have been reported to be effective alternatives. Immunosuppressant drugs such as azathioprine or methotrexate may also be used as monotherapy or steroid-sparing agents. As most patients are elderly and often frail it is important to monitor them carefully for adverse drug effects and to balance the risks of treatment against the benefits.

Mucous membrane pemphigoid
(cicatrical pemphigoid)

DEFINITION AND CLINICAL FEATURES

Mucous membrane pemphigoid is a chronic immunobullous disorder which causes erosion, ulceration, and scarring of the mucous membranes, particularly the conjunctivae. It may also affect the skin. This disease mainly occurs in middle-aged and elderly people but is less common than bullous pemphigoid.

Oral lesions occur in most patients as small blisters and ulcers which are slow to heal, erosions on the palate, and erosive gingivitis. Other sites of involvement include the upper respiratory tract, oesophagus, and anogenital mucosa, where scarring may result in strictures. Conjunctival involvement may lead to blindness (**103**).

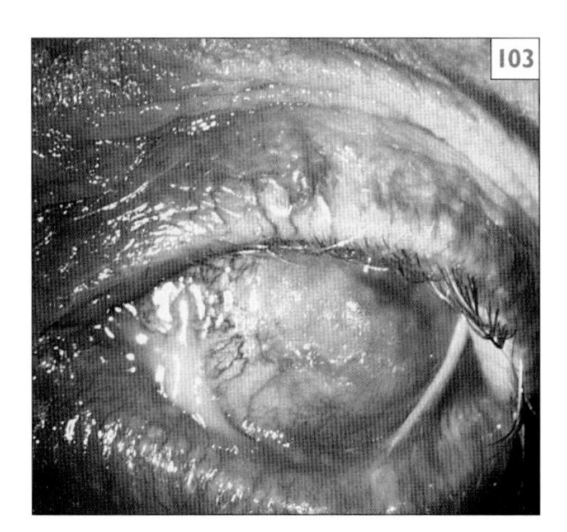

103 Mucous membrane pemphigoid.

DIFFERENTIAL DIAGNOSIS

Other subepidermal blistering diseases, erosive lichen planus.

INVESTIGATIONS

Skin biopsy shows subepidermal blistering with eosinophils and neutrophils. There may be dermal scarring. Direct IF of the buccal mucosa is positive in most patients. Circulating autoantibodies may be present in low titre.

TREATMENT

Treatment is often unsatisfactory and difficult to evaluate due to the fluctuating and scarring nature of this disease. Topical therapy may help reduce to disease activity but seldom achieves remission. Systemic treatment with corticosteroids and immunosuppressive drugs may be indicated for severe mucosal or laryngeal lesions and ocular disease requires management by an experienced ophthalmologist.

Pemphigoid gestationis

DEFINITION AND CLINICAL FEATURES

Pemphigoid gestationis is a rare immunobullous disorder associated with pregnancy or the post-partum period. It has occasionally been reported with trophoblastic tumours. It characteristically begins in the second or third trimester. Intensely itchy blisters develop on urticated areas initially round the umbilicus (**104**) and may spread to involve the rest of the body, especially the hands and feet (usually sparing the face and mucosal areas). Pemphigoid gestationis may occur in subsequent pregnancies, often with increased severity and can be exacerbated by the oral contraceptive pill. Transient blistering may occur in the neonate due to the transplacental passage of the autoantibody.

DIFFERENTIAL DIAGNOSIS

Especially in the pre-bullous phase, polymorphic eruption of pregnancy and eczema.

INVESTIGATIONS

Biopsy shows subepidermal blistering. All patients have complement binding activity at the BMZ as shown on direct and indirect IF, and about 50% have circulating autoantibodies. The target antigens are identical to those in bullous pemphigoid.

TREATMENT

Systemic corticosteroids are usually needed to control blistering and may be increased post-partum to prevent a flare. Oral antihistamines and potent topical corticosteroids can be used for mild disease.

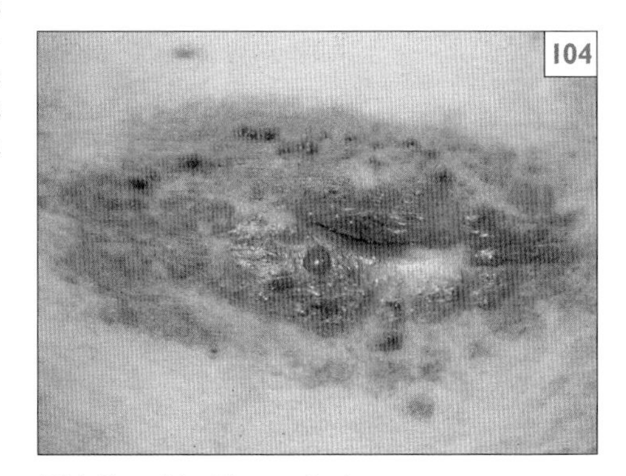

104 Pemphigoid gestationis.

Epidermolysis bullosa acquisita

DEFINITION AND CLINICAL FEATURES

Epidermolysis bullosa acquisita (EBA) is one of the rarest immunobullous diseases. The classic form is characterized by acquired fragility, blistering, and erosion of the skin and mucosa. Lesions heal with scarring and milia (**105**). An inflammatory bullous pemphigoid-like variant is also recognized. There is an association with inflammatory bowel disease and underlying malignancy. The target antigen has been identified as collagen VII of anchoring fibrils.

DIFFERENTIAL DIAGNOSIS

Porphyria cutanea tarda, dominant dystrophic epidermolysis bullosa, other immunobullous diseases.

INVESTIGATIONS

Biopsy usually shows subepidermal blistering. Direct IF is indistinguishable from bullous pemphigoid, but circulating IgG BMZ antibodies in EBA bind to the dermal side of the salt-split skin.

TREATMENT

Due to its rarity there is no established treatment. The mechanobullous variant is often resistant to therapy. Systemic corticosteroids and dapsone or sulfonamides may be tried.

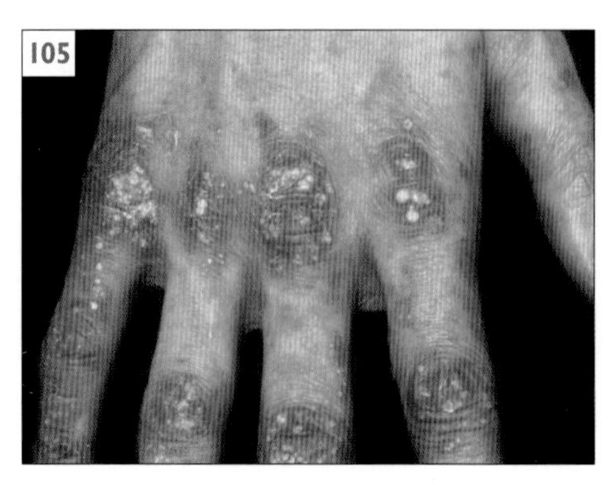

105 Epidermolysis bullosa acquisita.

Dermatitis herpetiformis

DEFINITION AND CLINICAL FEATURES

Dermatitis herpetiformis (DH) is a chronic autoimmune blistering skin disorder associated with an underlying gluten-sensitive enteropathy. It mainly affects Europeans and can present at any age. Intensely pruritic grouped papules and vesicles occur symmetrically on the extensor aspects of the elbows, knees (**106**), buttocks (**107**), shoulders, and scalp. Intact blisters may be destroyed by excoriation. The associated enteropathy is often asymptomatic.

DIFFERENTIAL DIAGNOSIS

Other pruritic dermatoses, such as eczema, scabies.

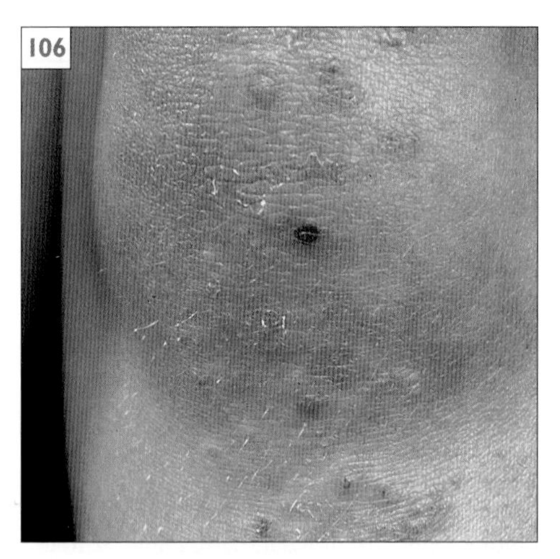

106 Dermatitis herpetiformis.

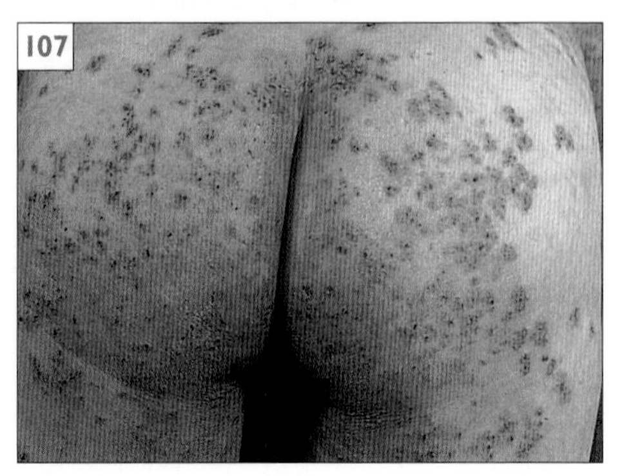

107 Dermatitis herpetiformis.

INVESTIGATIONS

Biopsy of intact blister or lesional skin shows subepidermal blistering and neutrophil-rich microabscesses at the tips of dermal papillae. Direct IF of normal, uninvolved skin shows granular deposits of IgA in the upper papillary dermis. There are no circulating antibodies to the BMZ or dermal papillae. However, 80% have endomysial antibodies which are a marker for the severity of underlying enteropathy. Autoantibodies against tissue transglutaminases may be identified in DH and coeliac disease, and are thought to play a pathogenic role. Small intestinal biopsy in DH usually shows partial or subtotal villous atrophy.

TREATMENT

Dapsone is the drug of choice and settles symptoms dramatically within a few days. The eruption also responds slowly to a gluten-free diet, which must be strictly followed if medication is to be tapered or discontinued. Sulphapyridine or sulphamethoxypyridazine are alternatives in patients who are intolerant of dapsone. There is an increased risk of small bowel lymphoma in patients with DH and a strict gluten-free diet has a protective effect against this.

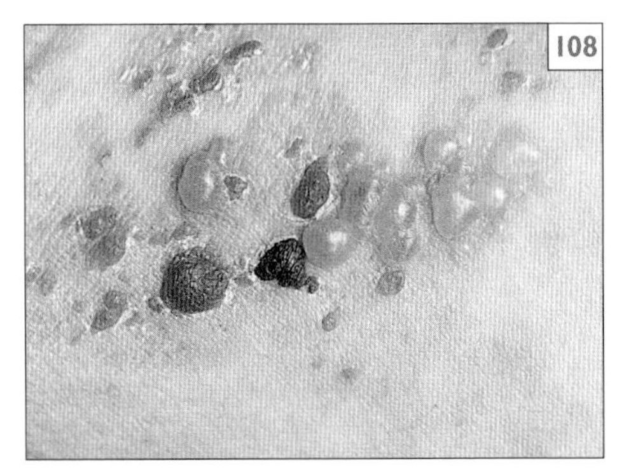

108 Linear IgA disease of adults.

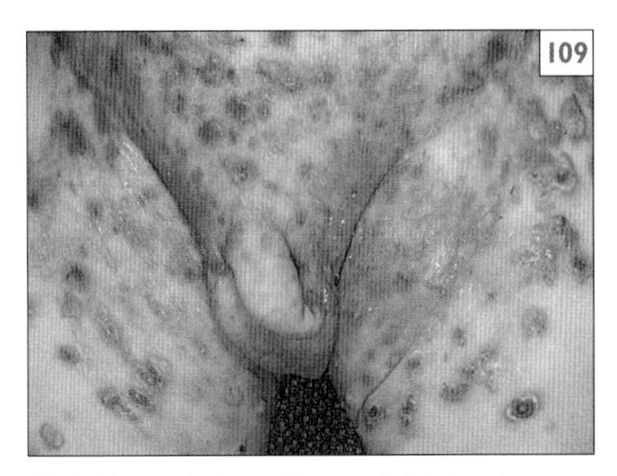

109 Chronic bullous disease of childhood.

Linear IgA disease

DEFINITION AND CLINICAL FEATURES

Linear IgA disease is a rare, acquired subepidermal blistering disease which is defined by its unique immunopathological finding of linear deposits of IgA along the cutaneous basement membrane. It encompasses a clinically heterogeneous group of patients divided into two main forms, linear IgA of adults (LAD) and chronic bullous disease of childhood (CBDC).

Clinically it resembles dermatitis herpetiformis but some lesions develop on the trunk and limbs similar to bullous pemphigoid (**108**). The trunk and limbs are almost always involved. However, in young children the perineum is a characteristic site (**109**). Mucosal involvement can be prominent and associated with scarring. Unlike dermatitis herpetiformis there is no associated gluten-sensitive enteropathy.

Linear IgA disease is less common in the West than either bullous pemphigoid or dermatitis herpetiformis. LAD may present throughout adult life with peaks at 30 and 65 years. The onset of CBDC is usually in the pre-school years and children often recover spontaneously.

DIFFERENTIAL DIAGNOSIS

Bullous impetigo, erythema multiforme, and other immunobullous diseases.

INVESTIGATIONS

Histology shows a subepidermal blister with eosinophils and neutrophils. Direct IF shows linear IgA deposition at the BMZ. Around 20% of LAD patients have circulating autoantibodies compared to 75% of CBDC patients.

TREATMENT

Dapsone or sulfonamides are usually prescribed. Other options include tetracycline, erythromycin, nicotinamide, and colchicine. Immunosuppressants may be used for recalcitrant disease.

Bullous systemic lupus erythmatosus

DEFINITION AND CLINICAL FEATURES

This is a rare autoimmune blistering eruption occurring in patients with underlying systemic lupus erythematosus (SLE). Blisters do not arise within specific LE lesions but, as in the primary blistering diseases, arise *de novo* on clinically normal-appearing skin which may be either sun- or non-sun-exposed. Primary lesions include widespread tense vesicles, bullae, and maculopapular erythema. Blisters may rupture leaving erosions and crust (**110**). Pruritus may be severe. Involvement of the oral mucous membranes occurs in about one-third of patients. Most patients do not have other cutaneous manifestations of SLE.

DIFFERENTIAL DIAGNOSIS

Photosensitivity, bullous drug eruptions.

INVESTIGATIONS

Histology shows subepidermal blister formation with a neutrophil-rich infiltrate in the upper dermis. Direct and indirect IF demonstrate IgG and IgA anti-BMZ antibodies that may target collagen VII as in epidermolysis bullosa acquisita.

TREATMENT

Dapsone may be very effective. Other patients respond to increased doses of oral corticosteroids used to control their SLE.

Bullous erythema multiforme

DEFINITION AND CLINICAL FEATURES

This is a variant of erythema multiforme (see p. 164) with blistering lesions. These appear as erythematous macules or plaques, often with a central blister or peripheral ring of vesicles (**111**). The mucous membranes are often involved with painful ulcers and erosions.

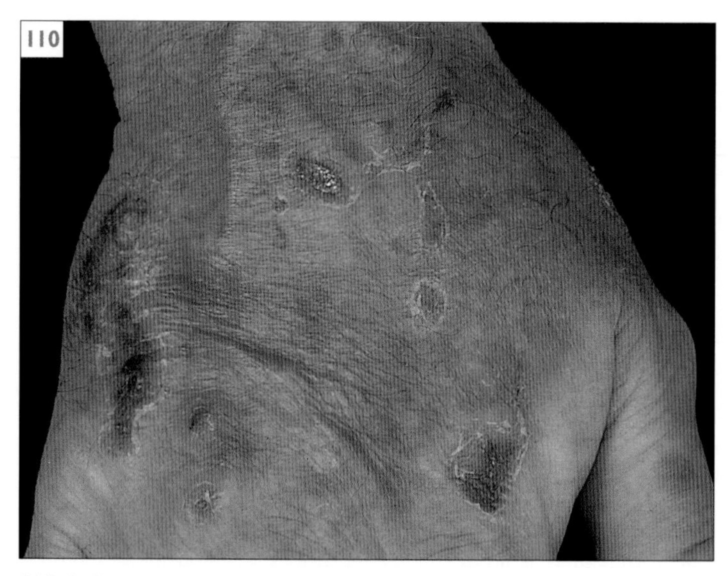

110 Bullous systemic lupus erythematosus.

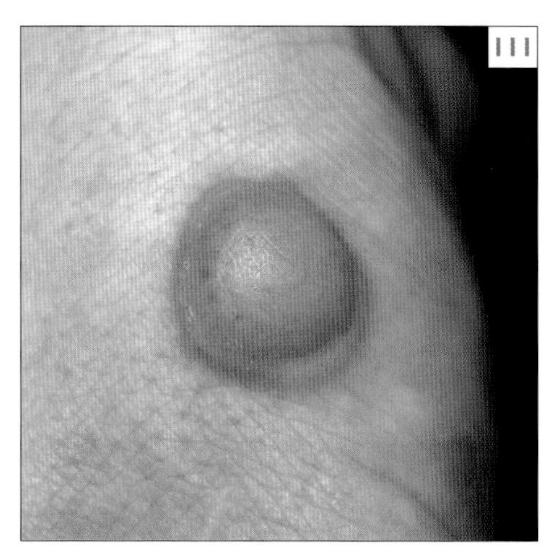

111 Bullous erythema multiforme.

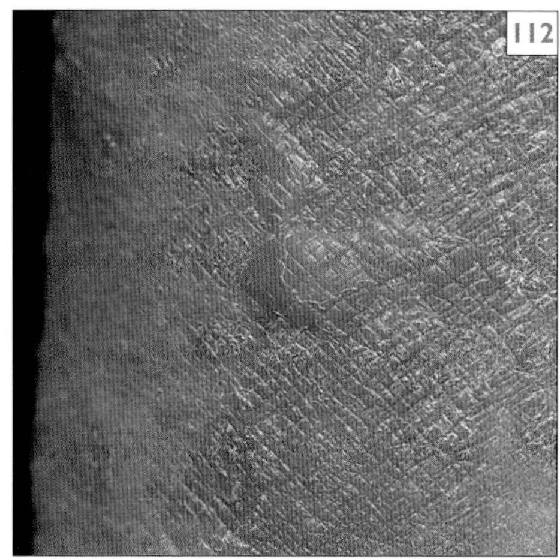

112 Blistering in lichen planus.

Bullous lichen planus and lichen planus pemphigoides

DEFINITION AND CLINICAL FEATURES

Blistering is an uncommon feature of lichen planus, and tends to occur within typical lesions on the lower legs (bullous lichen planus) (**113**), The gross blistering is thought to follow severe liquefaction degeneration of basal keratinocytes, which causes subepidermal splits. Blistering also occurs in lichen planus pemphigoides (LPP), a rare disorder with mixed features of bullous pemphigoid and lichen planus (**113**). It is speculated that antibasement membrane zone antibodies arise in LPP secondary to damage to the basal keratinocytes. LPP tends to occur in younger patients than bullous pemphigoid. Blistering is not confined to lichenoid lesions and may occur in apparently normal skin.

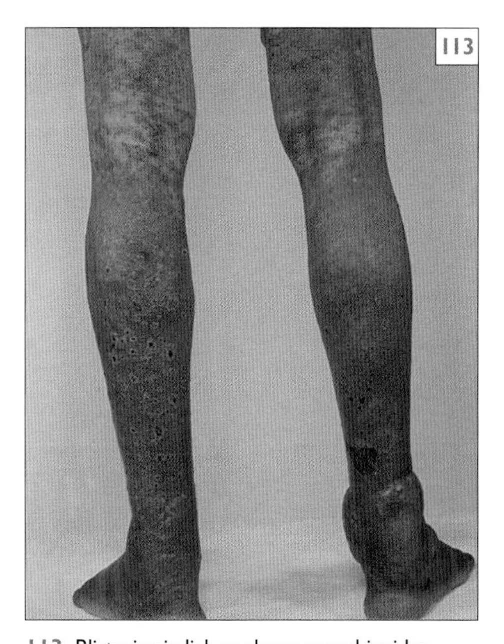

113 Blistering in lichen planus pemphigoides.

DIFFERENTIAL DIAGNOSIS

Other immunobullous disorders, bullous drug reaction.

INVESTIGATIONS

Histology of lesional skin may show a mixed infiltrate in LPP with subepidermal blistering, and direct IMF and indirect IMF are positive, with identical features to bullous pemphigoid.

TREATMENT

Blisters in lichen planus may be drained and lesions treated with superpotent topical corticosteroids. Systemic corticosteroids and immunosuppressant therapy are usually needed for disease control in LPP.

Epidermolysis bullosa

DEFINITION AND CLINICAL FEATURES

Epidermolysis bullosa (EB) is a rare group of inherited skin fragility disorders, caused by genetic mutation and characterized by blistering of the skin and mucous membranes, particularly in trauma-prone areas. Intensive study has helped identify the underlying genetic and molecular defects in these diseases, and this has furthered our understanding of normal skin structure and function. There are three major forms of inherited epidermolysis bullosa. They are classified by the structural level of the skin within which blisters spontaneously develop – suprabasal intraepidermal (EB simplex); lamina lucida subepidermal (EB junctional); and sublamina densa subepidermal (EB dystrophic) (**114**).

Epidermolysis bullosa simplex

Epidermolysis bullosa simplex (or EB simplex) is the commonest form. It is usually inherited as an autosomal dominant condition. Several variants exist, the most common of which is Weber–Cockayne disease with localized involvement of the palms and soles (**115**). More generalized variants include Köbner and Dowling–Meara. Trauma-induced blisters heal without scarring and tend to be worse in warm weather. In the generalized forms grouped blisters develop, especially on the trunk, with marked keratoderma on the palms and soles. Abnormalities in genes coding for keratins 5 and 14 have been identified. Most patients with EB simplex have no extracutaneous involvement or nail abnormalities.

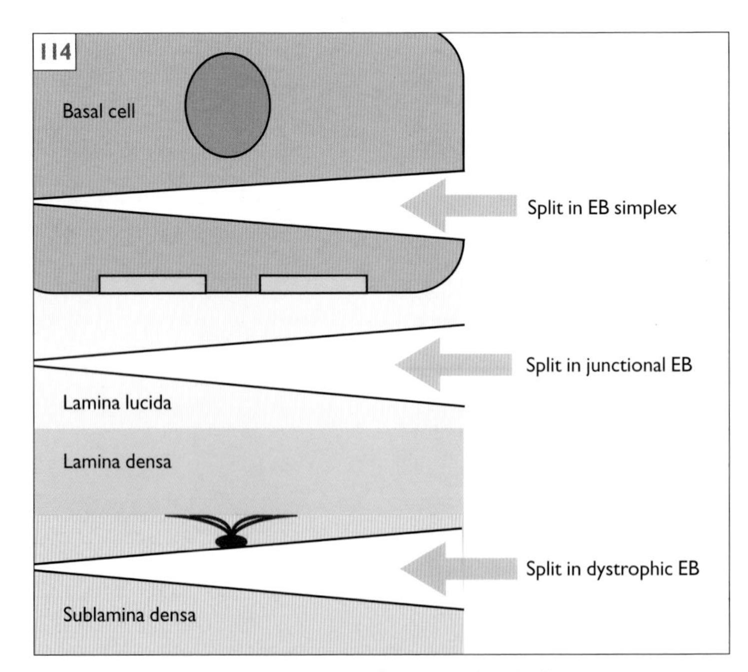

114 Level of split in inherited forms of epidermolysis bullosa.

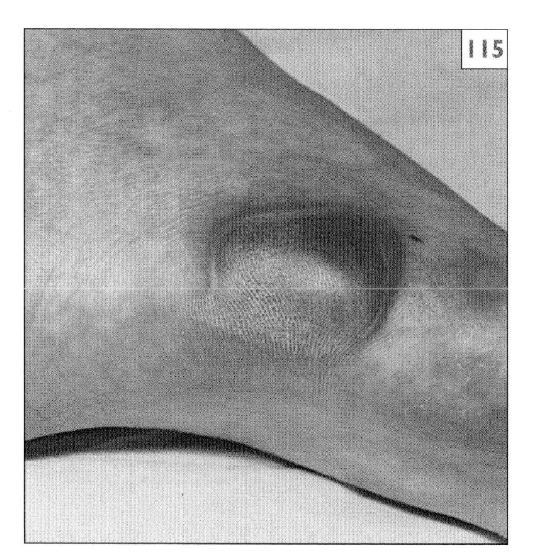

115 Weber–Cockayne disease.

Junctional epidermolysis bullosa

Junctional epidermolysis bullosa (JEB) is inherited as an autosomal recessive condition. At birth, large erosions develop around the mouth and anus which are slow to heal. Blisters and erosions heal with atrophic scars. Nails are abnormal or absent, dental enamel may be defective, and scarring alopecia may occur.

There are several variants that differ in disease extent and severity, extracutaneous involvement and the presence or absence of excessive granulation tissue. The most severe form is Herlitz (JEB-H), which is usually lethal – patients often do not survive infancy. The less severe non-Herlitz variant (JEB-nH) has two subsets, generalized and localized (**116**), and there are also inverse, and late-onset clinical subsets.

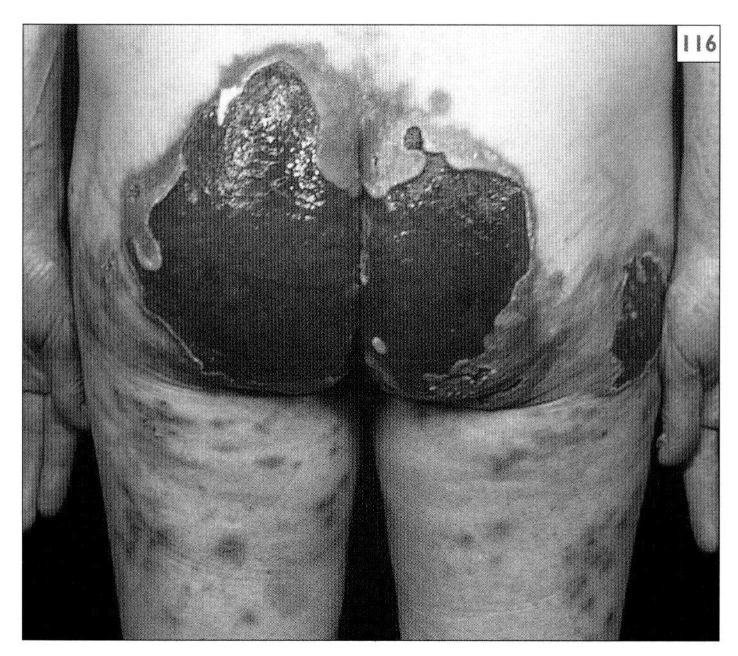

116 Junctional epidermolysis bullosa.

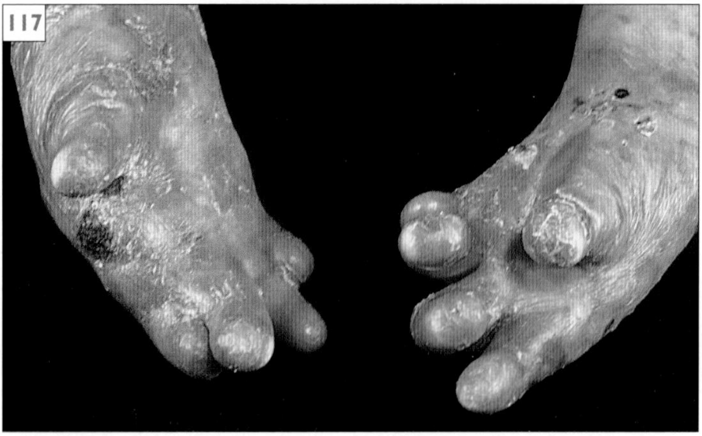

117 Dystrophic epidermolysis bullosa.

Dystrophic epidermolysis bullosa

There are two main variants of dystrophic epidermolysis bullosa (or dystrophic EB), autosomal dominant (DDEB) and autosomal recessive (RDEB). Those with the autosomal dominant variant usually have milder disease. Both diseases are due to abnormalities in collagen VII of anchoring fibrils. Patients suffer from widespread blistering with scarring and milia formation. Scarring alopecia may occur and the nails and teeth may be absent or abnormal. In RDEB fusion of the skin between the digits of the fingers and toes causes syndactyly and mitten deformities (**117**). Mucous membrane involvement may lead to oesophageal and anal strictures. Other complications include anaemia, growth retardation, and squamous cell carcinomas in areas of repeated blistering and scarring.

DIFFERENTIAL DIAGNOSIS

Staphylococcal scalded skin syndrome, bullous impetigo, neonatal herpes simplex, autoimmune bullous diseases, incontinentia pigmenti, aplasia cutis, focal dermal hypoplasia.

NVESTIGATIONS

Skin biopsy for histology, immunofluorescence, and electron microscopy to demonstrate the level of blistering. Specific antibody probes can be used to demonstrate a reduction or absence of certain antigens in the dermo–epidermal junction.

TREATMENT

There is no specific treatment for EB and management is based on protecting the skin against trauma and dealing with complications such as stricture formation. A multi-disciplinary approach is needed for patients with the more severe forms of EB. Prenatal diagnosis in the first trimester and pre-implantation genetic diagnosis have been used for couples at high risk of having affected children.

DISORDERS OF KERATINIZATION

Keratosis pilaris

DEFINITION AND CLINICAL FEATURES

Keratosis pilaris is a dry skin disorder due to abnormal keratinization of hair follicle epithelium. Mild forms are very common and start in early childhood, peaking in adolescence, and improving with age. Its features are prominent follicular hyperkeratosis with plugging that predominantly affects the extensor aspects of the upper arms (**118**) and legs and the buttocks. Perifollicular erythema (keratosis pilaris rubra) may occur. It may be associated with facial erythema and atrophy of the eyebrows (ulerythema ophryogenes) and pitted atrophic scars on the cheeks (atrophoderma vermiculata). A genetically distinct variant involves the scalp and leads to progressive scarring alopecia (keratosis follicularis spinulosa decalvans). Keratosis pilaris may be inherited as an autosomal dominant trait and is associated with ichthyosis vulgaris.

DIFFERENTIAL DIAGNOSIS

A rough skin resembling mild keratosis pilaris frequently occurs in people with a tendency to dry skin. Phrynoderma is a more extreme form of follicular keratosis which affects bony prominences and results from nutritional deficiency. Pityriasis rubra pilaris and the various forms of minute or digitate keratoses are easily distinguished.

INVESTIGATIONS

Histology of a lesion shows follicular hyperkeratosis and plugging.

TREATMENT

Emollients containing salicylic acid, lactic acid, or urea may help reduce the surface hyperkeratosis. There is usually a temporary improvement with sun exposure.

Perforating keratotic disorders

DEFINITION AND CLINICAL FEATURES

This ill-defined group of disorders present with keratotic papules, and may show epidermal extrusion (perforation/transepidermal elimination) of degenerate material derived from the dermis. All except elastosis perforans serpiginosa are associated with diabetes and renal failure. Kyrle's disease, or acquired perforating dermatosis, is characterized by larger keratotic nodules and papules on the limbs, while the lesions of Flegel's disease (**119**) are smaller and more widely distributed with a characteristic irregular margin (cornflake sign) and underlying erythematous base.

DIFFERENTIAL DIAGNOSIS

Lesions may resemble stucco-keratoses, actinic or arsenical keratoses, or disseminated actinic porokeratosis.

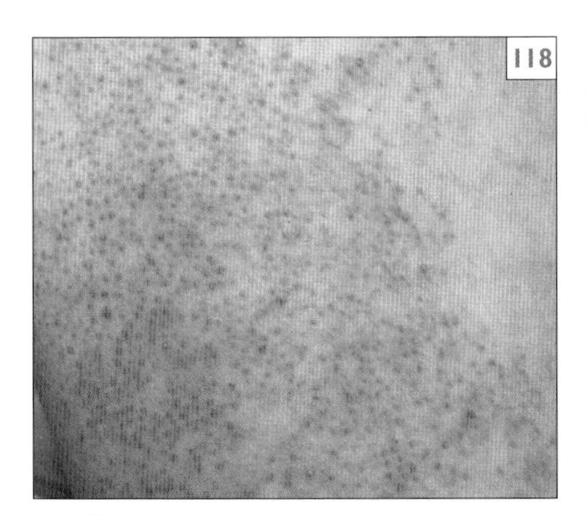

118 Keratosis pilaris.

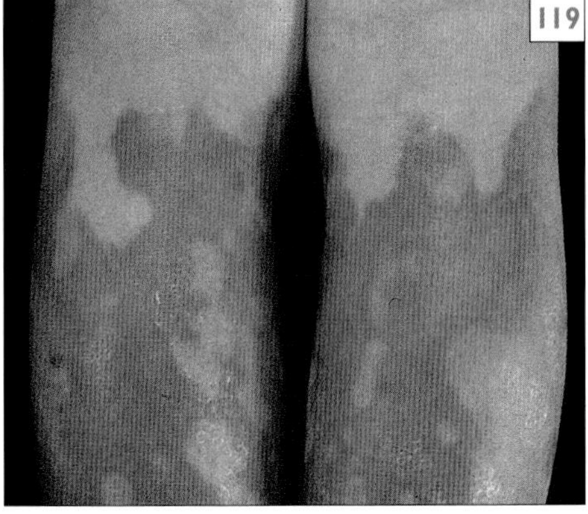

119 Flegel's disease.

INVESTIGATIONS

Histology of a lesion may show ortho- or parakeratosis in an otherwise atrophic epidermis. There is a variable band-like lymphocytic infiltrate and disruption of some follicular walls. Laboratory tests to exclude associated renal, liver, or endocrine diseases should be carried out.

Elastosis perforans serpiginosa is a distinctive condition characterized by annular or serpiginous patterns of small keratotic papules which extrude abnormal elastic tissue. It is associated with connective tissue disorders such as Ehlers–Danlos syndrome, Down's syndrome, and penicillamine therapy.

TREATMENT

Topical retinoids and destructive therapy such as cryotherapy or CO_2 lasers may be of help.

Erythrokeratodermas

DEFINITION AND CLINICAL FEATURES

Erythrokeratodermas are a group of rare disorders characterized by localized hyperkeratotic plaques and circumscribed but variable erythema. Mutations in genes coding for gap junction proteins have been identified in some families.

The features of erythrokeratoderma variabilis are transient migratory patches of polycyclic erythema which fade within weeks, and fixed scaly keratotic erythematous plaques over the extensor surfaces. There may be an associated palmoplantar keratoderma. Progressive symmetrical erythrokeratoderma lacks the migratory erythema, and is characterized by fixed symmetrical hyperkeratotic orange-red plaques with fine scale over the extensor surfaces, torso, ankles, and wrists (**120**). Onset is in infancy.

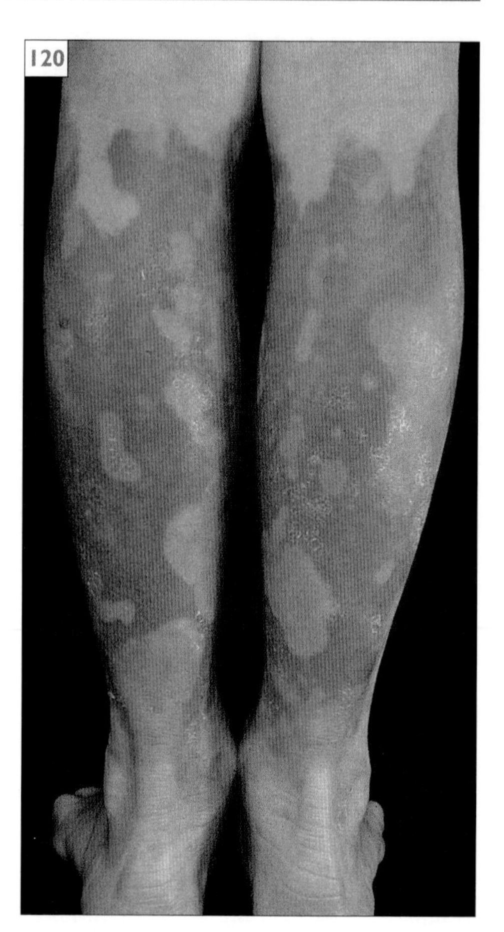

120 Erythrokeratoderma progressiva symmetrica.

DIFFERENTIAL DIAGNOSIS

Pityriasis rubra pilaris and psoriasis.

INVESTIGATIONS

Histology is non-specific.

TREATMENT

The oral retinoid acitretin and PUVA may be of help.

Darier's disease

DEFINITION AND CLINICAL FEATURES

First described in 1889, Darier's disease is a rare autosomal dominant disorder of keratinization. It is caused by a mutation in a gene on chromosome 12 which encodes serca-2, an ion pump that controls intracellular calcium levels. This leads to abnormalities in processing of cell membrane proteins and defective formation of desmosomes which are essential for normal cell adhesion. The clinical features are characteristic keratotic papules affecting the seborrhoeic areas in childhood or early adult life. Yellow-brown, warty, greasy papules arise on the upper chest and back, lower neck, scalp, and forehead and may coalesce into plaques (**121**). Occasionally hypertrophic plaques evolve in the major flexures and natal cleft and, rarely, bullous lesions can occur. Pruritus and body odour are common complaints and can cause considerable cosmetic and social disability. The dorsal hands and feet may show discrete skin-coloured papules (acrokeratosis verruciformis) and palmoplantar pits are very common. The nails are longitudinally ridged with notching at the free edges (**122**). Many patients have white patches on the oral mucosa. Bacterial and viral infections especially with *Staphylococcus* and herpes simplex are not uncommon. The condition is also aggravated by warmth and sunlight.

An increased incidence of neuropsychiatric problems including epilepsy have been noted in families with Darier's disease.

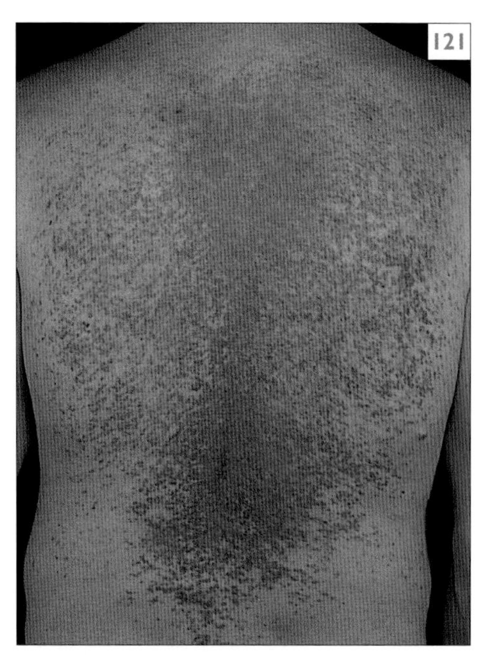

121 Darier's disease.

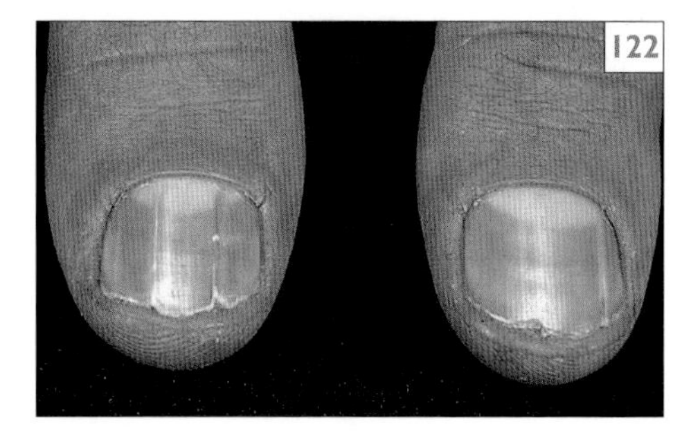

122 Nails in Darier's disease.

DIFFERENTIAL DIAGNOSIS

Clinically, early lesions may resemble seborrhoeic dermatitis or epidermal naevi. Histologically, other acantholytic disorders may cause confusion, in particular Hailey–Hailey disease and Grover's acantholytic dermatosis.

INVESTIGATIONS

Histology shows characteristic changes of dyskeratosis – abnormal keratinocytes with premature partial keratinization (corps ronds and grains), and acantholysis (separation) of suprabasal keratinocytes.

TREATMENT

Most patients with mild disease can control symptoms with emollients, good hygiene, and advice to avoid sun exposure and excess sweating. More severe disease usually responds to the oral retinoids, isotretinoin and acitretin.

Palmoplantar keratodermas

This diverse group is characterized by persistent hyperkeratosis of the palms and soles. They may be hereditary or acquired and can occur as an isolated abnormality or in association with other skin, ectodermal, or systemic abnormalities. Keratodermas are classified clinically as diffuse, focal, striate, or punctate. Genetic defects have been identified in some inherited keratodermas, but there is a lack of clear correlation between the abnormal gene and phenotypical features.

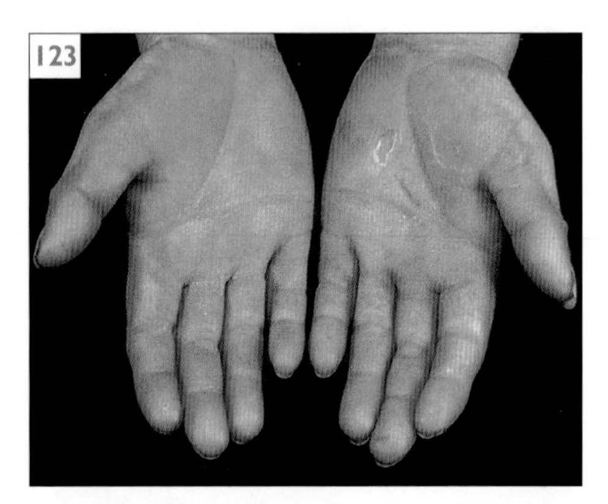

123 Thost–Unna PPK.

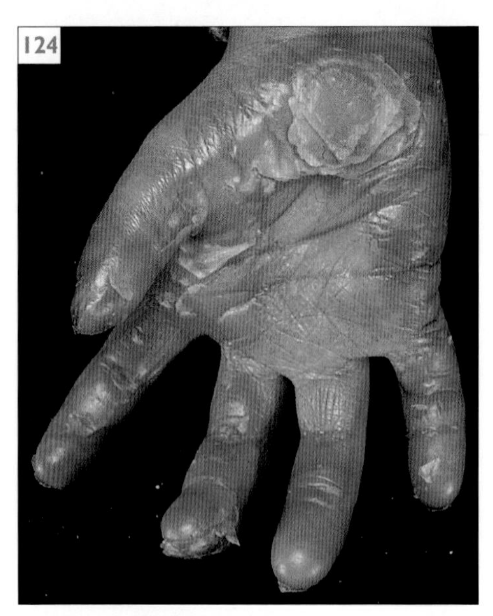

124 Vohwinkel PPK.

Hereditary palmoplantar keratoderma

DEFINITION AND CLINICAL FEATURES

A palmoplantar keratoderma (PPK) is a common associated feature of genetic disorders or syndromes such as hidrotic ectodermal dysplasia, epidermolysis bullosa simplex, ichthyosiform erythrodermas, pachyonychia congenita, dyskeratosis congenita, Rothmund–Thomson syndrome, and other poikilodermatous disorders.

The commonest inherited isolated PPKs are Thost–Unna (**123**) and Vorner keratoderma. These are diffuse keratodermas, and abnormalities in genes coding for type keratins 1 have been demonstrated. Histology of Vorner's keratoderma shows epidermolytic changes while Thost–Unna is non-epidermolytic. Transgradient keratodermas such as Vohwinkel's syndrome (**124**) are distinguished by involvement of the extensor surfaces of the hands, knees, and elbows. Many other keratodermas have been described in association with extracutaneous features including hair, nail, or tooth abnormalities, neurological, skeletal, and cardiac defects as well as internal malignancies. For example, Howell–Evans' syndrome or tylosis is a focal type of keratoderma associated with oesophageal cancer. In pachonychia congenita, a focal thickening of the palms and soles is accompanied by distinctive wedge-shaped nails due to subungual hyperkeratosis (**125**). Keratodermas of the feet may be associated with hyperhidrosis and malodour due to bacterial overgrowth, and can cause disability due to pain on walking.

DIFFERENTIAL DIAGNOSIS

Focal acral hyperkeratosis and punctate palmar keratoses are common autosomal dominant conditions characterized by discrete warty papules in Afro-Caribbeans (**126**). They are not regarded as palmoplantar keratodermas.

INVESTIGATIONS

Histology of Vorner's keratoderma is distinctive.

TREATMENT

Mild keratodermas may respond to emollients and keratolytics. Oral retinoids may be indicated for patients with functional impairment.

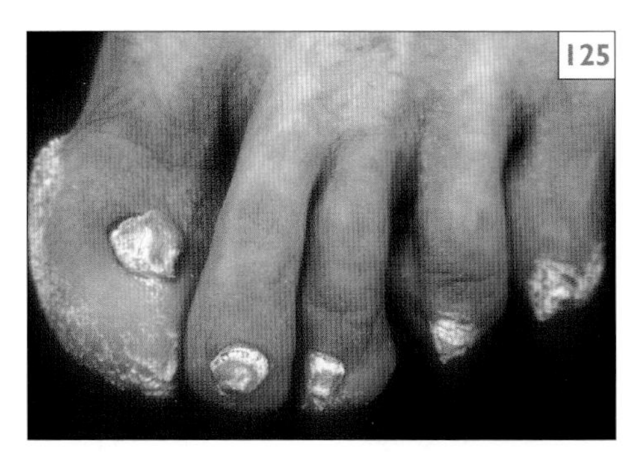

125 Subungual hyperkeratosis due to pachonychia congenita.

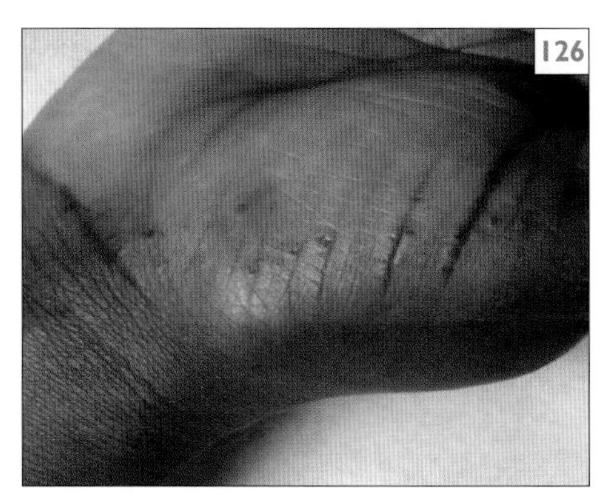

126 Focal acral hyperkeratosis.

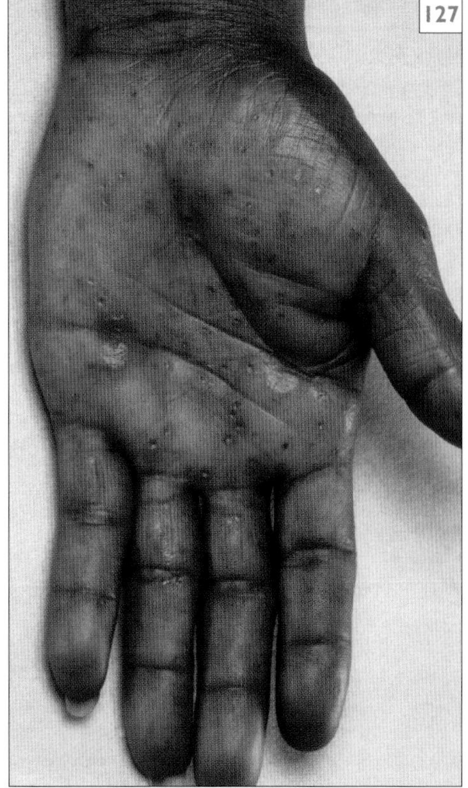

127 Punctate palmar keratoderma.

Acquired palmoplantar keratoderma

Acquired palmoplantar keratoderma may occur in association with various dermatosis including pityriasis rubra pilaris and Reiter's disease, psoriasis, eczemas, lichen planus, porokeratosis, viral warts, tinea manuum, lupus erythematosus, treponemal disease, and scabies. It may also occur in iododerma, hypothyroidism, internal malignancy, and HIV disease. A peri-menopausal plantar keratoderma (keratoderma climactericum) has been described in overweight women in their forties.

Punctate palmar keratoderma

DEFINITION AND CLINICAL FEATURES

Pinpoint hard keratotic papules appear on the palms and soles (**127**). Lesions are initially translucent then opaque and warty, and appear in adulthood. There may be associated punctate keratoses of the palmar creases. The latter are common in Afro-Caribbean people.

DIFFERENTIAL DIAGNOSIS

There is clinical overlap with other marginal keratodermas including focal acral hyperkeratosis.

INVESTIGATIONS

None needed.

TREATMENT

Topical therapy with keratolytics and retinoids has little effect. Systemic retinoids may be of benefit.

Ichthyoses

Ichthyosis (from *ichthys*, Greek for fish) describes dry, rough skin with persistent scaling which may resemble fish scale. It is a disorder of keratinization and differs from other scaly skin diseases such as eczema and psoriasis by being diffuse, uniform, and generally fixed in pattern. Mucosal surfaces are spared and hair, nails, and teeth are rarely affected. The inherited ichthyoses are a heterogeneous group comprising primary ichthyotic diseases and several ichthyosiform syndromes. Acquired ichthyosis may occur as a result of malabsorption, chronic hepatic or renal disease, hypothyroidism, sarcoidosis, leprosy, HIV disease, lymphoma, and other malignancies.

Ichthyosis vulgaris

DEFINITION AND CLINICAL FEATURES

This is the commonest hereditary ichthyosis and is an autosomal dominant condition with a reported incidence of 1 in 250 people. Scaling is usually obvious from 2 months onwards but may be delayed until childhood. The scale is white, flaky, and semi-adherent. It is most pronounced on the extensor surfaces of the arms (**128**) and lower legs and characteristically spares the flexures. The trunk, especially the abdominal wall, perioral skin, and the pinnae may also be involved. Palmoplantar hyperlinearity and keratosis pilaris are common associated features of both ichthyosis vulgaris and atopic eczema. The condition shows seasonal variation in most patients, improving in warm and sunny weather. Many patients improve in later life.

DIFFERENTIAL DIAGNOSIS

Acquired ichthyosis, severe xerosis, and recessive X-linked ichthyosis.

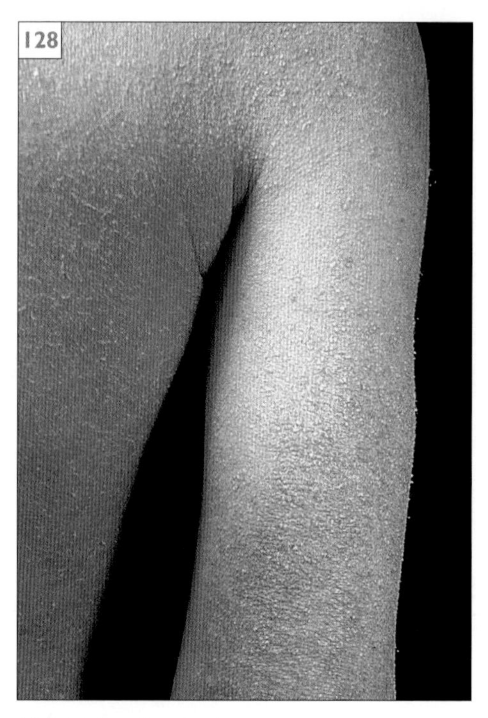

128 Ichthyosis vulgaris.

INVESTIGATIONS

Histology shows mild hyperkeratosis and a diminished or absent granular layer. Electron microscopy reveals scanty and fragmented keratohyaline granules in the granular cells.

TREATMENT

Avoidance of low humidity and regular use of emollients is of benefit. Urea or alpha hydroxy acid-containing preparations have keratolytic actions and reduce surface scaling.

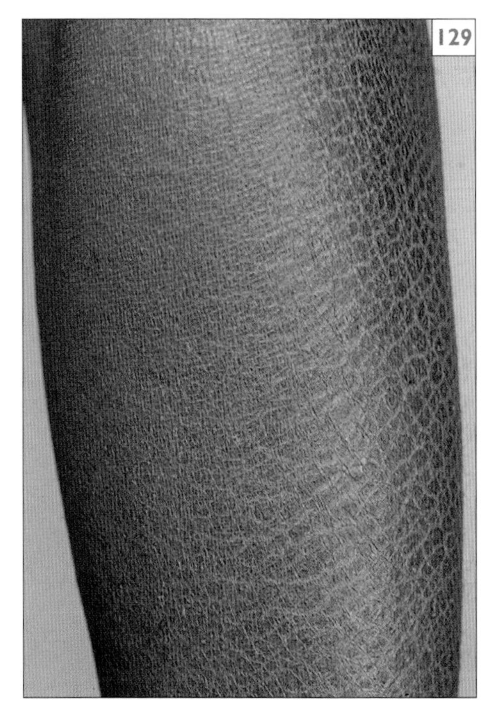

129 Recessive X-linked ichthyosis.

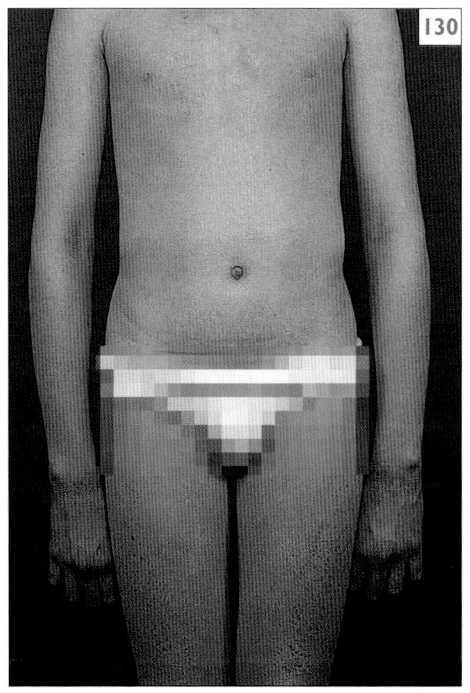

130 Recessive X-linked ichthyosis.

Recessive X-linked ichthyosis

DEFINITION AND CLINICAL FEATURES

An X-linked ichthyotic disorder affecting males which is caused by a defect in the enzyme steroid sulphatase. This causes defective disintegration of stratum corneum intercellular lipids and impaired desquamation. Scaling is generally evident within the first month of life and increases throughout childhood, stabilizing in the teens. The scale typically is polygonal, adherent and light brown in colour (**129**). It affects the extensor surfaces of the upper arms, the outer thighs, and around the lower legs. The neck, abdomen (**130**), and preauricular facial skin are also commonly affected. The palms and soles are spared. Placental steroid sulfatase deficiency coexists and may lead to prolonged and complicated labour, with increased risk of neonatal birth trauma. Affected males also have an increased incidence of testicular maldescent, cryptorchidism, and testicular cancer.

DIFFERENTIAL DIAGNOSIS

Ichthyosis vulgaris.

INVESTIGATIONS

Histology of affected skin shows hyperkeratosis and a variable granular cell layer. Steroid (cholesterol) sulfatase deficiency can be demonstrated in fibroblast and leucocyte cultures. Raised serum cholesterol sulphate can be detected on serum lipoprotein electrophoresis. Serum cholesterol levels are normal.

TREATMENT

As for ichthyosis vulgaris (see above).

Non-bullous ichthyosiform erythroderma (NBIE)

DEFINITION AND CLINICAL FEATURES

A rare and usually severe autosomal recessive ichthyosis. Over 90% of cases present at birth with a collodion membrane – a yellow, shiny, tight film like a sausage skin. Ectropion and constricting bands may occur and the membrane sheds over a period of weeks, revealing a generalized scaly erythroderma. Scaling can affect all areas (**131**) including the scalp, ears, face, flexures, palms, and soles and is white, light, superficial and semi-adherent. Scalp involvement often causes pityriasis amiantacea (see p. 41) and may lead to patchy cicatricial alopecia. Ectropion (**132**), which generally improves, digital constriction, and nail dystrophy are features of severe disease. Hypohidrosis occurs due to obstruction of sweat ducts by the hyperkeratotic stratum corneum.

DIFFERENTIAL DIAGNOSIS

Lamellar ichthyosis, Netherton's syndrome, trichothiodystrophy, psoriasis.

INVESTIGATIONS

Histological features support the clinical diagnosis. Electron microscopy shows abnormal lamellar bodies which are retained in the stratum corneum.

TREATMENT

Emollients and keratolytics as for other ichthyoses. Oral retinoids may help reduce scaling, pruritus, and erythema.

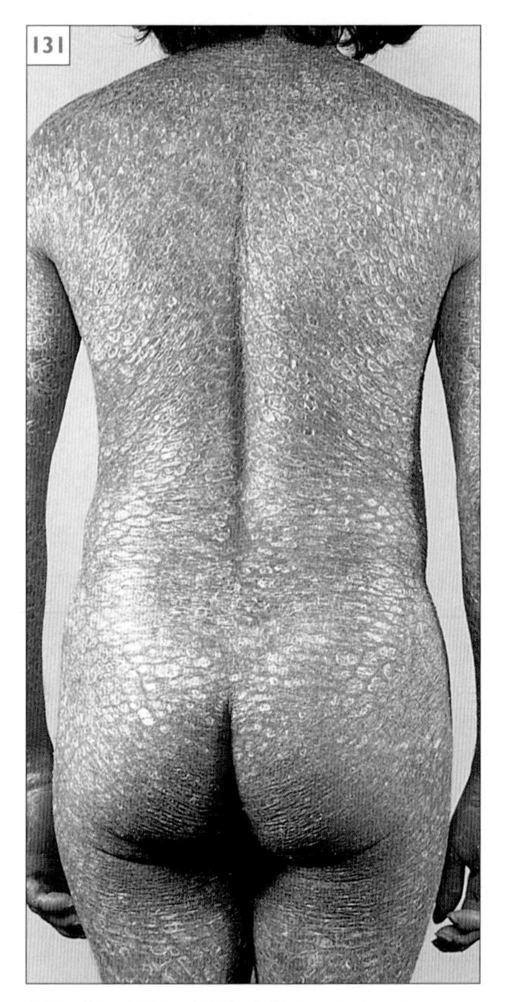

131 Non-bullous ichthyosiform erythroderma.

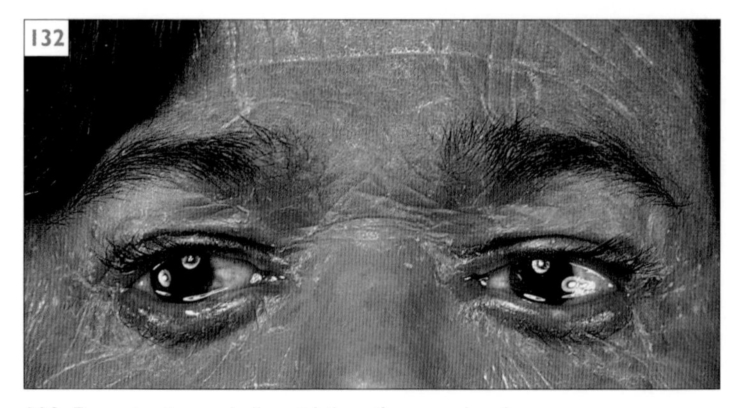

132 Ectropion in non-bullous ichthyosiform erythroderma.

Bullous ichthyosiform erythroderma

DEFINITION AND CLINICAL FEATURES

A rare autosomal dominant disorder of keratinization that in its early phase is associated with blistering caused by mutations in the genes for keratins 1 and 10. Extensive, flaccid blistering, and skin fragility are apparent within hours of birth. These heal without scarring and blistering and erythroderma diminish in childhood as a characteristic grey, waxy scale increases. Linear hyperkeratosis is most prominent in the flexures, scalp, anterior neck, abdominal wall, and infragluteal folds (**133**). Erosions and recurring skin infections occur with malodorous skin. Palmoplantar hyperkeratosis develops in many patients (**134**). This condition tends to improve with age.

DIFFERENTIAL DIAGNOSIS

In the neonate: epidermolysis bullosa, staphylococcal scalded skin syndrome, herpetic infections, and incontinentia pigmenti. In older children: other ichthyoses.

INVESTIGATIONS

Histology of skin shows characteristic changes of epidermolytic hyperkeratosis. Electron microscopy reveals clumped keratin filaments around granular keratinocyte nuclei.

TREATMENT

At least half of the cases have no family history of the disease and are due to new keratin mutations, but parents of affected children should be examined carefully for focal keratotic lesions as these indicate that future siblings will be affected. Emollients are of limited use, as the scaling is greasy, and keratolytics may be irritating. Topical antiseptics can reduce microbial overgrowth and oral retinoids may help, although they increase skin fragility.

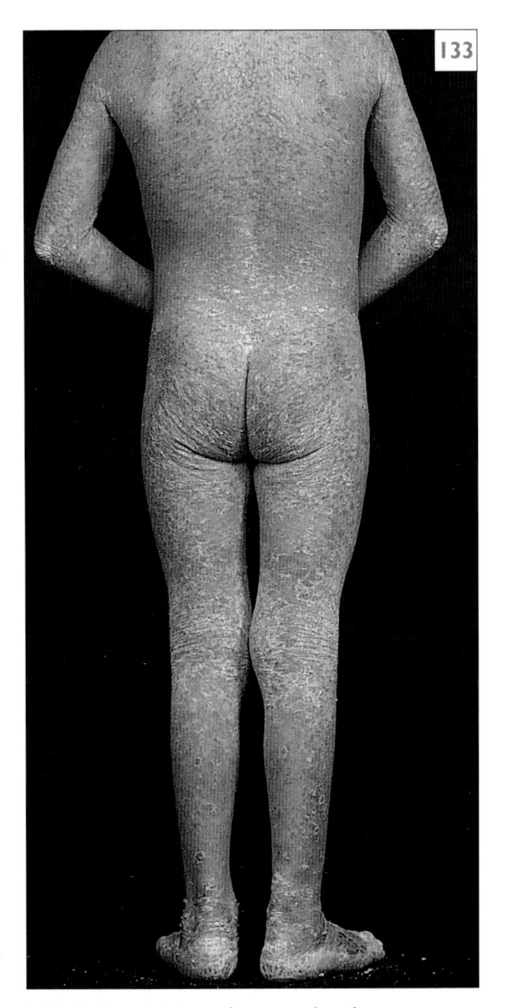

133 Bullous ichthyosiform erythroderma.

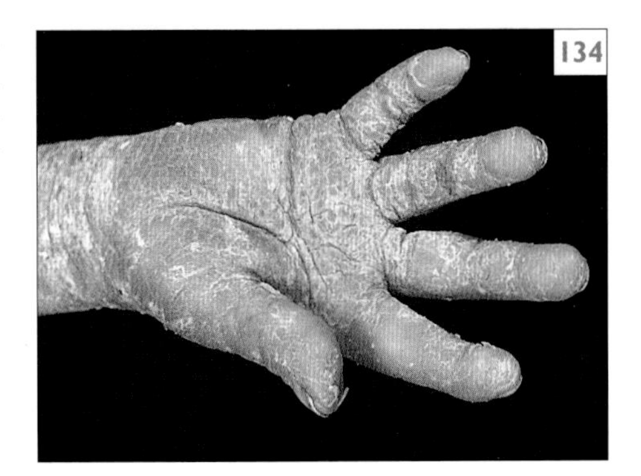

134 Palmar hyperkeratosis in bullous ichthyosiform erythroderma.

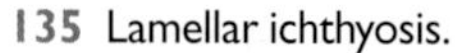

135 Lamellar ichthyosis.

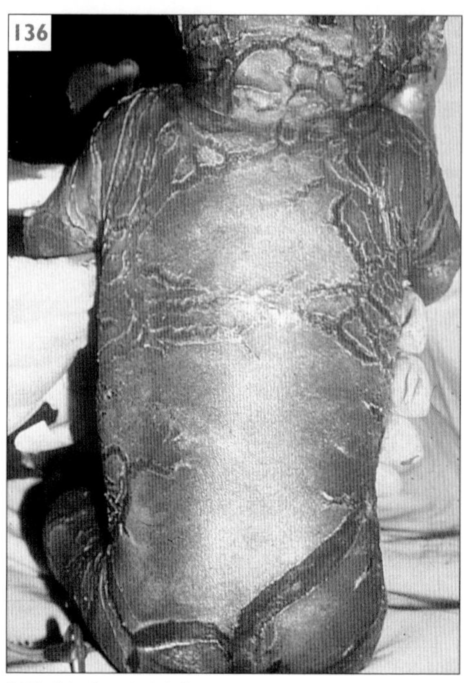

136 Harlequin ichthyosis.

Lamellar ichthyosis

DEFINITION AND CLINICAL FEATURES

A rare autosomal recessive ichthyosis. Infants usually present as collodion babies, but the erythroderma is less intense than in infants with NBIE. Thick, plate-like, pigmented, adherent scale (**135**) over most of the skin ensues but mild variants occur. Additional problems include pruritus, hypohidrosis, ectropion, and crumpled pinnae.

DIFFERENTIAL DIAGNOSIS

X-linked recessive ichthyosis, other ichthyosiform erythrodermas.

INVESTIGATIONS

Light microscopy shows massive orthohyperkeratosis; the remainder of the epidermis may be of normal thickness. Electron microscopy shows various epidermal abnormalities.

TREATMENT

Emollients and keratolytics. Oral retinoids may be used for severe disease.

Harlequin ichthyosis

DEFINITION AND CLINICAL FEATURES

Harlequin ichthyosis is a very rare severe erythrodermic ichthyosis that causes a striking appearance at birth. The affected infant, usually premature, is encased in grossly hyperkeratotic, thick, yellow, firmly adherent plaques covering the whole body surface and severely restricting movement (**136**). Soon after birth deep red fissures appear, producing the harlequin pattern. Severe ectropion, eclabium, rudimentary nose and ears, and conjunctival oedema contribute to the typical facies. Respiratory insufficiency, poor temperature control, and feeding difficulties commonly lead to a rapid demise. It is an autosomal recessive condition and although the phenotype is uniform, various genetic defects have been identified.

DIFFERENTIAL DIAGNOSIS

Collodion baby (usually due to other ichthyosiform erythrodermas – see NBIE).

INVESTIGATIONS

Skin biopsy shows massive orthohyperkeratosis extending down into the hair follicles and pilo-sebaceous units. In some cases vacuoles are seen in the stratum corneum and EM shows abnormal lamellar bodies.

TREATMENT

Intensive neonatal care can improve the chances of survival. Acitretin therapy hastens shedding of hyperkeratotic scale. Parents should be offered detailed genetic counselling and prenatal diagnostic for subsequent pregnancies.

Ichthyosiform syndromes

Netherton's syndrome

This autosomal recessive syndrome comprises an ichthyosiform dermatosis, hair shaft defects, and atopic features. It may initially escape diagnosis due to a gradual evolution of the major manifestations. Mutations in the gene coding a serine protease inhibitor SPINK5 have been identified in several patients. The triad of congenital erythroderma, failure to thrive in infancy, and poor hair growth suggest the diagnosis. Many patients develop recurrent crops of erythematous, scaly, migrating lesions with an incomplete double edge of peeling scale, so-called ichthyosis linearis circumflexa (**137**). Another pathognomonic feature is a ball-and-socket hair-shaft defect known as trichorrhexis invaginata. Raised total and specific IgE levels and childhood food allergies are characteristic.

DIFFERENTIAL DIAGNOSIS

Erythrodermic atopic eczema, psoriasis, staphylococcal or candidal infection, immunodeficiency states.

Other very rare ichthyosiform syndromes include Sjögren–Larsson and Refsum's disease which are associated with neurological impairments, IBIDS (ichthyosis, brittle hair, impaired intelligence, decreased fertility, and short stature).

INVESTIGATIONS

Hair shaft analysis for trichorrhexis invaginata.

TREATMENT

Regular emollients and topical or systemic antibiotics for skin and respiratory infections. Retinoids should be avoided. Future treatment may include use of protease inhibitors.

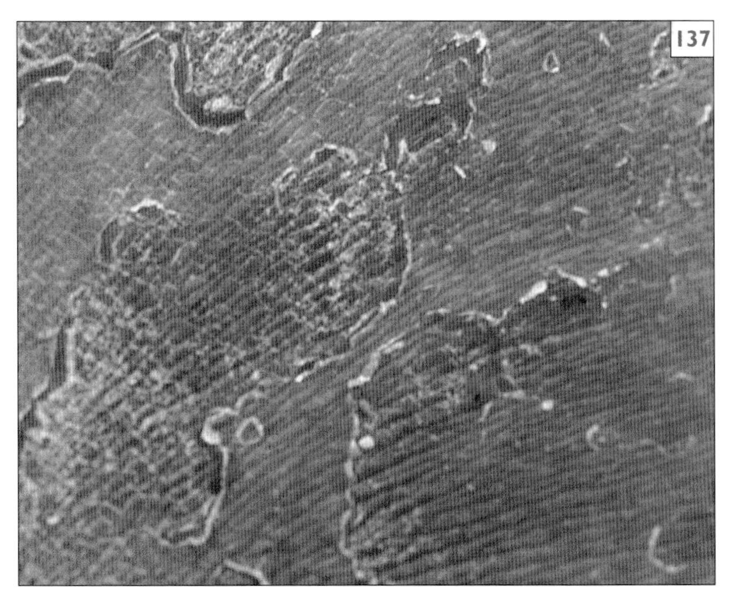

137 Ichthyosis linearis circumflexa (Netherton's syndrome).

ACNE AND RELATED DISORDERS

Acne vulgaris

DEFINITION AND CLINICAL FEATURES

A common inflammatory disorder of the pilosebaceous unit characterized by excessive production of sebum and the presence of comedones, papules, pustules, and cysts. Lesions almost always occur on the face though the upper back and chest are involved in around 70% of cases. The condition usually starts in adolescence and its peak prevalence is between the ages of 14 and 19. However, acne may persist into adult life and may present first after the age of 25 (late onset acne). Increased production of sebum, hypercornification of the pilosebaceous ducts, and colonization with *Propionibacterium acnes* are all important aetiological factors. The increased sebum production (seborrhoea) occurs in response to raised levels of androgens and gives the skin a shiny appearance (**138**). Comedonal lesions (**139**) usually precede inflammatory lesions (**140**) by several years. In dark-skinned individuals, resolution of lesions may be followed by disfiguring long-lasting postinflammatory hyperpigmentation.

Deep nodules and cysts may occur (nodulocystic acne) (**141**) resulting in disfiguring hypertrophic scars (**140**). Nodulocystic acne is often a recalcitrant disease with widespread involvement of the trunk (**142**), and requires prompt treatment to prevent extensive scarring. Acne conglobata is an uncommon severe variant of nodulocystic acne with multiple draining sinuses (**143**). In rare cases it may present acutely with malaise, fever, and arthralgia (acne fulminans).

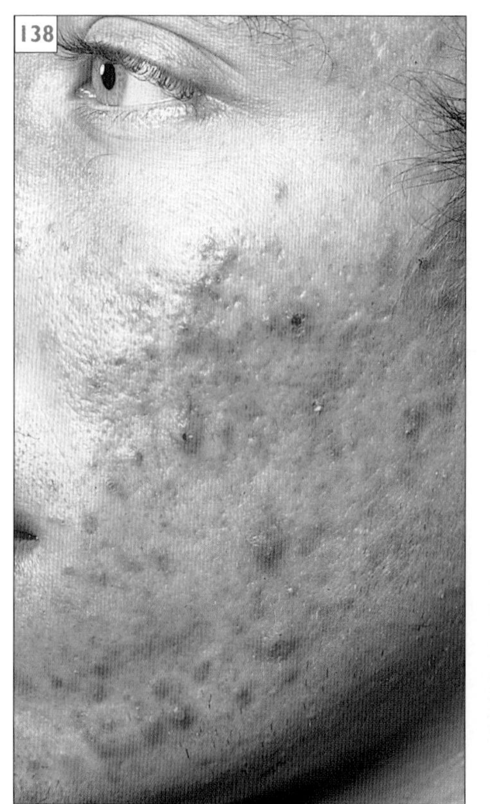

138 Acne vulgaris.

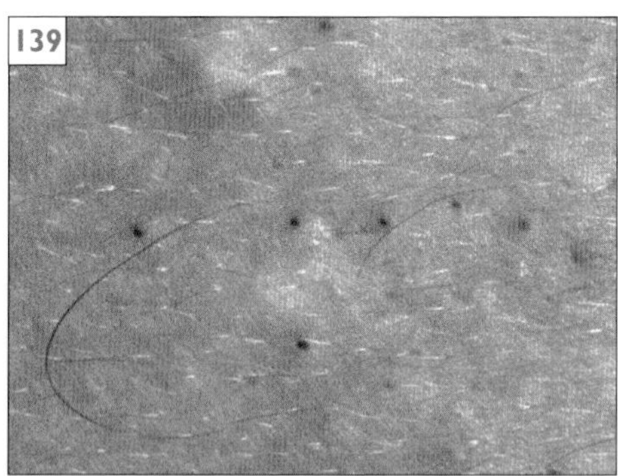

139 Comedones (blackheads) in acne vulgaris.

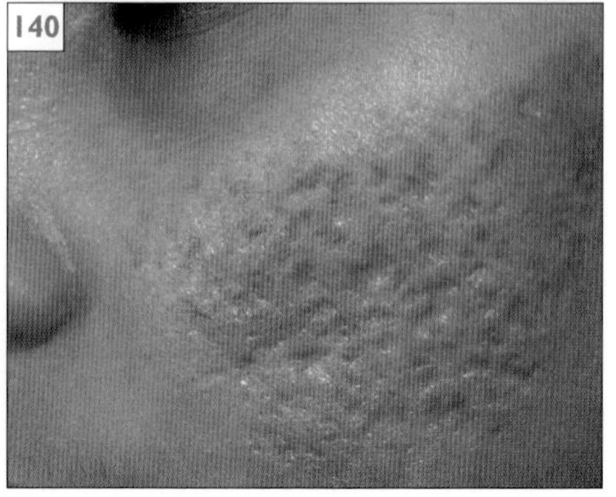

140 Scarring in acne vulgaris.

DIFFERENTIAL DIAGNOSIS

Acne is rarely misdiagnosed. Rosacea usually starts in adulthood and lacks comedones and scarring. Inflammatory papules and pustules occur in perioral dermatitis but comedones are not present. Chloracne (see page 29).

INVESTIGATIONS

None are usually required. Rarely acne may occur as part of an endocrine disorder such as polycystic disease of the ovaries, Cushing's disease, or adrenogenital syndrome.

TREATMENT

Acne can be a source of considerable psychological distress. It should be treated actively to lessen this burden and prevent scarring. Oily cosmetics should be discontinued as these may encourage comedone formation. Topical retinoids, keratolytics, and antibiotics are used as monotherapy or in combination for mild acne. More severe disease may require a prolonged course of oral antibacterial therapy, but increasing levels of antibiotic-resistant *P. acnes* have emerged in recent years. Hormonal therapy with the combined oral contraceptive pill and the antiandrogen cyproterone acetate may be helpful in females who require contraception and menstrual control. Oral isotretinoin is the most effective antiacne drug and is indicated for severe acne, and in milder cases where other treatment has failed or there is profound psychological distress. Pregnancy must be avoided as this drug is a known teratogen.

Drug-induced acne

A number of drugs including isoniazid, oral corticosteroids and gonadotrophins, lithium, phenytoin, and iodides may give rise to a monomorphic acne which responds poorly to conventional treatment. Acne in body builders may occasionally indicate use of androgens such as anabolic steroids.

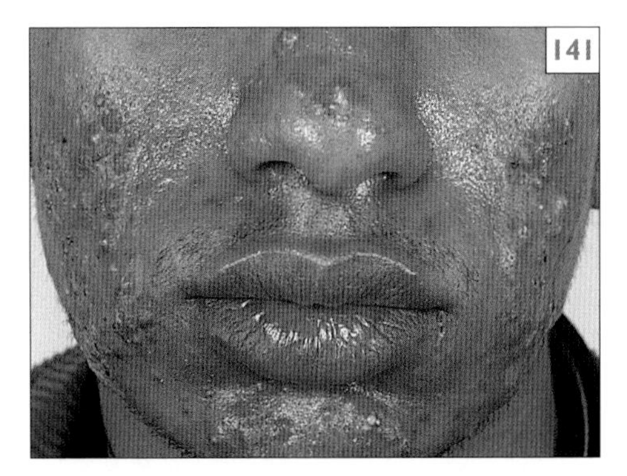

141 Nodulocystic acne.

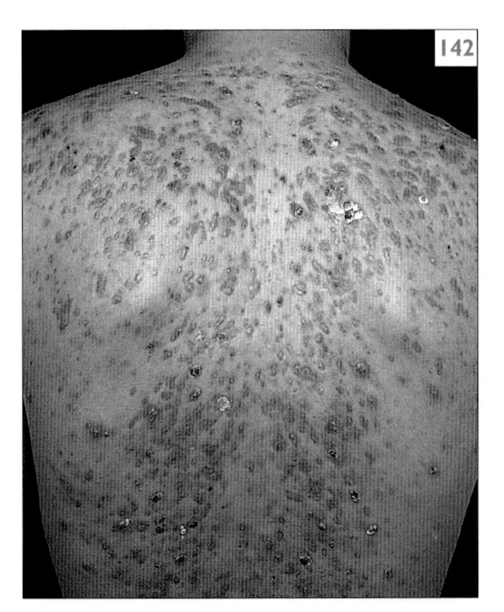

142 Nodulocystic acne.

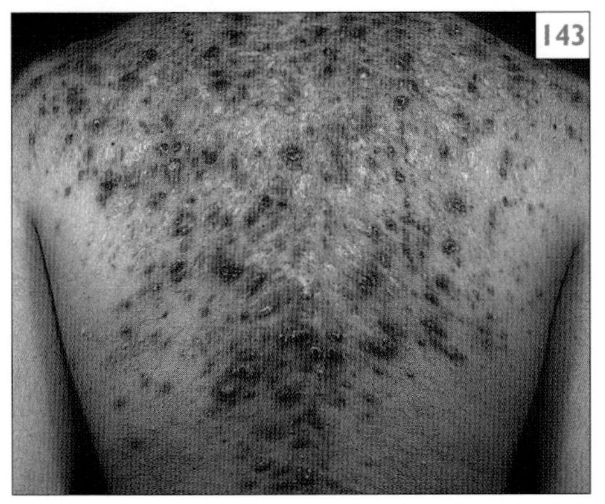

143 Acne conglobata.

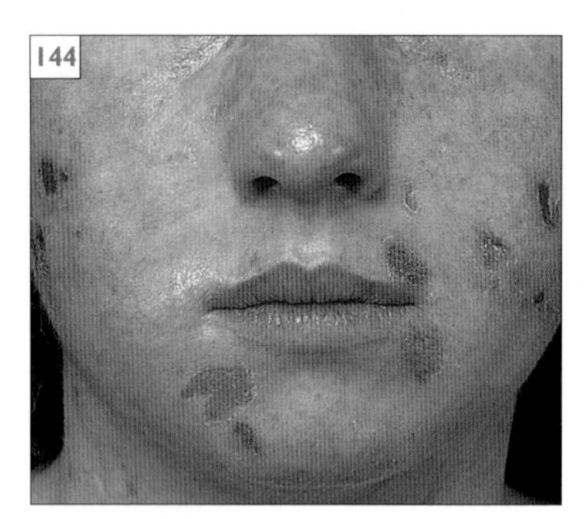

144 Acne excoriée.

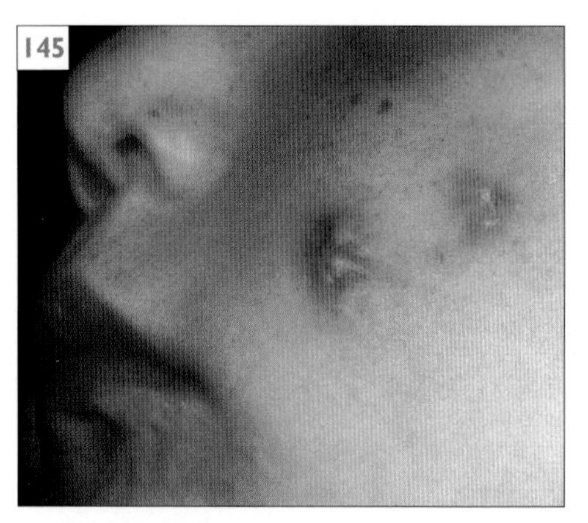

145 Infantile acne.

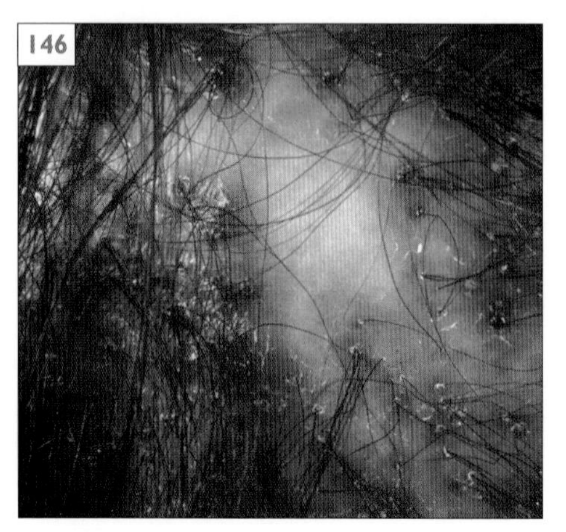

146 Folliculitis decalvans.

Acne excoriée

This condition occurs predominantly in females and is caused by repeated picking of minor acne lesions which delays healing and causes linear excoriations and erosions (**144**). Lesions are usually present on the chin and cheeks. Patients often have an underlying psychological problem such as depression.

Infantile acne

This rare form of acne mainly affects baby boys and is characterized by papular and pustular lesions on the cheeks which may leave scars. The onset is usually between 3 months to 2 years of age, and is thought to occur due to transplacental stimulation of the adrenal gland (**145**).

Acne-associated scalp folliculitis

DEFINITION AND CLINICAL FEATURES

Various forms of pustular folliculitis on the hair-bearing scalp may occur in association with acne. Folliculitis decalvans is a chronic progressive scalp folliculitis that leads to scarring and atrophy (**146**). It may occur in association with severe acne and hidradenitis suppurativa, and collectively these are called the follicular occlusion triad. Dissecting folliculitis of the scalp is similar to nodular acne with suppurative, painful discharging nodules. It is commonest in Afro-Caribbean men.

DIFFERENTIAL DIAGNOSIS

Folliculitis keloidalis nuchae has a predilection for the nape of the neck. Erosive pustular dermatosis and tufted folliculitis.

TREATMENT

Oral antibiotics and oral isotretinoin may help but both conditions can respond poorly to treatment.

Rosacea

DEFINITION AND CLINICAL FEATURES

This is a chronic inflammatory skin disorder, characterized by papules and pustules on a background of erythema and fine telangiectasia, in which the convexities of the face are chiefly involved (**147**). During inflammatory episodes, papules and pustules are evident (**148**), and facial swelling may occur (**149**). Minor degrees of ocular involvement occur in around 50% of rosacea sufferers. Conjunctivitis and blepharitis are the most frequent ocular complaints, and rosaceal keratitis can lead to corneal scarring. Rosacea typically begins in the third or fourth decade and may be commoner in females. It is seen less frequently in those with pigmented skins, and a fair skin complexion combined with chronic sun exposure may be important in its aetiology. Occasionally, persistent tissue thickening due to oedema, fibrosis, and sebaceous hyperplasia develops giving rise to phymas. These are almost exclusive to males and the commonest is rhinophyma which gives a bulbous craggy appearance to the nose (**150**).

DIFFERENTIAL DIAGNOSIS

Acne occurs in younger individuals and is distinguished by the presence of comedones. The central facial distribution of seborrhoeic dermatitis is similar to rosacea, but pustules and papules do not occur.

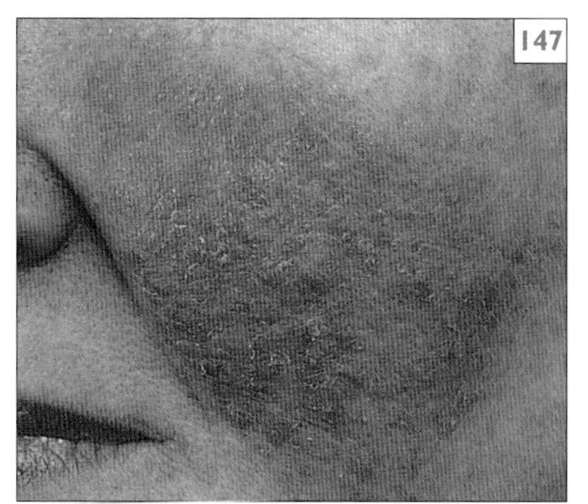

147 Rosacea.

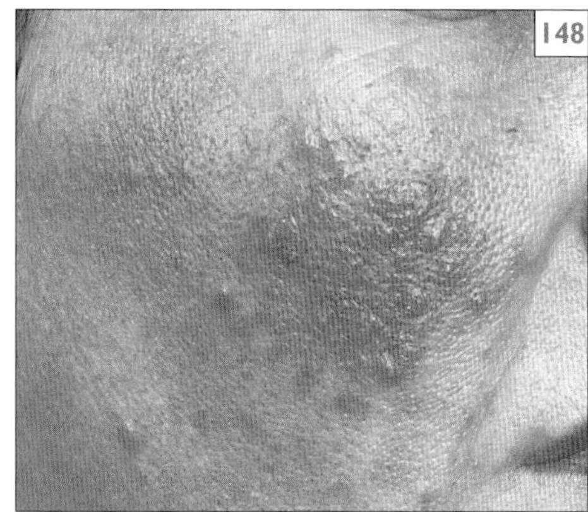

148 Papules and pustules of rosacea.

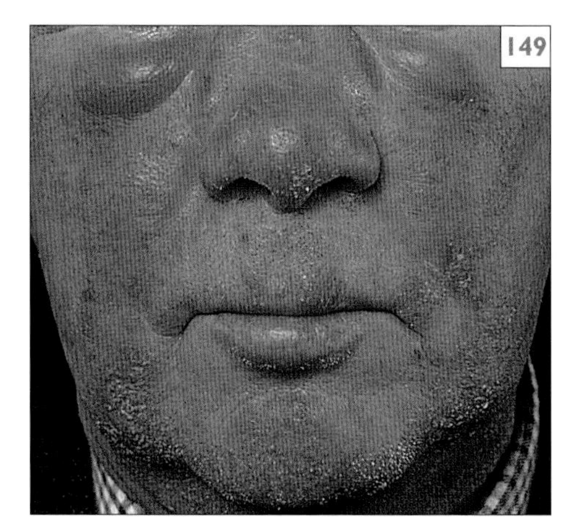

149 Facial swelling in rosacea.

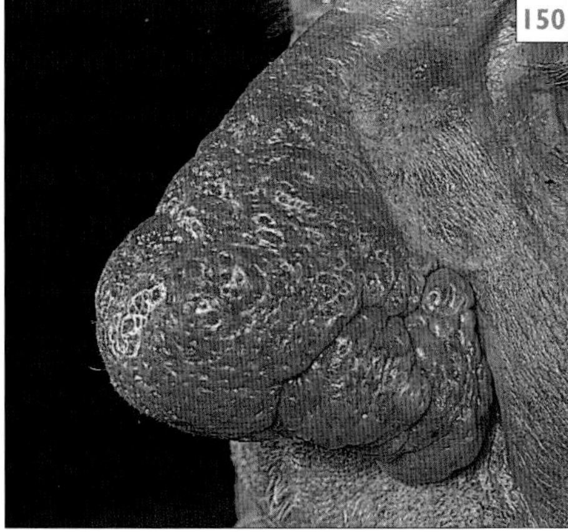

150 Rhinophyma.

INVESTIGATIONS
None are usually indicated.

TREATMENT
Mild cases of papulopustular rosacea usually respond well to topical metronidazole. Oral tetracyclines or oral isotretinoin are indicated for more severe or recalcitrant disease. The underlying telangiectasia and erythema may persist, and can be improved with vascular laser therapy. Facial erythema is often accompanied by a sensitivity to minor irritants including cosmetics. Sun blocks are recommended. Phymas can be remodelled surgically.

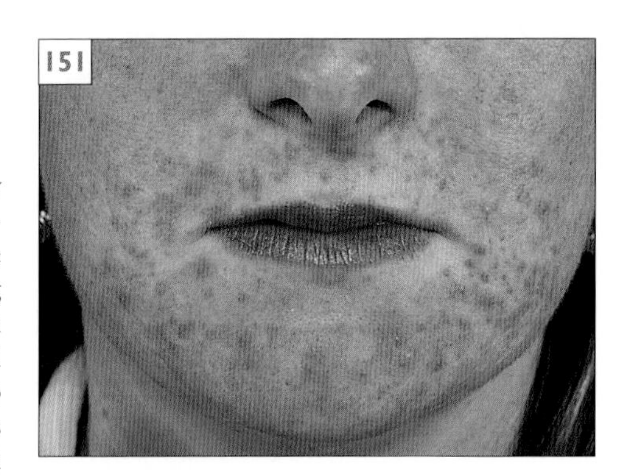

151 Perioral dermatitis.

Perioral dermatitis

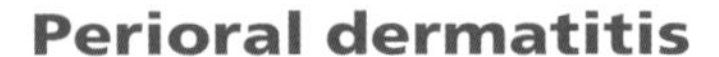

DEFINITION AND CLINICAL FEATURES
An eruption of multiple tiny papulovesicles around the mouth. The perioral distribution of this eruption is characteristic (**151**), with predominance in the nasolabial folds and sparing of a small area around the vermilion of the lip (**152**). The periocular area may also be involved (**153**). This condition typically occurs in young women. The cause is unknown, but occlusive cosmetics have been incriminated and the eruption may follow use of topical corticosteroids.

DIFFERENTIAL DIAGNOSIS
Rosacea tends to affect the upper face; the background erythema is striking. Contact dermatitis from lipstick or toothpaste is more localized and involves the lip vermilion. Irritant contact dermatitis secondary to lip licking is eczematous and not papular.

INVESTIGATIONS
None.

TREATMENT
Topical corticosteroids should be stopped. This may trigger an initial flare, but there is usually a good response to a 6-week course of an oral tetracycline.

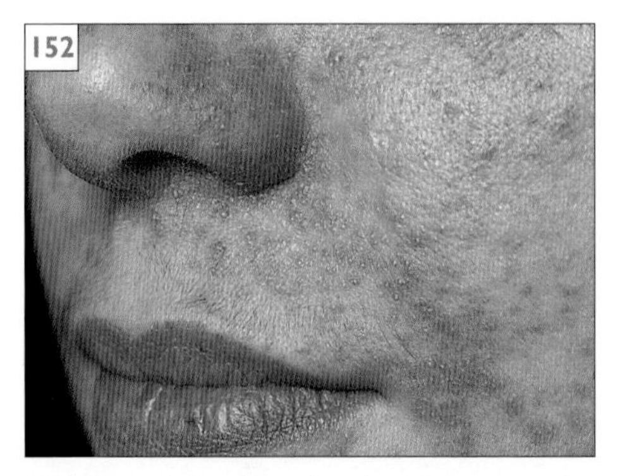

152 Perioral dermatitis showing sparing around the lips.

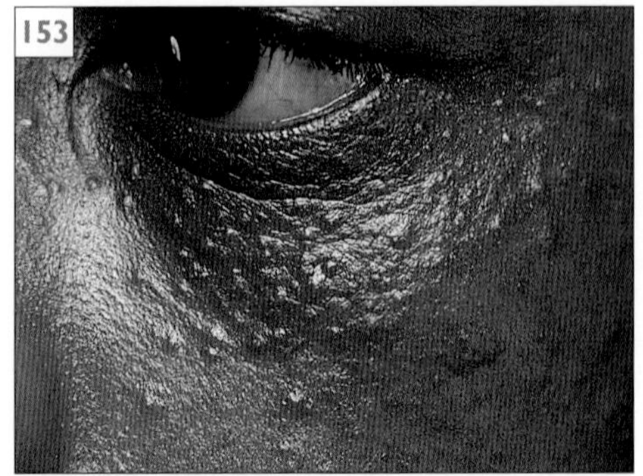

153 Periocular dermatitis.

GENITAL AND PERIANAL DERMATOSES

The genital and perianal skin can be affected by many of the dermatoses that characteristically occur at other sites, but some conditions have a predilection for this anatomical region. Difficulties arise in diagnosis as the classical morphology is altered due to the effect of occlusion at these flexural sites. A brief review of the embryology and anatomy of this area is important in understanding the nature and distribution of the dermatoses that do occur.

EMBRYOLOGY AND ANATOMY

The external genitalia begin to form at about 4 weeks, shortly after the cloaca has developed, but sexual differentiation is not apparent until 12 weeks. At 7 weeks, the primitive perineum is formed (**154**) when the urorectal septum has reached the cloacal membrane, dividing it into the anterior urogenital membrane and posterior anal membrane. Subsequent masculinization (**155**) or feminization (**156**) is a consequence of tissue response to the presence or absence of androgens.

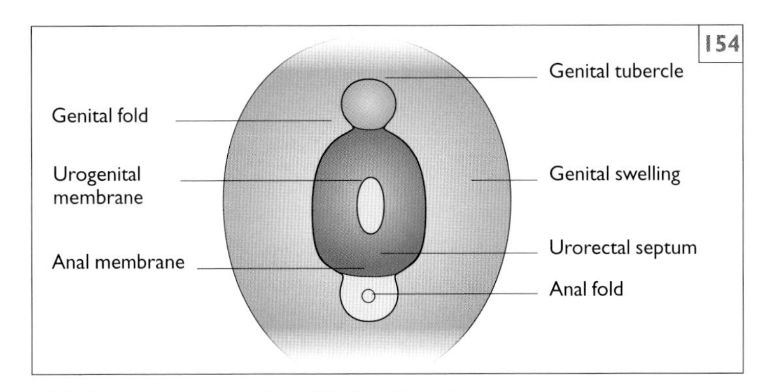

154 Primitive perineum (simplified) at 7 weeks.

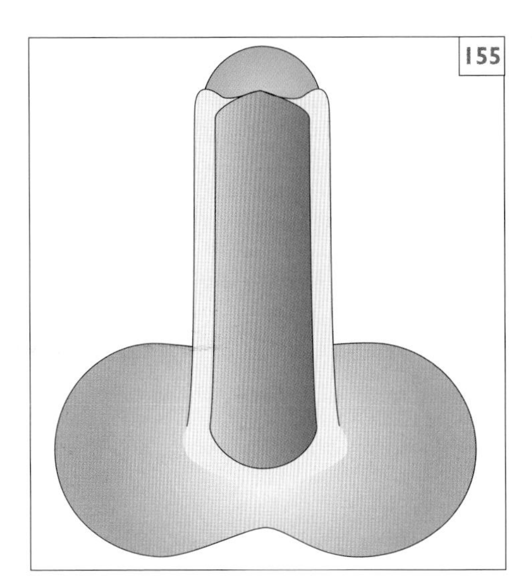

155 Adult male external genitalia (simplified).

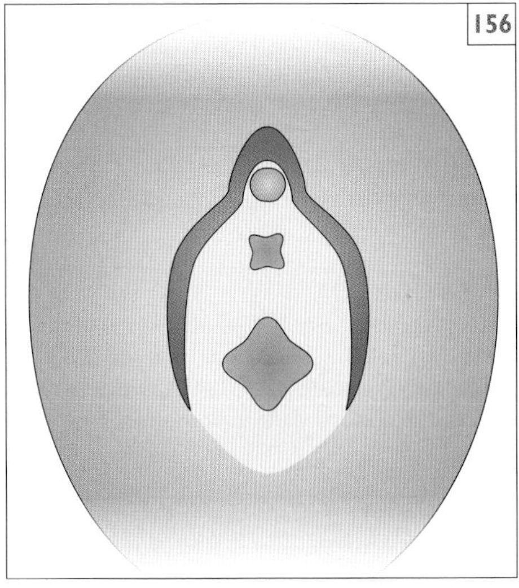

156 Adult female external genitalia (simplified).

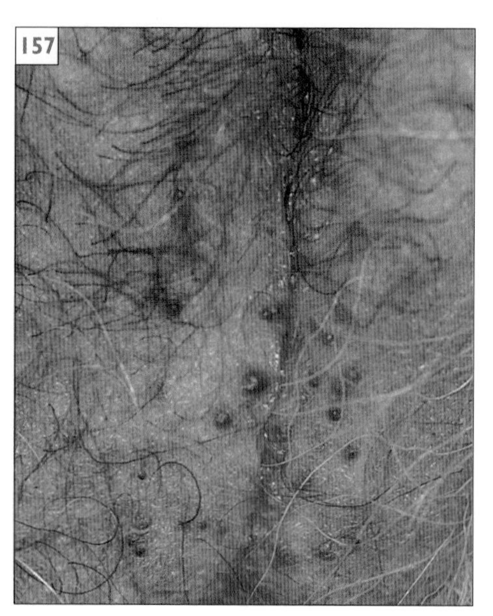

157 Angiokeratomas.

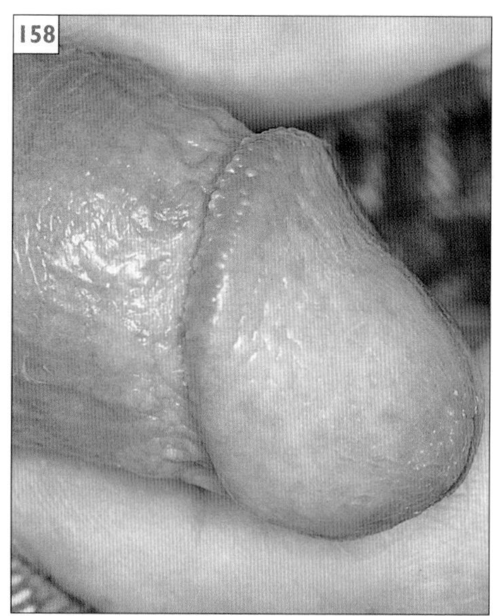

158 Penile pearly papules.

Angiokeratomas

DEFINITION AND CLINICAL FEATURES

Acquired, ectatic, thin-walled vessels covered by hyperkeratotic epithelium, affecting the scrotum or labia majora. They appear as bright red papules (**157**), which darken with age. They develop most commonly in middle age and are considered to be a degenerative phenomenon. Lesions are usually asymptomatic, but occasionally bleed following trauma. Rarely, they may be extensive, affecting the penis and upper thighs.

DIFFERENTIAL DIAGNOSIS

Angiokeratoma corporis diffusum (Anderson–Fabry's disease) (see page 132).

INVESTIGATIONS

Histopathology may help differentiate between these angiokeratomas and those seen in Anderson–Fabry's disease, as vacuoles may be seen in the endothelial and smooth muscle cells in the latter.

TREATMENT

Reassurance may suffice. Hyfrecation, electrocautery or laser ablation may be performed but lesions tend to recur.

Papillomatosis

DEFINITION AND CLINICAL FEATURES

Benign papillary projections of the epithelium. These are thought to be a normal variant and are unrelated to papilloma virus infection. They occur as shiny, opalescent micropapules encircling the coronal sulcus in men and are known as penile pearly papules (**158**). They also occur in women, sited symmetrically on the inner aspects of the labia minora or the vulval vestibule (**159**). They may be very tiny projections giving the affected epithelium a granular appearance but occasionally they may be long and filiform. The lesions are normally asymptomatic.

DIFFERENTIAL DIAGNOSIS

Viral warts.

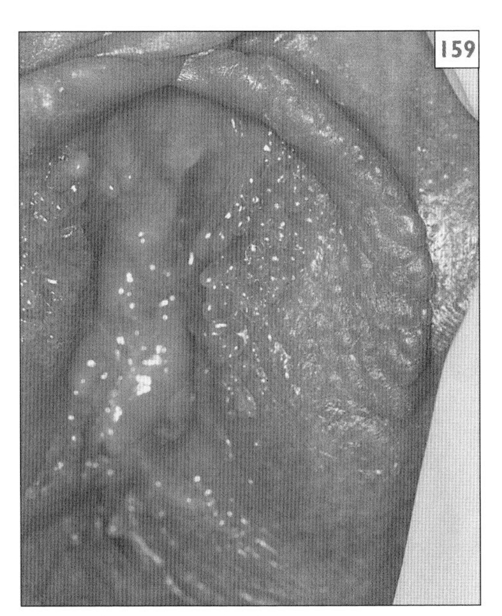

159 Vestibular papillomatosis.

INVESTIGATIONS

This is not usually necessary. However, histology shows identical features to angiofibromas with epithelial projections with a core of normal connective tissue and a dense vascular network.

SPECIAL POINTS

No treatment is necessary other than reassurance.

Fordyce spots

DEFINITION AND CLINICAL FEATURES

Sebaceous gland hyperplasia on the mucosal surfaces where the glands do not have an associated hair unit and open directly onto the surface. They appear on the inner labia majora and minora, penile shaft, and buccal mucosal and are considered a normal variant. Fordyce spots appear after puberty as numerous small yellow papules and are more noticeable when the skin is stretched (**160**). Sometimes they are so numerous that they appear as confluent patches (**161**). They are usually asymptomatic but in some female patients they may be associated with pruritus.

DIFFERENTIAL DIAGNOSIS

Epidermoid cysts, milia. Sebaceous gland adenoma.

INVESTIGATIONS

None necessary.

TREATMENT

Reassurance.

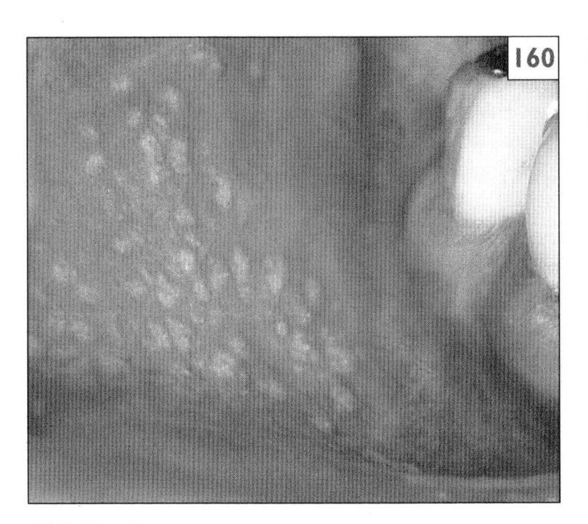

160 Fordyce spots.

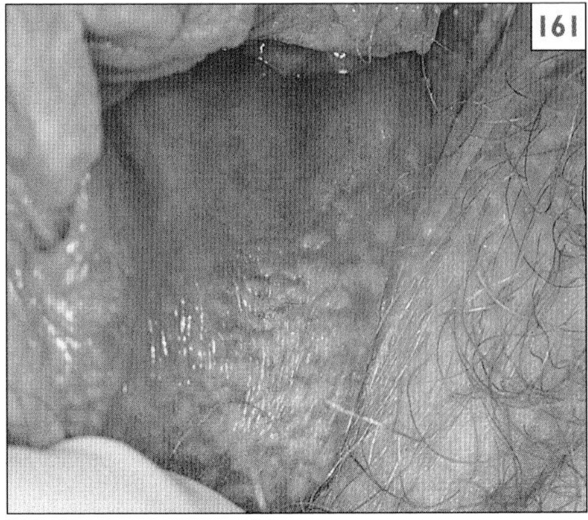

161 Fordyce spots.

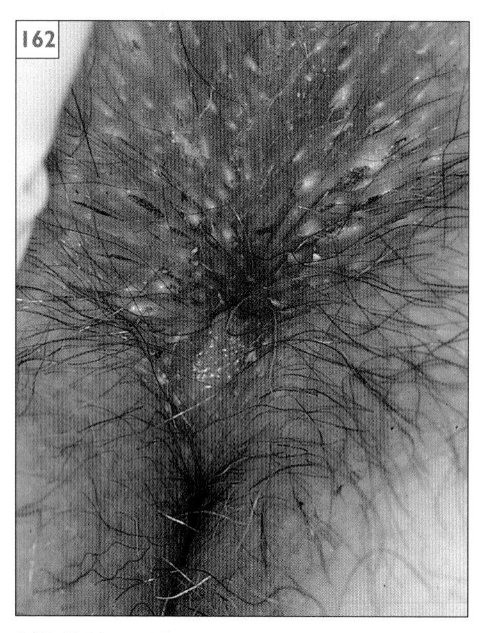

162 Epidermoid cysts.

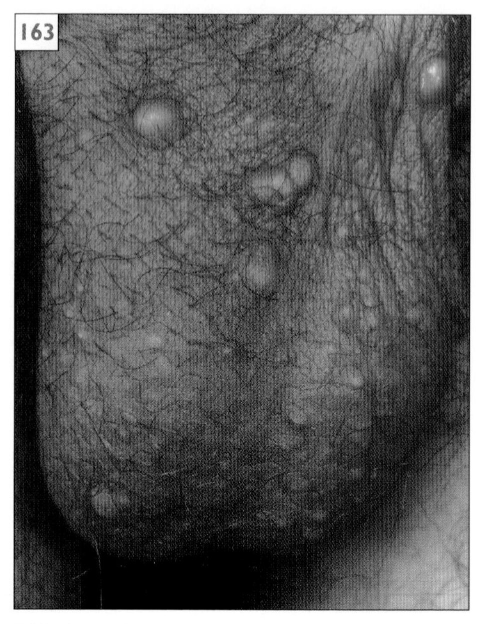

163 Scrotal calcinosis.

Epidermoid cysts

DEFINITION AND CLINICAL FEATURES

A dermal cyst lined with stratified squamous epithelium and filled with keratin and its breakdown products. Epidermoid cysts usually arise on the cornified squamous epithelium of the anogenital skin and are not seen on the glans penis or vulval vestibule (**162**). They are common and are often multiple. Lesions appear as dome-shaped yellow or white papules. A central punctum can sometimes be seen. The cysts enlarge slowly and occasionally can become inflamed.

DIFFERENTIAL DIAGNOSIS

Steatocystoma multiplex, eccrine gland tumours.

INVESTIGATIONS

Histology shows features of an epidermoid cyst. A hair may be present within the cyst, and there is often an associated chronic inflammatory or surrounding foreign body reaction.

TREATMENT

Symptomatic lesions may be excised.

Scrotal calcinosis

DEFINITION AND CLINICAL FEATURES

An idiopathic disorder characterized by multiple hard white papules and nodules on the scrotum (**163**) and, rarely, the penis. Similar lesions may rarely occur on the vulva. Their origin is unclear but they may arise from other benign cysts or the eccrine ducts.

DIFFERENTIAL DIAGNOSIS

Epidermoid cysts, onchocerciasis nodules (in endemic areas).

INVESTIGATIONS

None usually necessary.

TREATMENT

Symptomatic or unsightly cysts may be incised and extruded under local anaesthetic.

Lichen sclerosus

DEFINITION AND CLINICAL FEATURES

A chronic, scarring, inflammatory dermatosis that has a predilection for the genital and perianal skin. Typically, at extragenital sites, the lesions are porcelain white papules and plaques (**164**) with plugged follicles and sweat ducts. The individual lesions may coalesce to form sheets of atrophic skin, often with extensive areas of purpura. Bullous lesions can occur. In the anogenital area there are usually confluent, white, atrophic patches (**165**), occurring in a figure-of-eight pattern. There is usually architectural distortion, with either partial or complete loss of the labia minora, burying of the clitoris and introital narrowing in females, and partial or complete phimosis and meatal stenosis in males (**166**).

The cause is unknown but there is an association with autoimmune diseases and the condition is commoner in females. The peak incidence in females is in childhood or around the menopause, so hormonal factors may be important. It is more difficult to assess the incidence in boys, as, very often, they are circumcised for phimosis but the tissue is not routinely examined histologically, so may go undiagnosed.

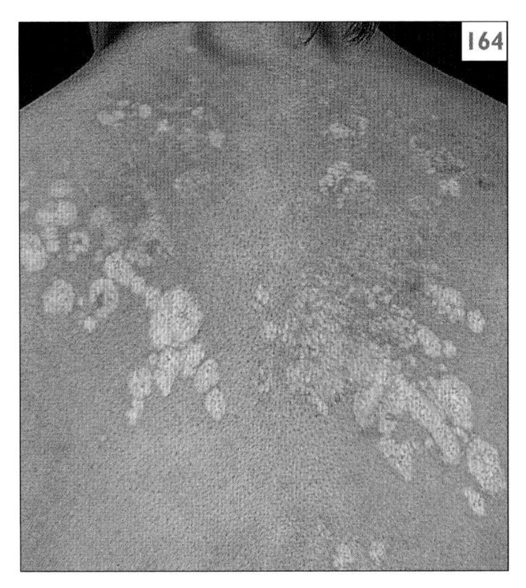

164 Lichen sclerosus.

DIFFERENTIAL DIAGNOSIS

Other dermatoses that can produce atrophy and scarring, i.e. lichen planus, cicatricial pemphigoid, and pemphigus.

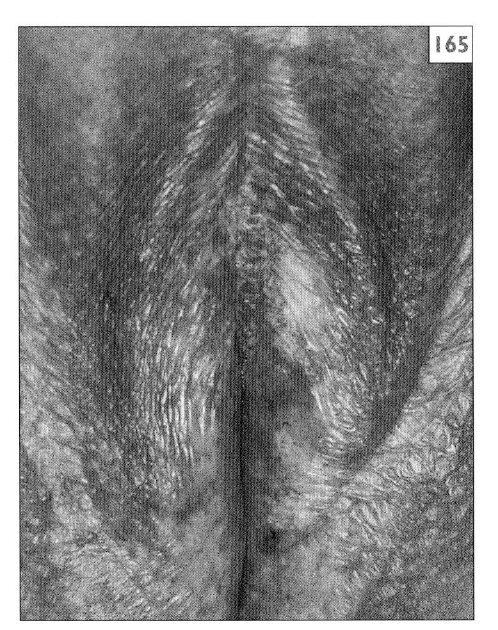

165 Lichen sclerosus.

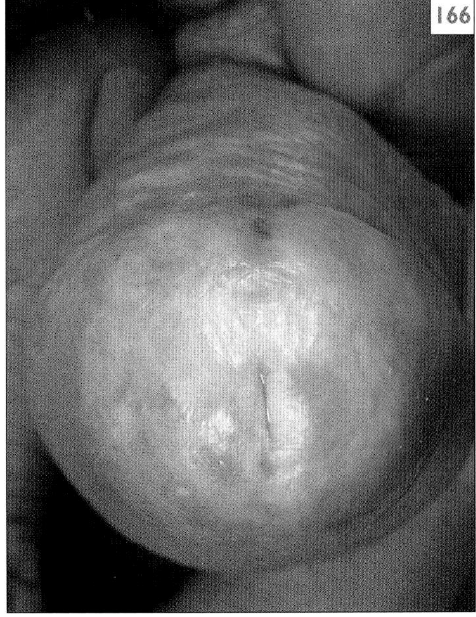

166 Balanitis.

INVESTIGATIONS

A skin biopsy will show epidermal atrophy with hyalinization of the underlying papillary dermis, and a lymphocytic infiltrate. Screening for other autoimmune diseases in particular thyroid disease if clinically indicated.

TREATMENT

For genital lesions potent topical corticosteroids give symptomatic relief and can improve clinical signs and prevent scarring. Topical sex hormones are also prescribed but there is less evidence to support their use. Soap substitutes and emollients are also usually recommended Circumcision may be needed in males and, if the foreskin alone is involved, can be curative. Extragenital lesions may respond to calcipotriol or low-dose UVA1. Adult patients with genital lichen sclerosus should be monitored for development of premalignant areas and squamous cell carcinoma. This usually arises in sclerotic areas in approximately 5% of patients.

Lichen planus

DEFINITION AND CLINICAL FEATURES

A lymphocyte-mediated, inflammatory, mucocutaneous disease with characteristic lesions on the skin and mucous membranes of the mouth and genitalia (see pp. 47-49).

Lichen planus can present in the anogenital area with the classical lesions of flat-topped, shiny, violaceous papules and Wickham's striae (**167**). Annular lesions may occur, particularly on the penis (**168**). However, lichen planus may present either as erosive disease (**169**) or with hypertrophic, hyperkeratotic plaques. In either of these variants there may be associated atrophy and scarring. Erosive disease may affect the gingiva (**170**), vagina (**171**), and vulval vestibule, which is known as the vulvo–vaginal–gingival syndrome. This is typically a treatment resistant, chronic disease and it may lead to severe vaginal stenosis. Postinflammatory hyperpigmentation may also be seen.

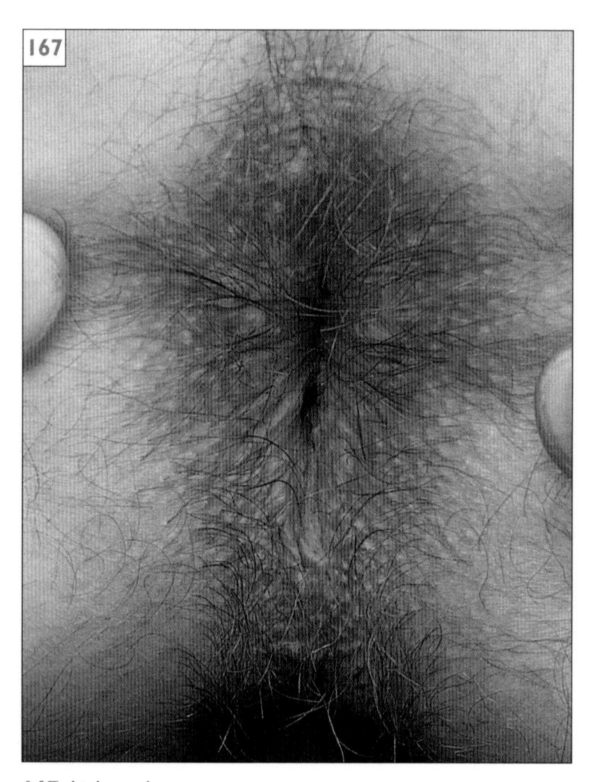

167 Lichen planus.

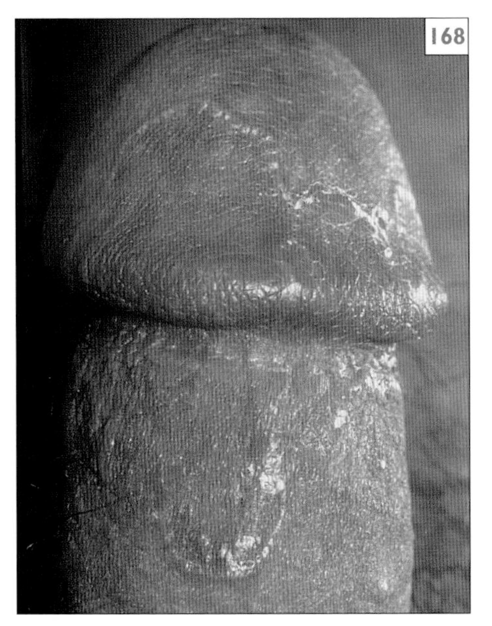

168 Annular lichen planus.

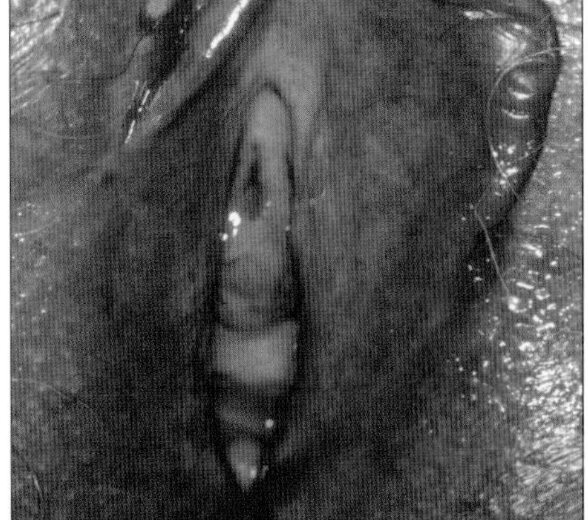

169 Erosive lichen planus.

DIFFERENTIAL DIAGNOSIS

Lichen sclerosus, perianal lichen simplex chronicus, cicatricial phemphigoid, and pemphigus.

INVESTIGATIONS

A skin biopsy should confirm the diagnosis. There is a dense, lymphocytic, band-like infiltrate along the dermo-epidermal junction with vacuolar degeneration of the basal layer.

TREATMENT

Potent topical corticosteroids are usually given for symptomatic oral or genital lesions. A range of systemic drugs have been used for severe erosive disease with inconsistent results, including retinoids, ciclosporin, and immunosuppressants. There is a rare association with the development of squamous cell carcinoma.

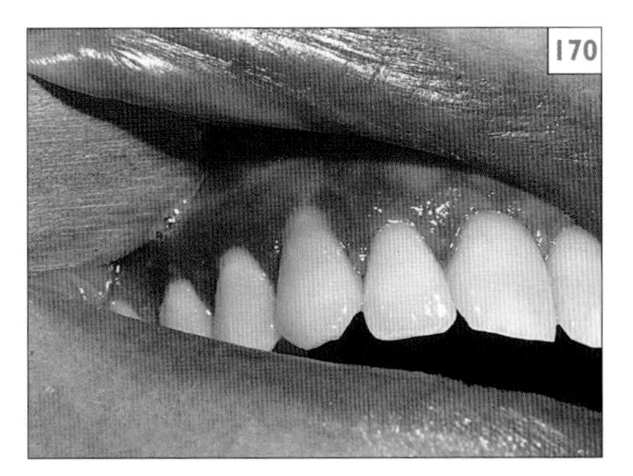

170 Erosive lichen planus.

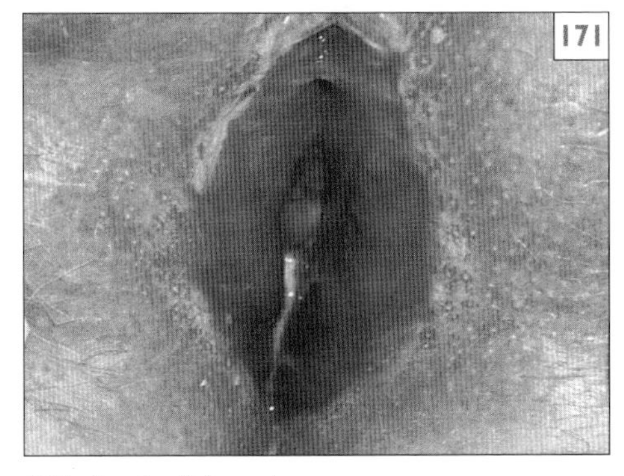

171 Erosive lichen planus.

Reiter's syndrome

DEFINITION AND CLINICAL FEATURES

This is a triad of urethritis, conjunctivitis, and arthritis. Its aetiology is uncertain but it may follow infectious gastroenteritis or chlamydial urethritis. There is a strong association with HLA B27 and the disease occurs most commonly in young men. The main cutaneous lesions seen in Reiter's are keratoderma blenorrhagica, and circinate balanitis. Keratoderma blenorrhagica describes psoriasiform, hyperkeratotic papules on the volar aspects of the hands and feet (**172**), which may occasionally be pustular. The lesions may extend to affect the extensor surfaces of the limbs and dorsal aspects of the toes and fingers. The nails may also be affected by changes similar to those seen in psoriasis. Erythematous scaly or eroded annular lesions on the glans penis which spread outwards are described as circinate balanitis (**173**).

DIFFERENTIAL DIAGNOSIS

Psoriasis.

INVESTIGATIONS

There is no diagnostic test for Reiter's. Microscopy and culture of urethral smears, urine, and stools may help to establish a relevant infection. Skin biopsies are of little value as the histopathological features are similar to those seen in psoriasis.

TREATMENT

Any underlying infection should be treated. NSAIDs are usually given for arthritis. Skin lesions may be treated topically as for psoriasis.

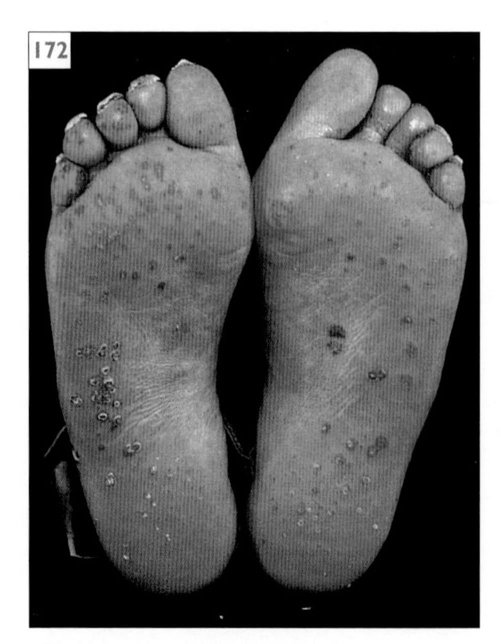

172 Keratoderma blenorrhagica.

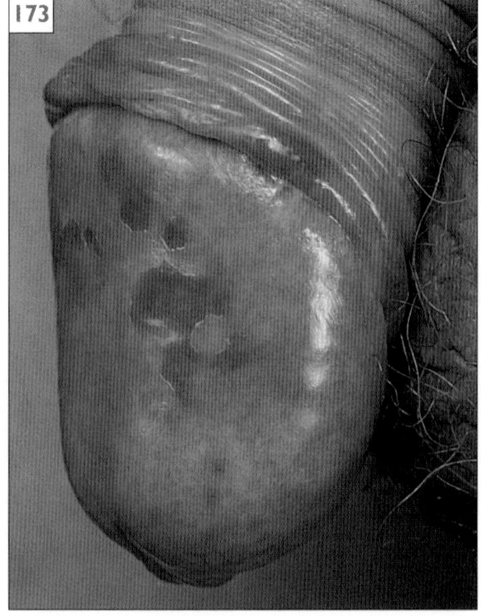

173 Circinate balanitis.

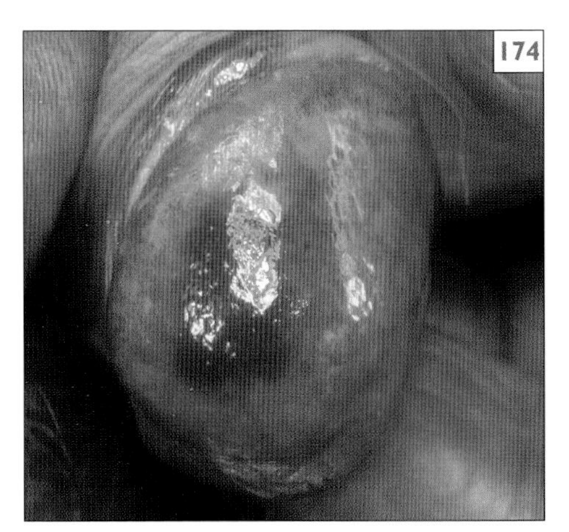

174 Balanitis of Zoon.

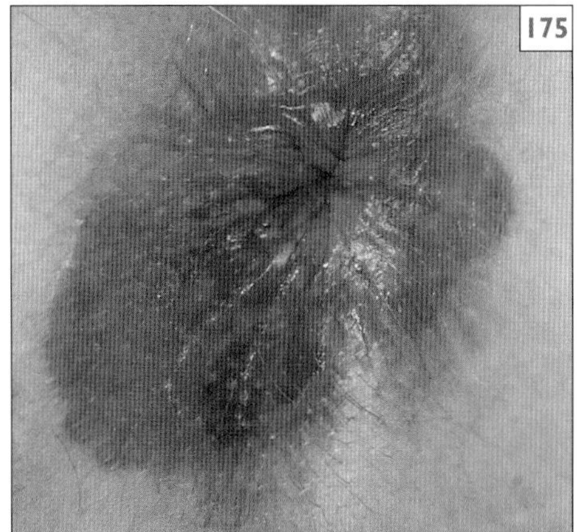

175 Extramammary Paget's disease.

Balanitis of Zoon

DEFINITION AND CLINICAL FEATURES

A chronic reactive balanitis characterized by well-demarcated glazed erythematous or orange-brown patches of the glans and mucosal prepuce (**174**). It usually occurs in middle-aged men with a poorly retractile foreskin and is thought to represent a chronic irritant process. A similar entity may occur on the vulva.

DIFFERENTIAL DIAGNOSIS

Lichen planus, Bowen's disease, psoriasis, seborrhoeic dermatitis, secondary syphilis, Kaposi's sarcoma.

INVESTIGATIONS

A skin biopsy should be performed to confirm the diagnosis. Histology shows a characteristic dermal band of plasma cells with extravasited erythrocytes haemosiderin and vascular proliferation.

TREATMENT

Improved washing with soap substitutes and application of moderate or potent topical corticosteroids with or without added anticandidal agents may help, but the condition usually runs a relapsing course. Circumcision is the definitive treatment.

Extramammary Paget's disease

DEFINITION AND CLINICAL FEATURES

A localized plaque resembling Paget's disease of the nipple clinically and histologically but occurring at sites rich in apocrine glands such as the axillae and anogenital area. The vulva is the commonest site for extramammary Paget's disease. The condition may arise primarily in the epidermis or secondary to an underlying adenocarcinoma. The lesion appears as a sharply demarcated eroded or scaly red plaque (**175**) and pruritus is prominent so there may be secondary lichenification.

DIFFERENTIAL DIAGNOSIS

Psoriasis, intraepithelial neoplasia, basal cell carcinoma, lichen simplex.

INVESTIGATION

A skin biopsy will show invasion of the epidermis with pale vacuolated Paget cells. The patient should be examined for an underlying adenocarcinoma of the cervix or rectum.

TREATMENT

Any underlying malignancy should be excised with all clinically abnormal epithelium. Moh's micrographic surgery may help define tumour margins as inadequate excision can lead to tumour recurrence. Topical 5-fluorouracil, imiquimod, bleomycin, and photodynamic therapy have also been used.

Hidradenitis suppurativa
(apocrine acne)

DEFINITION AND CLINICAL FEATURES
A chronic inflammatory and suppurative condition of apocrine gland follicles. Tender, inflamed, papules, pustules, and cysts arise in the axillae, submammary flexures, inguinal areas, and perineum (**176**). The initial lesions may develop sinuses and fistulous tracts with considerable scarring (**177**). Double-pored or polyporous comedones are often present in the affected areas. The cause is unknown, but occlusion of the apocrine gland follicle unit and obstruction of apocrine gland secretion may be the initiating event ('apocrine acne'). It occurs after puberty when the apocrine glands are fully developed and is commoner in women, suggesting hormonal influences. Hidradenitis suppurativa usually occurs alone but may be associated with acne conglobata and dissecting cellulitis of the scalp, the so-called follicular occlusion triad.

DIFFERENTIAL DIAGNOSIS
Furunculosis, Crohn's disease, granuloma inguinale, and lymphogranuloma venereum.

INVESTIGATIONS
Pus swabs should be taken for microbiological assessment to determine antibiotic sensitivities, but pathogens are often not isolated. Skin biopsy of chronic ulcers in long-standing disease to exclude malignancy.

TREATMENT
The disease often runs a chronic course. Weight loss in the obese with improved local hygiene, and the use of antiseptic washes may help. Long-term oral antibiotics as used for acne rather than penicillins are usually given. Oral clindamycin may be considered for more severe disease. Intralesional corticosteroids can reduce inflammation in localized disease. Surgical intervention ranges from simple excision of cysts and laying open of sinus tracts, to radical excision of all affected tissue.

Acrodermatitis enteropathica

DEFINITION AND CLINICAL FEATURES
A rare condition of abnormal zinc absorption, characterized by dermatitis, diarrhoea, failure to thrive, and alopecia. It is thought to be inherited as an autosomal recessive trait. Typically, the infant develops symptoms and signs at about 6 weeks after weaning (**178, 179** or earlier if not breast fed. Erythematous, scaly areas develop periorificially, around the eyes, mouth, and nappy area. Lesions also develop on the hands and feet. There may be vesicobullous areas. The scalp hair becomes sparse and is lost. Zinc absorption usually improves in adulthood. Chronic zinc deficiency may also occur in adults with alcoholic liver disease and pancreatitis and typically causes skin lesions on pressure prone sites with seborrhoeic dermatitis-like changes on the face, and a non-itchy scaly dermatitis on the trunk.

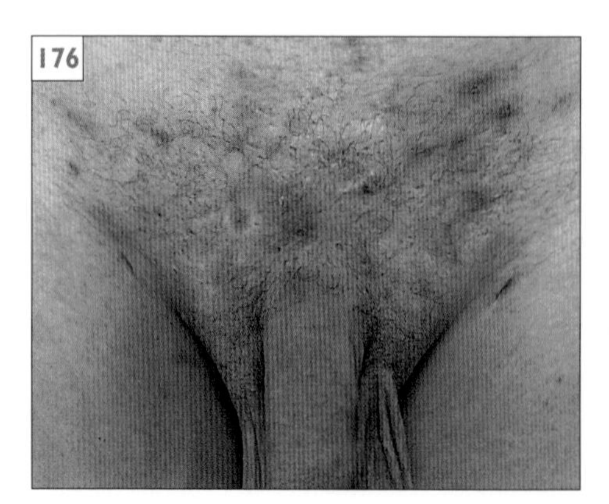

176 Hidradenitis suppurativa.

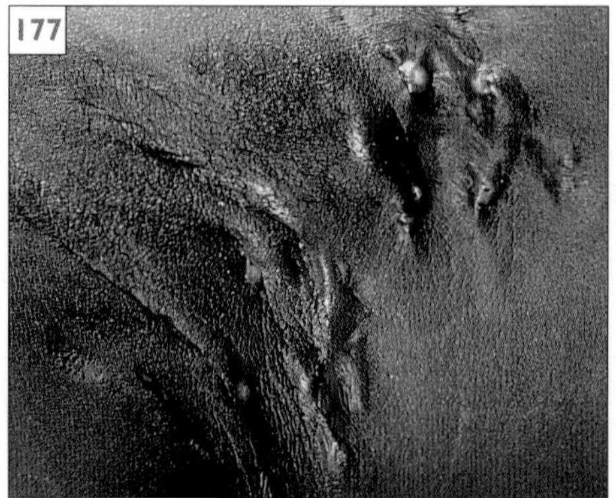

177 Hidradenitis suppurativa.

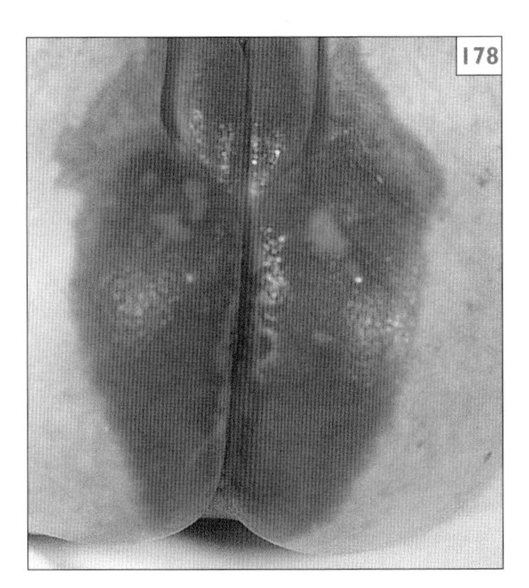

178 Acrodermatitis enteropathica.

DIFFERENTIAL DIAGNOSIS

Eczema, psoriasis, and candidiasis.

INVESTIGATIONS

Measurement of plasma or serum zinc level. However, plasma albumin binds zinc, so levels may be falsely low in hypoalbuminaemia. Alkaline phosphatase levels are also low.

SPECIAL POINTS

Oral zinc clears the clinical lesions within 2 weeks but must be continued at least until adult life.

Cutaneous Crohn's disease

DEFINITION AND CLINICAL FEATURES

Chronic inflammatory changes of flexural skin, characterized by lymphoedema or ulcerative necrosis, occurring in association with either active or inactive Crohn's disease. Skin disease usually occurs in association with gut disease, but may precede the onset of symptoms by several years and does not correlate with the degree of active bowel disease. The commonest site is the perianal area, where chronic sinuses and ulcers develop which can lead to fistulas and ischiorectal abscesses. There is also marked oedema and tag formation. Vulval involvement usually presents with severe, generalized oedema of the labia, but it may be unilateral. There is often intense erythema and oedema. There may be deep, linear fissuring along the skin folds (**180**).

DIFFERENTIAL DIAGNOSIS

Apocrine acne (hidradenitis suppurativa), deep fungal infection, lymphogranuloma venereum, amoebiasis, Behçet's syndrome, and sarcoidosis.

INVESTIGATIONS

Skin biopsy may show characteristic granulomatous inflammation or lymphangiectasia. If relevant, investigation of gastrointestinal function.

TREATMENT

Topical and intralesional corticosteroids and drugs used to control bowel disease including sulfasalazine, mesalazine and, recently, anti-tumour necrosis factor antibodies.

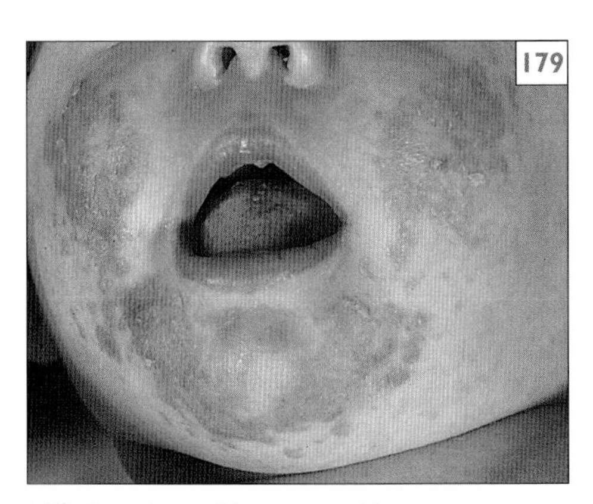

179 Acrodermatitis enteropathica.

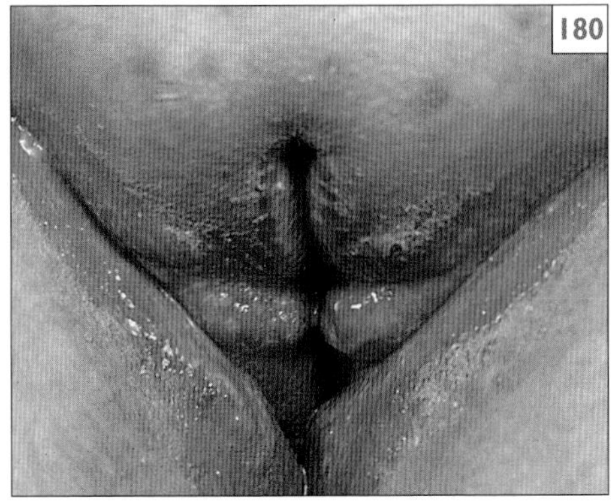

180 Cutaneous Crohn's disease.

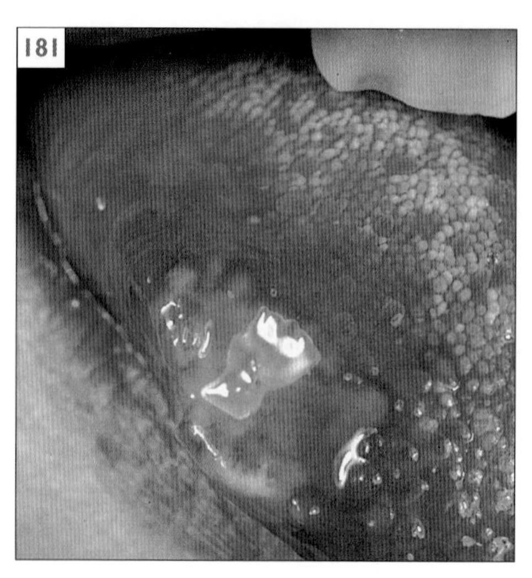

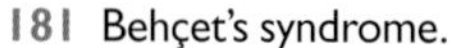

181 Behçet's syndrome.

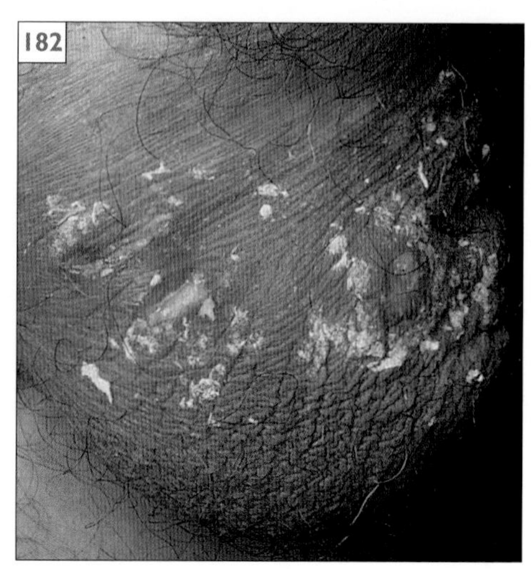

182 Behçet's syndrome.

Behçet's syndrome

DEFINITION AND CLINICAL FEATURES

Behçet's syndrome is the association of recurrent aphthous stomatitis with genital ulceration and eye disease. In addition, there may be other cutaneous and systemic manifestations. The majority of the patients are male and of Mediterranean or Eastern origin and there is an association with certain HLA types. The cause is unknown but there is usually an underlying leukocytoclastic vasculitis and immune complexes can be identified. Oral and genital ulcers are usually large and classified as major aphthae. They are painful and recurrent. Over 90% of patients have eye involvement, including iridocyclitis, anterior and posterior uveitis, retinal vasculitis, and optic atrophy (**181, 182**). An associated arthralgia, erythema nodosum, and papulopustular nodules may occur. There may also be profound, systemic symptoms; neurological involvement is a serious complication.

DIFFERENTIAL DIAGNOSIS

Aphthous ulceration, herpes simplex, cytomegalovirus infection, secondary syphilis, Crohn's, erythema multiforme.

INVESTIGATIONS

There is no diagnostic test and it is a diagnosis of exclusion. Therefore, investigations must be directed to exclude other causes of genital ulceration. Pathergy, the tendency to pustulate at a site of trauma, is a characteristic feature. Histology of papulopustular lesions may support the diagnosis.

TREATMENT

The disease runs a chronic course and causes considerable morbidity. Potent topical corticosteroids and colchicine can help mucocutaneous disease. Other systemic treatments include dapsone, ciclosporin, methotrexate, and oral corticosteroids.

Intraepithelial neoplasia

DEFINITION AND CLINICAL FEATURES

Loss of the normal orientation and architecture of the epithelium with cellular atypia. The terminology and classification of genital epithelial neoplasia has been subject to controversy and change. The newer terminology for vulval intraepithelial neoplasia recommends distinguishing mild basal atypia (previously termed VIN1), which is often regenerative, from atypia involving two-thirds to full thickness of the epithelium – now called undifferentiated VIN (previously VIN 2 and 3), or severe basal atypia with differentiated upper layers – now called differentiated VIN. VIN may be multifocal and may also involve the vagina, cervix, perianal area, and anal canal. There is a strong association between multifocal anogenital disease and oncogenic papilloma virus, particularly HPV 16 and 18. Similar variants of intraepithelial neoplasia can also affect the penile area (PIN). Full thickness PIN occurs in various clinical patterns previously termed erythroplasia of Queyrat, Bowen's disease of the penis, and bowenoid papulosis.

Morphologically, there is great variation in these lesions. Solitary lesions may arise, which clinically can appear as erythematous scaly plaques, erosions, or white patches (**183**). Multifocal disease may demonstrate a variety of lesions with different morphological features in the same patient. These range from pigmented papules and plaques, resembling seborrhoeic keratoses (previously bowenoid papulosis) (**184**).

DIFFERENTIAL DIAGNOSIS

Psoriasis, lichen planus, lichen sclerosus, basal cell papillomas, viral warts, and squamous cell carcinoma.

INVESTIGATIONS

Histology. Screening for HPV and other sexually transmitted infections. Cervical screening for affected women, and all those whose sexual partners have lesions.

TREATMENT

Treatment depends on the sex of the patient, site of involvement, and severity. Options include excision of small lesions, topical 5-fluorouracil, topical imiquimod, and superficial destructive treatment such as cryosurgery, curettage, and cautery laser ablation and photodynamic therapy. Circumcision may be indicated. Patients require long-term follow up as they are at risk of invasive carcinoma. Thicker or polypoid lesions on the vulva should be excised.

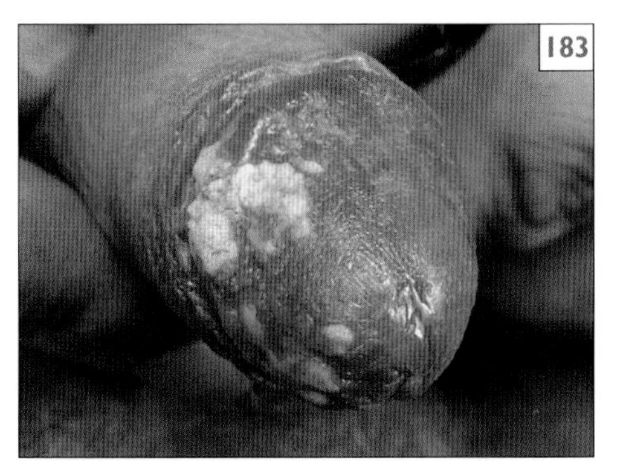

183 Intraepithelial neoplasia.

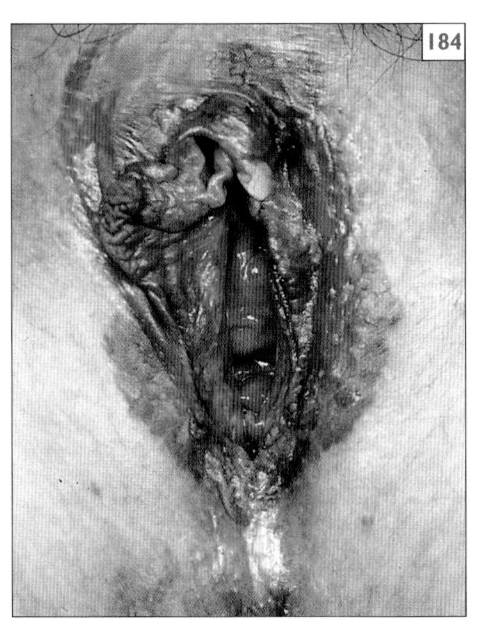

184 Multifocal undifferentiated VIN.

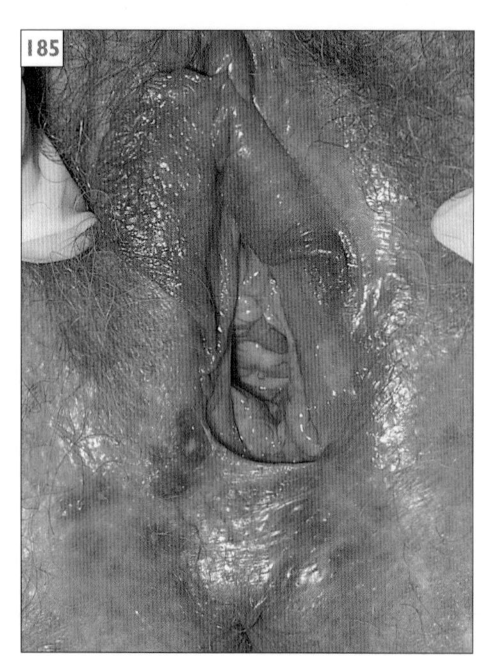

185 Vulval herpes simplex.

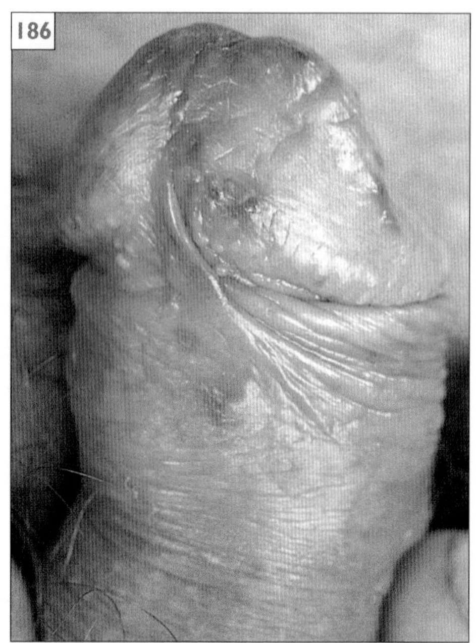

186 Recurrent penile herpes simplex.

Herpes genitalis

DEFINITION AND CLINICAL FEATURES

Infection of the genital area with herpes simplex viruses (HSV) Type I or Type 2 which is usually sexually transmitted (see p. 232). HSV-2 is the commonest type in this area. Ulcers may be preceded by malaise and are most frequent on the glans, prepuce, and shaft of the penis, and in females the vagina and cervix may be involved in addition to the vulva. Primary infection results in multiple turbid vesicles that are usually bilateral and coalesce to produce eroded areas which are very painful (**185**). There may be marked oedema and secondary urinary retention. Recurrent disease is due to reactivation of the virus, and presents with smaller closely grouped vesicles (**186**) without constitutional symptoms. Chronic ulcerative disease may occur in patients with HIV infection (see pp. 238–239).

DIFFERENTIAL DIAGNOSIS

Impetigo, herpes zoster.

INVESTIGATIONS

Culture of virus from vesicle fluid or direct visualization by electron microscopy. Screening for other sexually transmitted disease.

TREATMENT

Antiviral therapy is indicated in severe primary infection or troublesome recurrent disease. Aciclovir has been widely used but has low bioavailability; valaciclovir and famciclovir are newer alternatives. Other drugs which may be used for severe infection with aciclovir-resistant HSV include foscarnet and cidofovir.

Candidiasis

DEFINITION AND CLINICAL FEATURES

An opportunistic infection with yeasts of the *Candida* genus that can occur on any epithelium but has a predilection for mucosal surfaces. Various sites in the anogenital area may be affected in isolation or together. Vulval candidiasis is usually associated with vaginal infection and a curdy, white vaginal discharge. The vulval skin is red, oedematous, and sometimes studded with subcorneal pustules (**187**). In chronic cases the mucosa may become glazed and atrophic. Candidal balanitis usually affects uncircumcised men and is characterized by small papules or pustules which rupture, leaving very superficial erosions on the glans. Flexural candidiasis affects the genitocrural folds, perianal area, and natal cleft. The classical features of this intertrigo are erythema and maceration which spread on to the surrounding skin where satellite pustules develop.

Over 70% of infections are caused by *Candida albicans* (see p.226) The healthy vagina may be colonized by yeast in a minority of women. Its overgrowth may be triggered by pregnancy, high-dose oral contraceptive, diabetes, oral antibiotics, inflamed macerated dermatoses, and immunosuppression due to disease or drugs.

DIFFERENTIAL DIAGNOSIS

Bacterial or tinea intertrigo, trichomonas, Hailey–Hailey disease, psoriasis, seborrhoeic eczema, contact eczema.

INVESTIGATIONS

Direct microscopy of smears with 10% potassium hydroxide (KOH). Culture of swabs. Exclude diabetes mellitus.

TREATMENT

In many cases topical antifungal therapy with a polyene or azole antifungal will suffice. Single-dose oral azole therapy may also be used for acute vulvovaginitis. Courses of systemic therapy are needed for immunocompromised patients.

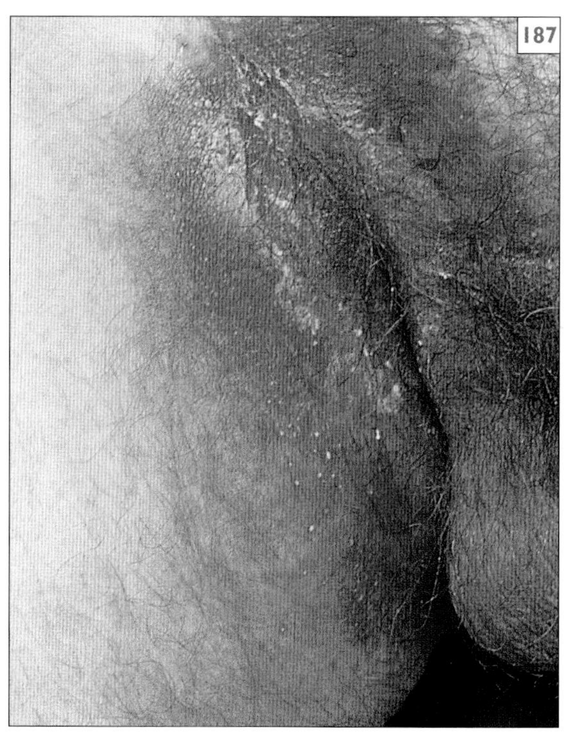

187 Vulval candidiasis.

Syphilis

DEFINITION AND CLINICAL FEATURES

An infectious disease caused by the spirochaete *Treponema pallidum*. Syphilis is a contagious, sexually acquired infection, which, if untreated, is characterized by a variety of cutaneous and systemic signs and symptoms. The incubation period ranges from 9–90 days. Primary syphilis (**188**) is characterized by a chancre, which is a well-defined, painless ulcer at the site of contact, most frequently in the anogenital area. It is usually solitary but there may be multiple lesions.

With secondary syphilis (**189**) in the untreated patient, a maculopapular eruption occurs on the face, trunk, and limbs which has a psoriasiform appearance with distinctive lesions on the palms and soles (**190**). In flexural sites of the anogenital area, clusters of papules develop which vary from being smooth and shiny to wart-like and are known as condylomata lata (**191**).

There has been an increase in the incidence of syphilis in homosexual men with a high proportion of HIV coinfection. Congenital syphilis is now very rare due to routine screening for syphilis in pregnancy.

DIFFERENTIAL DIAGNOSIS

Primary chancre: any ulcer, e.g. Behçet's, Sutton's, major aphthous. Secondary: psoriasis, pityriasis rosea. Condylomata lata: viral warts.

INVESTIGATIONS

Smears of primary and secondary lesions with dark field microscopy. Serology for antibody detection. Histopathology. Screening for other sexually transmitted infections.

TREATMENT

Primary prevention is based upon safe sexual practices and consistent condom use. Parenteral penicillin G is the preferred drug at all stages of syphilis and the dose and duration depend on the clinical stage and disease manifestations. Tetracyclines and macrolides are alternatives in penicillin-allergic individuals. Follow up and identification of sexual contacts is an important part of management.

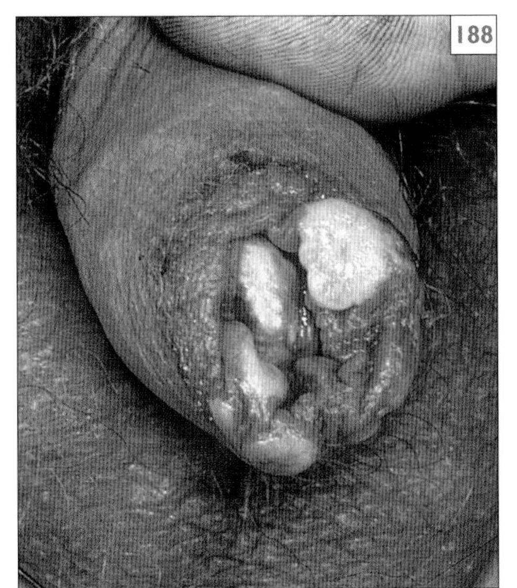

188 Primary syphilis.

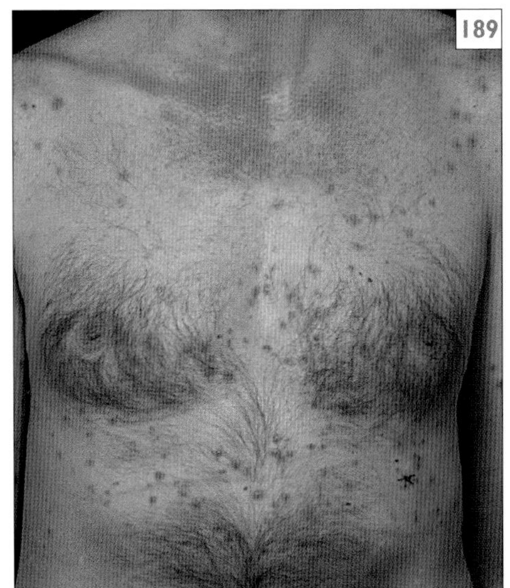

189 Secondary syphilis.

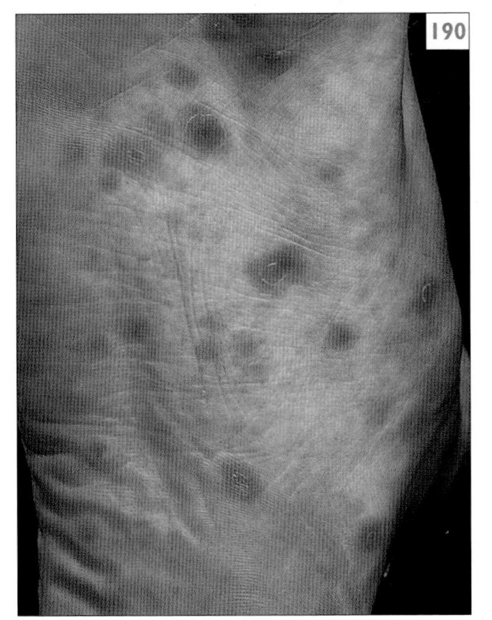

190 Secondary syphilis.

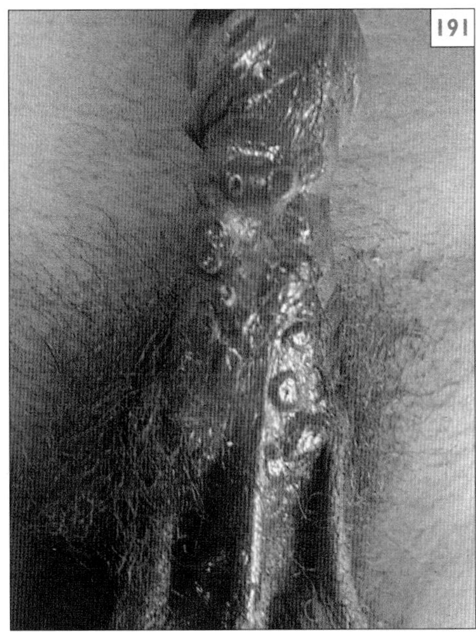

191 Condylomata lata.

HAIR DISORDERS

Alopecia areata

DEFINITION AND CLINICAL FEATURES

A chronic non-scarring autoimmune disorder affecting the hair follicle. Typically, there is a sudden onset of solitary or multiple circular or oval bald areas, usually affecting the scalp (**192**) but any hair-bearing area may be affected. The residual hair follicles are visible confirming a lack of scarring. Diagnostic exclamation mark hairs may be visible at the margins of the lesion. The affected scalp is usually normal in colour but may be erythematous. Hairs at the edge of the patch may be easily removed with gentle traction. Spontaneous regrowth frequently occurs, but the areas may spread peripherally and may eventually involve the whole scalp (alopecia totalis) and even facial (**193**) and body hair (alopecia universalis). Rarely, a diffuse alopecia may occur without discrete bald patches. Regrowing hairs are usually white. Nail changes may also occur, particularly in extensive disease, as fine regular pitting or a roughened, sandpaper appearance (trachyonychia) (**194**). Alopecia areata is a common disorder affecting all races and either sex equally. It occurs at any age, with the highest incidence between 10 and 30 years.

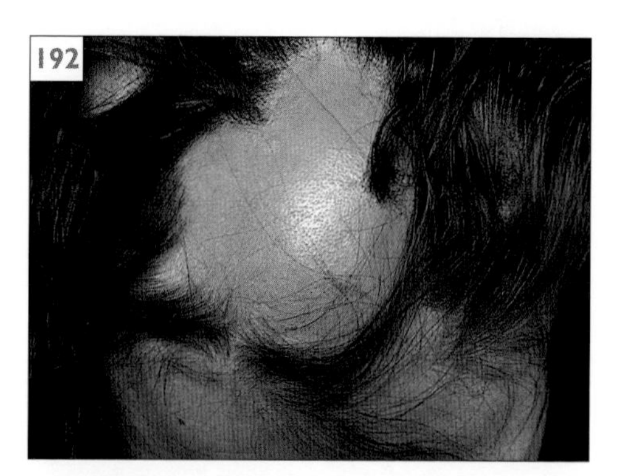

192 Alopecia areata.

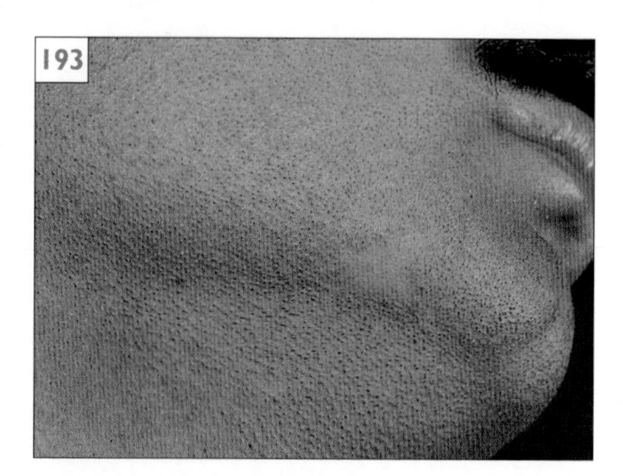

193 Facial alopecia areata.

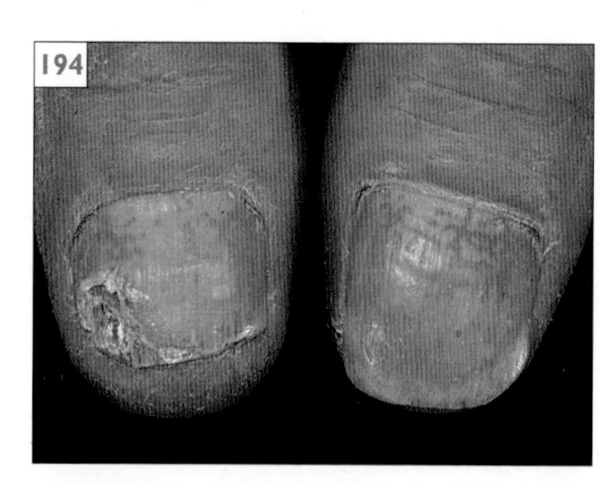

194 The nails in alopecia areata.

DIFFERENTIAL DIAGNOSIS

Scalp fungal infections in children may be confirmed on mycological examination and Wood's light. Trichotillomania shows broken hairs of varying lengths. In older patients, scarring alopecia due to lichen planus or discoid lupus erythematosus may also cause patchy alopecia. Telogen effluvium also causes diffuse non-scarring alopecia.

INVESTIGATIONS

Organ-specific autoantibodies may be demonstrated. Scalp biopsy may be required to exclude other disorders.

TREATMENT

Spontaneous regrowth usually occurs in localized disease. Topical, intralesional, and systemic corticosteroids can produce temporary regrowth. Contact sensitization therapy using irritants (dithranol) or allergens (diphencyprone) and PUVA are also used. The more extensive the hair loss, the less likely the prospect of regrowth. Extensive involvement, atopy, other autoimmune diseases, nail involvement, and onset in childhood are poor prognostic factors. Patients with extensive hair loss may need considerable psychological support.

Telogen effluvium

DEFINITION AND CLINICAL FEATURES

Increased shedding of club (telogen) hairs due to an increase in the number of hairs in the resting phase of the hair cycle. It may follow a variety of triggers. Acute telogen effluvium presenting with sudden extensive hair shedding may occuring 4–8 weeks after a severe illness or systemic upset. Loss of several hundred hairs per day produces a diffuse alopecia affecting the entire scalp (**195**). Other hair-bearing areas may also be involved. Pre-existing androgenetic alopecia may become more evident, the scalp appears normal, and duration is variable (but recovery is usually complete within 6 months). Chronic telogen effluvium refers to idiopathic telogen hair shedding persisting for longer than 6 months. Chronic diffuse hair loss may also be secondary to starvation, malnutrition, connective tissue diseases, thyroid dysfunction, iron deficiency anaemia, syphilis, and drug treatment.

DIFFERENTIAL DIAGNOSIS

Diffuse hair shedding can also occur in the early stages of female androgenetic alopecia. Anagen effluvium occurs within 1–2 weeks of the precipitating drug or event.

INVESTIGATIONS

Trichogram (plucked scalp hairs) will show an increase in the number of telogen hairs and reduction in anagen hairs. Scalp biopsy in chronic telogen effluvium shows an anagen: telogen ratio of 1:8 compared with 1:14 in a normal scalp. In patients with chronic telogen hair loss investigations to exclude systemic disease, e.g. FBC, ferritin, TSH, ANA, syphilis serology should be considered.

TREATMENT

Acute telogen effluvium should resolve spontaneously. Any underlying cause should be treated in chronic diffuse telogen loss.

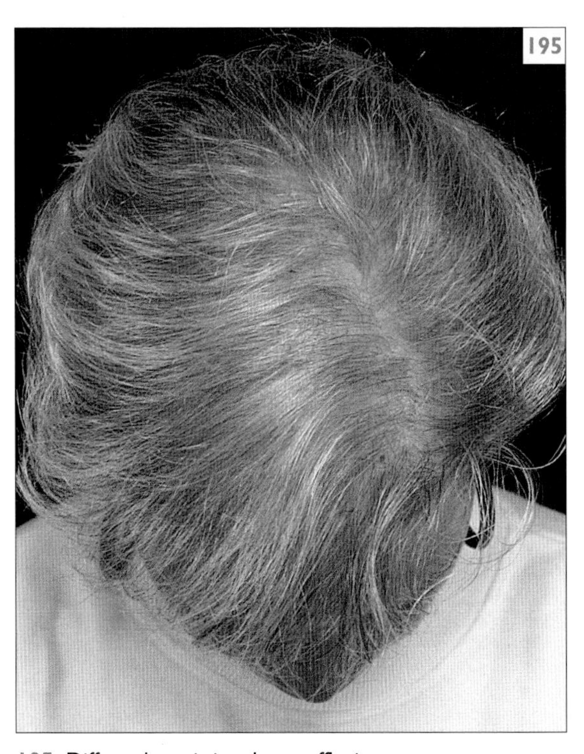

195 Diffuse alopecia in telogen effluvium.

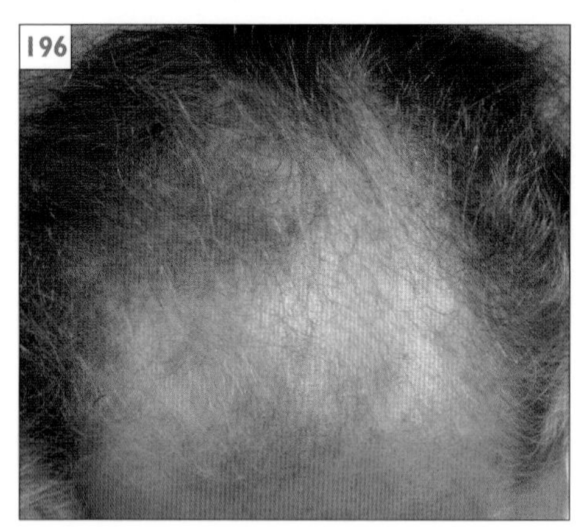

196 Androgenetic alopecia (male pattern baldness).

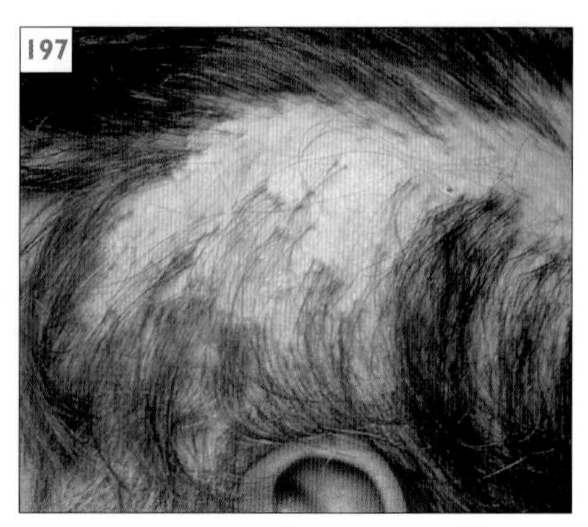

197 Scarring alopecia.

Androgenetic alopecia

DEFINITION AND CLINICAL FEATURES

Miniaturization of the hair follicles through successive cycles affecting the fronto-vertex and crown of the scalp, producing a gradual conversion of terminal to vellus hairs. The scalp hair loss begins with recession at the temples and the frontal hairline in men (Hamilton pattern) (**196**) and thinning over the crown and vertex. This progresses slowly over several years; in severe cases hair remains at the occiput and sides of the scalp alone. Vellus hairs may remain on the vertex. In women (Ludwig pattern) the frontal hairline is maintained but a diffuse thinning occurs over the top of the scalp with widening of the parting. Although increased shedding may occur initially, the history is usually one of gradual thinning. The androgen dihydrotestosterone is thought to play a causal role in shortening the duration of anagen and causing miniturization of susceptible follicles.

DIFFERENTIAL DIAGNOSIS

Telogen effluvium may produce diffuse alopecia but usually affects the back and sides of the scalp as well as the fronto-vertex. Hairstyles producing traction may cause recession of the anterior hair margin.

INVESTIGATIONS

Severe hair loss in women with associated menstrual irregularities should be investigated to exclude an androgen-secreting tumour.

TREATMENT

Topical minoxidil increases the duration of anagen and may improve hair coverage but cessation of treatment results in loss of all new hairs. Oral finasteride inhibits the synthesis of dihydrotestosterone and is effective in men. Systemic antiandrogens such as cyproterone acetate or spironolactone may be used in women, but pregnancy must be avoided as these drugs can cause feminization of a male foetus. Surgical options include excision of bald areas with tissue expansion and hair transplantation.

Scarring alopecia

DEFINITION AND CLINICAL FEATURES

Permanent destruction of hair follicles secondary to inflammatory and scarring cutaneous disorders. Scarred patches of alopecia without visible hair follicles occur irregularly throughout the scalp (**197**) or other hair-bearing area. The skin is usually scarred and atrophic. There may be signs of active cutaneous disease, such as lichen planus elsewhere or discoid lupus erythematosus with erythematous indurated scaling plaques

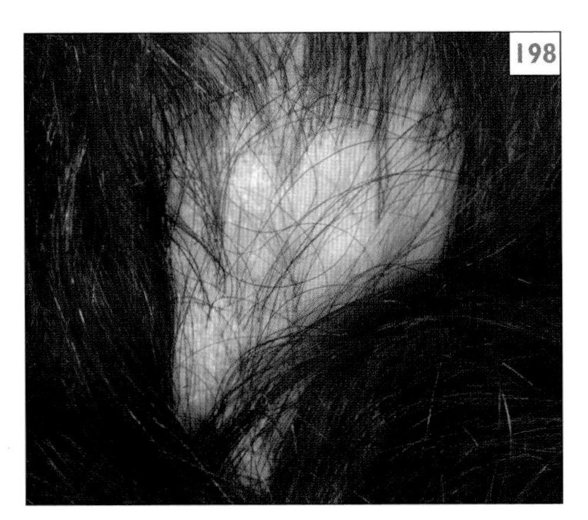

198 Pseudopelade.

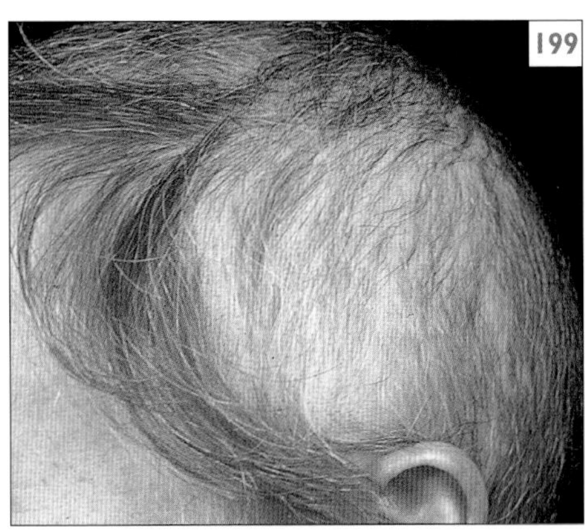

199 Trichotillomania (traumatic alopecia).

and follicular plugging. Pseudopelade (**198**) is a noninflammatory form of scarring alopecia of unknown cause, characterized by pale, waxy, patchy areas of skin atrophy. Folliculitis decalvans is a slow, progressive form of the disorder, with pustules around the hairs and chronic staphylococcal infection (see p. 78). Other scarring disorders include burns, X-ray therapy, trauma, staphylococcal infection, fungal infections, and neoplasms.

DIFFERENTIAL DIAGNOSIS

Patchy alopecia may be produced by alopecia areata, which is non-scarring.

INVESTIGATIONS

Scalp biopsy will confirm the presence of scarring, with destruction of hair follicles and sebaceous glands, and may provide evidence of the underlying inflammatory dermatosis.

TREATMENT

Hair loss in areas of scarring alopecia is permanent. Therapy includes treating any underlying disorder, e.g. with corticosteroids, antimalarial drugs, or long-term antibiotics. Cosmetic plastic surgery may be useful at a later stage.

Trichotillomania

DEFINITION AND CLINICAL FEATURES

Self-induced alopecia produced by deliberate trauma to the hair. A diffuse area of thinned hair with a poorly defined margin (**199**). Scalp skin is normal. Affected hairs show breakage of varying lengths. The area may be solitary or multiple. A normal, tonsural, long-haired margin often remains. Patients may exhibit other evidence of self-mutilation (see dermatitis artefacta, p. 28). Trichotillomania occurs more frequently in females and may occur at any age. It is usually a sign of underlying psychological distress.

DIFFERENTIAL DIAGNOSIS

Alopecia areata produces more discrete, completely bald areas of alopecia. Tinea capitis can produce broken hairs, and scaling and inflammation may be present. Mycological examination confirms the diagnosis.

INVESTIGATIONS

Hair microscopy will reveal broken hairs of various lengths. Mycology to exclude fungal infection.

TREATMENT

Occlusion of the area often allows recovery. Children frequently outgrow the habit, while in adults psychiatric therapy may be required.

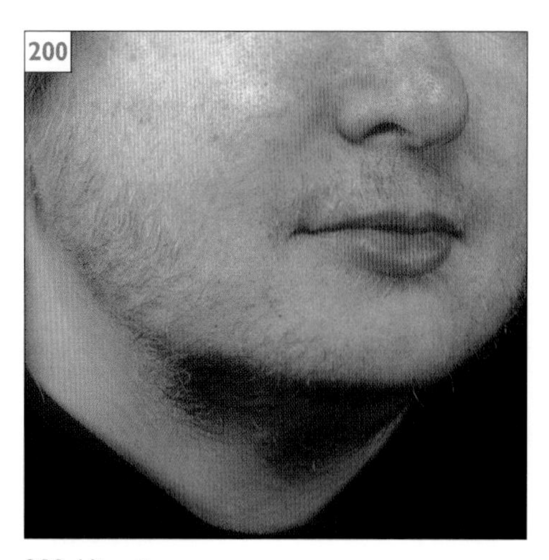

200 Hirsutism.

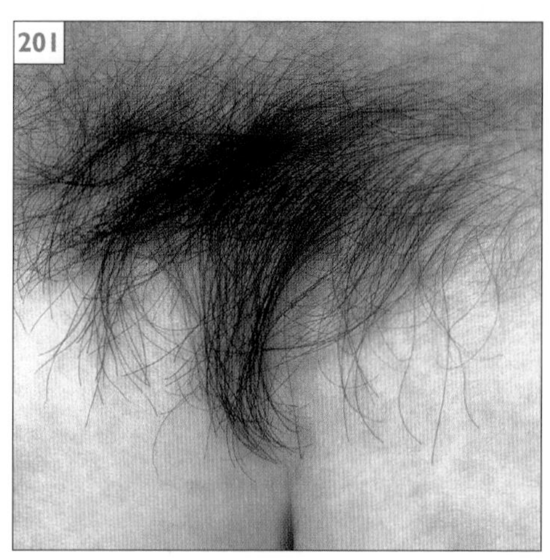

201 Localized hypertrichosis.

Hirsutism

DEFINITION AND CLINICAL FEATURES

Excessive growth of coarse terminal hairs in women in an androgen-dependent pattern (face breasts, upper back, lower abdomen) (**200**). The perception of what is normal or desirable hair growth depends on social, cultural and racial influences. The degree of hirsutism may be scored using the grading system of Ferriman and Gallwey.

INVESTIGATIONS

If there are associated menstrual irregularities the patient's androgen profile should be checked to exclude an underlying endocrine abnormality or virilizing ovarian tumour. Many hirsute women have subtle underlying polycystic ovarian syndrome, but in some there is no apparent abnormality.

TREATMENT

Excess hair may be bleached, plucked, waxed, sugared, or shaved. Topical eflornithine decarboxylase may improve cosmesis by slowing and thinning terminal hair growth. Laser hair removal is a newer option, but several treatments are necessary as only follicles in anagen respond. The hair reduction is not permanent, but repeated treatment may lead to a gradual reduction in hair density.

Hypertrichosis

DEFINITION AND CLINICAL FEATURES

Excessive growth of hair, typically vellus, in a non-androgen pattern. It may be localized or generalized. Congenital hypertrichosis occurs in several rare hereditary syndromes and if localized to the lumbosacral area may be associated with underlying spinal cord problems (**201**). Acute diffuse hypertrichosis may occur in thyroid disease, porphyrias, malnutrition, anorexia nervosa and, very rarely, with underlying malignancy. It may also be induced by several drugs including ciclosporin, minoxidil, diazoxide, corticosteroids, psoralens, and minocycline.

DIFFERENTIAL DIAGNOSIS

Hirsutism.

TREATMENT

Discontinue offending drug if possible and consider hair removal as for hirsutism.

PIGMENTATION DISORDERS

Hypermelanosis

Postinflammatory hyperpigmentation

DEFINITION AND CLINICAL FEATURES

A brown or purple-brown discolouration from the accumulation of haem, iron, and melanin pigments in the dermis, with or without increased melanin in the epidermis. Postinflammatory hyperpigmentation occurs after trauma, thermal injury, or inflammatory dermatoses such as atopic eczema, lichen planus, acne, and SLE. The discolouration intensifies and persists after the primary lesions have resolved (**202**, **203**). It is particularly likely to occur in dark-skinned individuals.

DIFFERENTIAL DIAGNOSIS

Other causes of hyperpigmentation including melasma, ochronosis, and so on. Exogenous material may stain the skin or be implanted during trauma to produce a dark macule or tattoo. Identification of the cause of postinflammatory hyperpigmentation relies on a history of a pre-existing condition and on examination of coexisting lesions.

INVESTIGATIONS

Histology may be helpful in lichen planus but is often unable to identify the pre-existing inflammatory condition.

TREATMENT

Postinflammatory pigmentation usually resolves spontaneously, although this may take many months. The primary dermatoses should be adequately controlled in order to prevent further pigmentary changes.

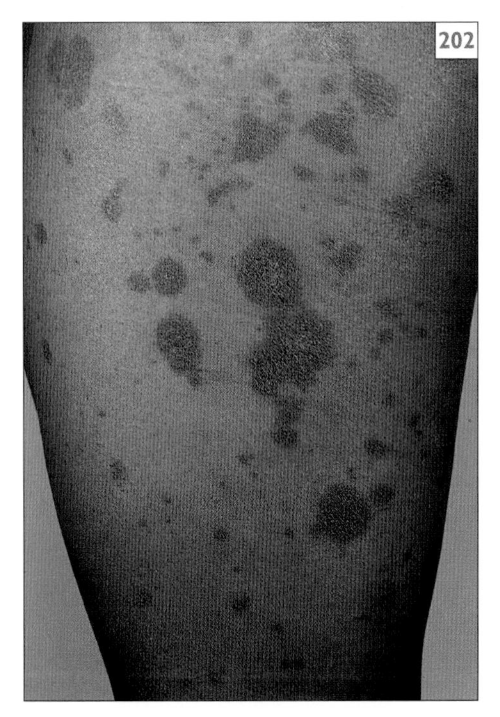

202 Postinflammatory hyperpigmentation.

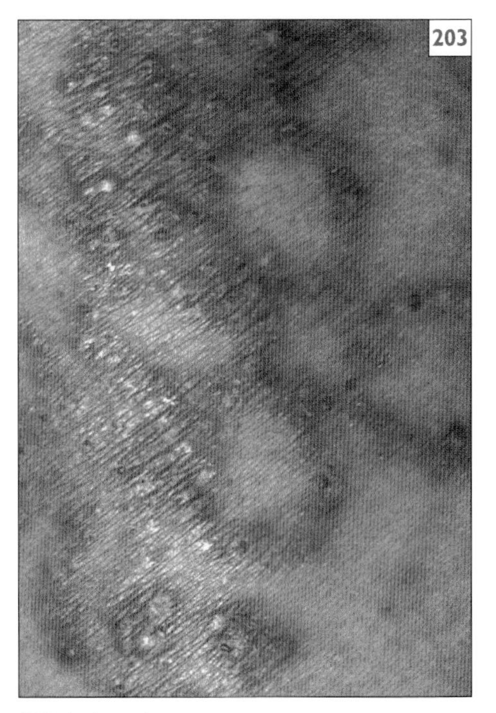

203 Lichen planus.

Café-au-lait macules

DEFINITION AND CLINICAL FEATURES

Café-au-lait ('white coffee') macules are hyperpigmented areas occurring on any cutaneous surface, unrelated to UV exposure. Characteristically homogeneous in colour, typically light brown, they vary in size (from 1 mm to many centimetres) and number and may be present at birth or acquired in early childhood. They are sharply demarcated from the surrounding skin by a smooth contour (**204, 205**). Café-au-lait macules occur as solitary lesions in 10–15% of the normal population, but the presence of six or more café-au-lait macules greater than 5 mm in diameter is usually a sign of neurofibromatosis. This is usually the earliest cutaneous sign of this genetic disorder. Other diagnostic signs include axillary (**206**) and inguinal freckling, and presence of two or more neurofibromas (**207, 208**).

Larger more irregular melanotic macules are also seen in Albright's syndrome, in which there is fibrous dysplasia of bone and endocrine dysfunction. The full syndrome with precocious puberty occurs only in girls. The dark macules of the syndrome are usually larger and few in number, and they tend to be unilateral and may be arranged in a linear or segmental pattern (**209**) with irregular edges.

DIFFERENTIAL DIAGNOSIS

Congenital melanocytic naevi.

INVESTIGATIONS

Ophthalmic examination reveals Lisch nodules and iris harmatomas in most patients with neurofibromatosis. The diagnosis of neurofibromatosis is usually made on clinical grounds, but molecular genetic testing is feasible as the abnormal gene has been identified.

TREATMENT

Café-au-lait macules do not require treatment. Patients with suspected neurofibromatosis should receive genetic counselling. Treatment is symptomatic.

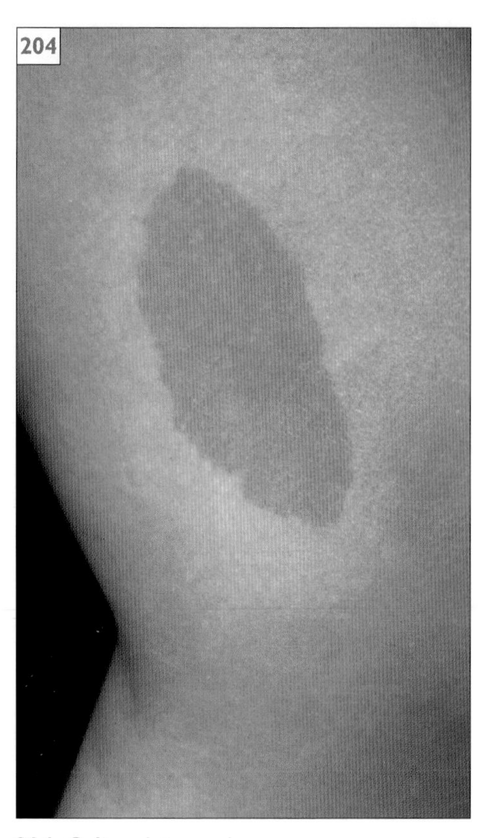

204 Café-au-lait macule.

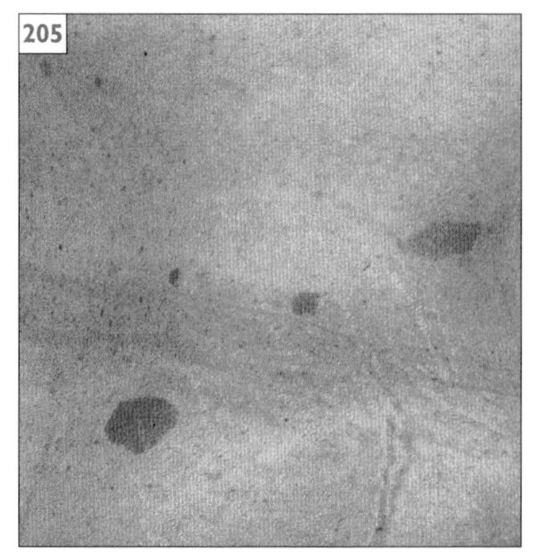

205 Café-au-lait macules.

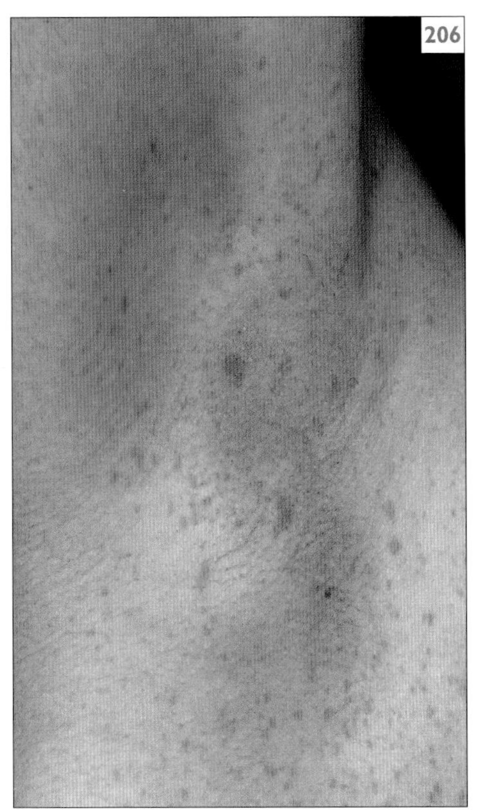

206 Axilliary freckling in neurofibromatosis.

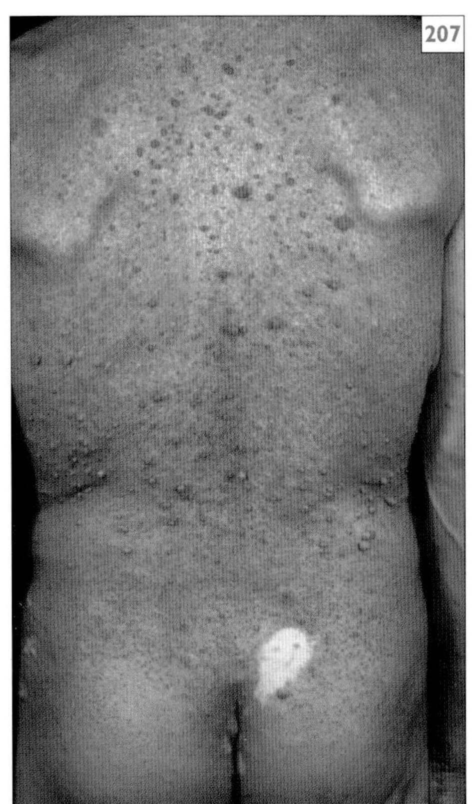

207 Multiple neurofibromas in neurofibromatosis.

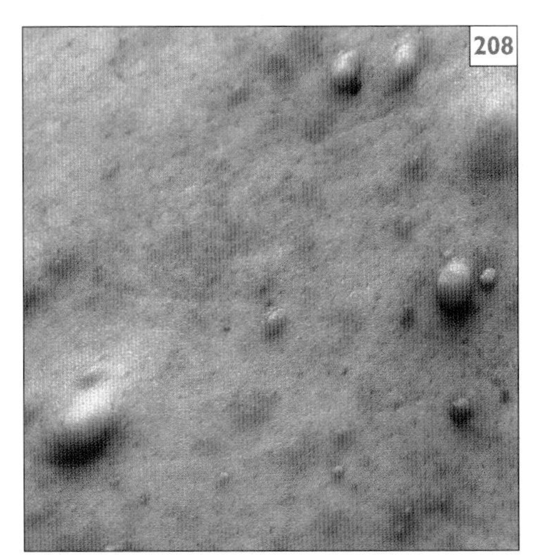

208 Multiple neurofibromas in neurofibromatosis.

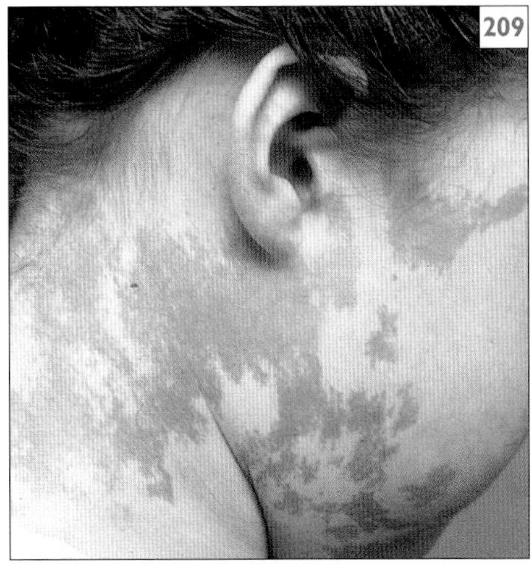

209 Albright's syndrome.

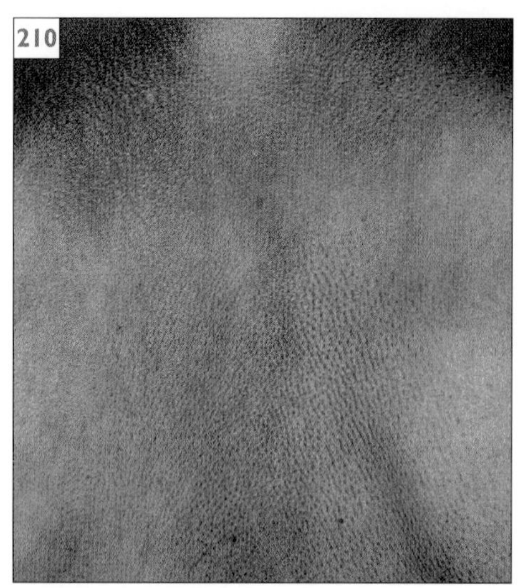

210 Macular amyloid.

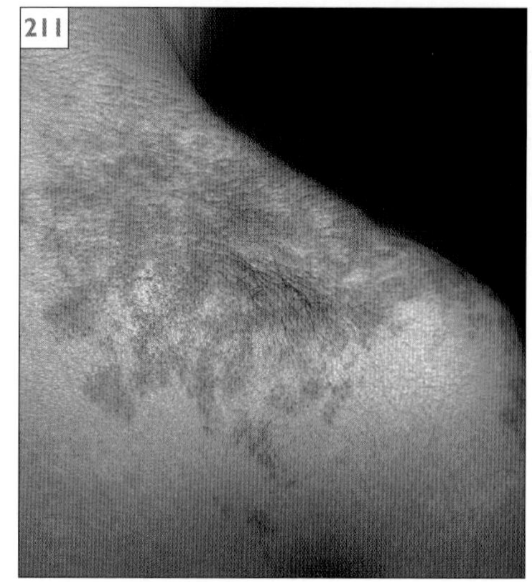

211 Becker's naevus.

Macular amyloid and lichen amyloidosus

DEFINITION AND CLINICAL FEATURES

A chronic hyperpigmented eruption consisting of pruritic macules or papules with histological evidence of amyloid deposition in the papillary dermis. Macular amyloid often involves the upper back and chest and appears as clusters of small pigmented macules which may coalesce into a reticulate or rippled pattern (**210**). It may follow prolonged friction and hypopigmented areas may develop. Papular amyloid usually presents as a pigmented pruritic eruption on the lower limbs, especially the shins.

DIFFERENTIAL DIAGNOSIS

Lichen planus, postinflammatory hyperpigmentation.

INVESTIGATION

Skin biopsy and special stains for amyloid.

TREATMENT

Potent topical corticosteroids may be tried with or without occlusion, but improvement is often only temporary. Calcipotriol and phototherapy are other options.

Becker's naevus

DEFINITION AND CLINICAL FEATURES

An acquired area of hyperpigmented skin which may show evidence of increased androgen sensitivity. Becker's naevus is a relatively common anomaly affecting 0.5% of young men. It usually develops in adolescence as an irregular asymmetrical area of hyperpigmentation which may later thicken and develop coarse dark hairs (**211**). Lesions usually arise on the upper chest or shoulders. The melanocyte density within lesions may be normal or increased but ultrastructurally there is evidence of increased melanogenesis. It is thought to arise from an abnormal skin clone with hypersensitivity to androgens.

DIFFERENTIAL DIAGNOSIS

Café-au-lait macule, linear and whorled naevoid hyperpigmentation.

INVESTIGATION

None usually necessary. Histological changes may be subtle.

Incontinentia pigmenti

DEFINITION AND CLINICAL FEATURES

Incontinentia pigmenti is a complex developmental syndrome due to an X-linked dominant trait that is usually lethal in males; 95% of cases are females. Vesicular, verrucous, and pigmented skin lesions are associated with developmental defects of the eye, skeleton, and central nervous syndrome. Skin changes are present at or soon after birth. Three clinical stages are recognized: blisters, warty papules and irregular pigmentation. Linear groups of clear, tense blisters develop on the limbs and/or trunk in recurrent crops (**212**). They are accompanied or followed by smooth red or bluish-purple nodules or plaques. Linear warty lesions may appear on the backs of the fingers or toes. Sometimes pigmentation is the only abnormality. Brown or blue-grey pigmentation may be present from the outset or may develop as the inflammatory lesions are subsiding. A bizarre 'splashed' or 'Chinese figure' distribution is diagnostic (**213**). The pigmentation slowly fades, becoming imperceptible by the third decade.

DIFFERENTIAL DIAGNOSIS

During a purely bullous phase, childhood bullous pemphigoid must be excluded.

INVESTIGATIONS

Skin biopsy shows subepidermal blistering and eosinophilia in the bullous phase, but direct immunofluorescence is negative.

TREATMENT

No specific treatment is available, but genetic counselling should be offered to the affected family.

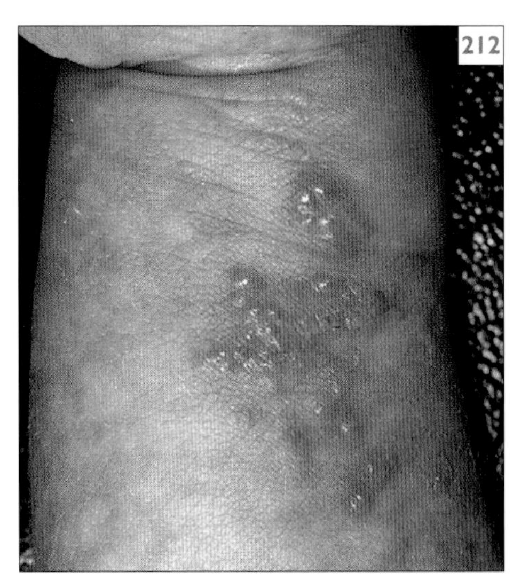

212 Incontinentia pigmenti.

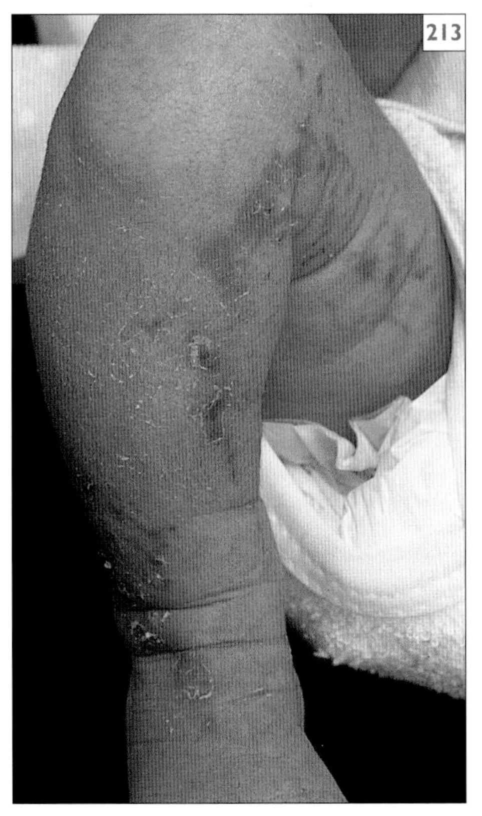

213 'Chinese figure' distribution in incontinentia pigmenti.

Melasma

DEFINITION AND CLINICAL FEATURES

Melasma or chloasma is a common hypermelanosis on the sun-exposed skin of the face that typically occurs in women during pregnancy or when taking the oral contraceptive pill. The aetiology is not clear but raised oestrogen levels may play a role. Only rarely is melasma seen in postmenopausal women, or in men. The hyperpigmentation affects the cheeks, forehead, upper lip, and chin (**214**), and becomes more marked following sun exposure. The pigmentation is usually symmetrical with a ragged border and is accentuated by examination under Wood's light.

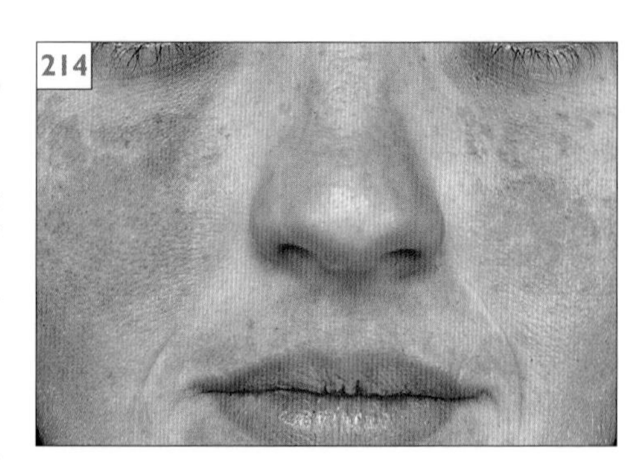

214 Melasma (chloasma).

DIFFERENTIAL DIAGNOSIS

The appearance is usually diagnostic. Postinflammatory hyperpigmentation.

INVESTIGATIONS

None usually necessary.

TREATMENT

Pregnancy-induced melasma usually fades postpartum. Discontinuing hormonal contraception may help. Melasma usually fades in winter weather and strict sun protection measures should be taken. Topical treatment includes hydroquinone 2–4%, retinoic acid, azelaic acid, and chemical peels.

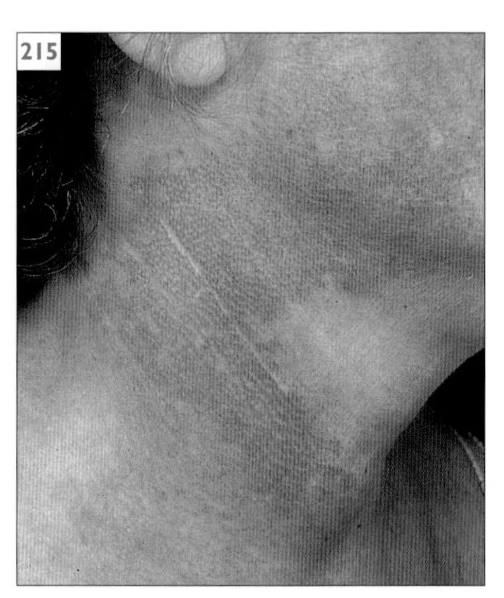

215 Poikiloderma of Civatte.

Poikiloderma of Civatte

DEFINITION AND CLINICAL FEATURES

Pigmentation and telangiectasia in a characteristic distribution on the lateral cheeks and side of the neck in middle-aged women. Milder forms are common and often not brought to medical attention. A reddish-brown, reticulate pigmentation with telangiectasia and atrophy develops in irregular but symmetrical patches on the lateral cheeks and sides of the neck (**215**). Areas shaded by the chin are spared, implicating chronic sun sunlight as an aetiological factor. Photoactive substances in cosmetics may also be important.

DIFFERENTIAL DIAGNOSIS

Postinflammatory hyperpigmentation.

INVESTIGATIONS

None usually necessary.

TREATMENT

There is no established treatment but sunscreens may be indicated and vascular laser therapy can reduce the telangiectasia, although care needs to be taken to avoid scarring.

Dermal melanocytosis

DEFINITION AND CLINICAL FEATURES

Hyperpigmentation of the skin due to the presence of functional dermal melanocytes which have failed to migrate fully to the skin during development. Lesions present as brown-blue-grey macules. Mongolian blue spots are very common in oriental babies and usually affect the lumbosacral area (**216**). They usually fade in early childhood. In naevus of Ota, the hyperpigmentation affect the upper face (**217**) and naevus of Ito affects the upper neck and back. These naevi tend to persist throughout life.

DIFFERENTIAL DIAGNOSIS

Mongolian blue spots may be misdiagnosed as bruises.

INVESTIGATIONS

None required.

TREATMENT

Laser treatment, e.g. with Q-switched ruby laser, may help reduce facial hyperpigmentation.

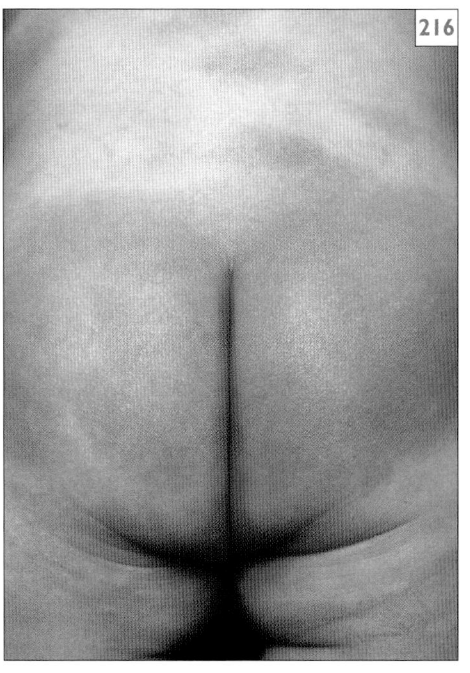

216 Mongolian blue spots.

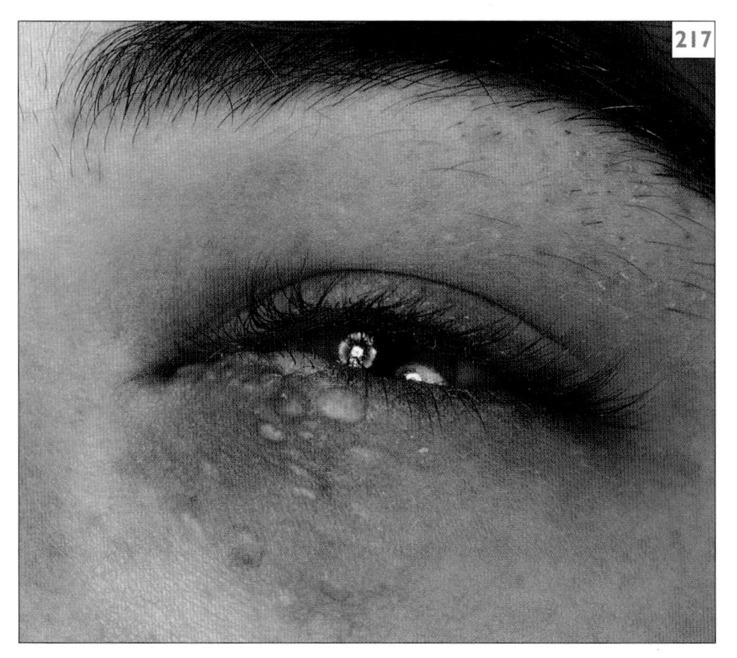

217 Naevus of Ota.

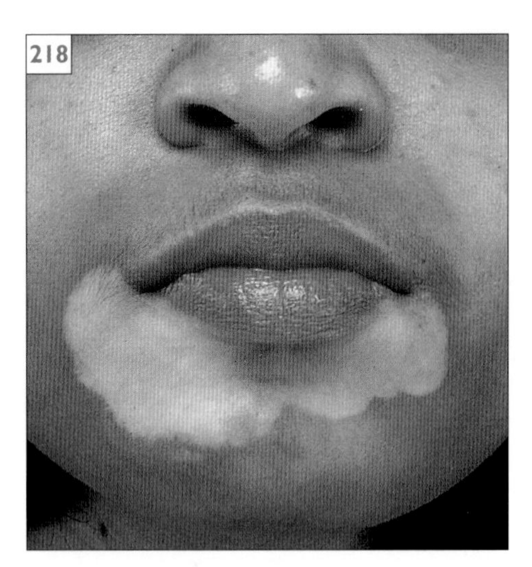

218 Perioral vitiligo.

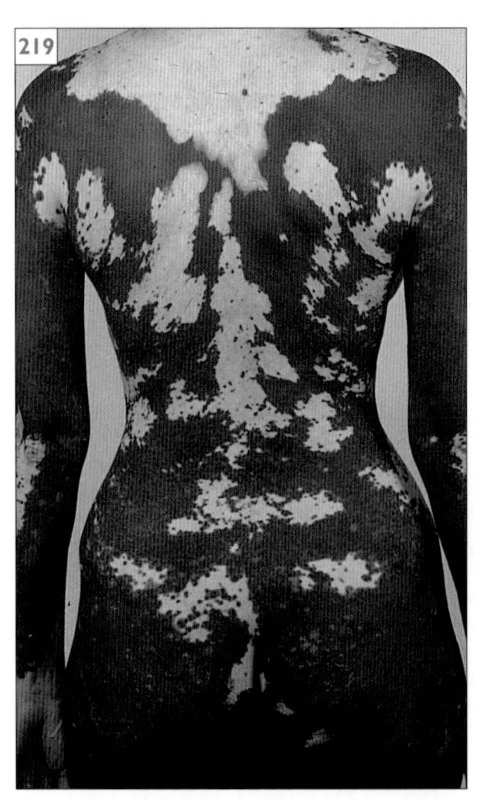

219 Vitiligo.

Hypomelanosis

Vitiligo

DEFINITION AND CLINICAL FEATURES

Vitiligo is an acquired, idiopathic, progressive whitening of the skin and hair characterized by the total absence of melanocytes in affected skin. It is common, with an incidence of about 1% of the population, and is thought to have an autoimmune basis.

Vitiligo usually presents with discrete, well-circumscribed, chalk-white macules on the extensor surfaces and in periorificial areas, which are typically symmetrical (**218**). Spontaneous remission can occur but is not usual. Progression can lead to widespread depigmentation and a cosmetically debilitating condition, especially in darker-skinned persons (**219**). Patients with vitiligo have an increased risk of developing other autoimmune diseases, including thyroid disease, diabetes mellitus, pernicious anaemia, and Addison's disease.

DIFFERENTIAL DIAGNOSIS

Chemically induced leukoderma, which is usually occupational, may become clinically indistinguishable from idiopathic vitiligo, so an occupational history should always be taken. Piebaldism is present at birth.

INVESTIGATIONS

Consider screening for other autoimmune diseases with fasting glucose, thyroid autoantibodies and TSH, antinuclear antibodies.

TREATMENT

There is no curative therapy. Cosmetic camouflage can safely and effectively conceal affected areas. Sunscreens should be used on depigmented areas in sunny climates. Potent topical corticosteroids or topical tacrolimus may encourage repigmentation of localized areas. For more widespread disease, topical or systemic psoralen-UVA (PUVA) therapy can be used. Repigmentation may take many months to achieve and is often incomplete. Other treatments include the 308 nm excimer laser and skin grafting.

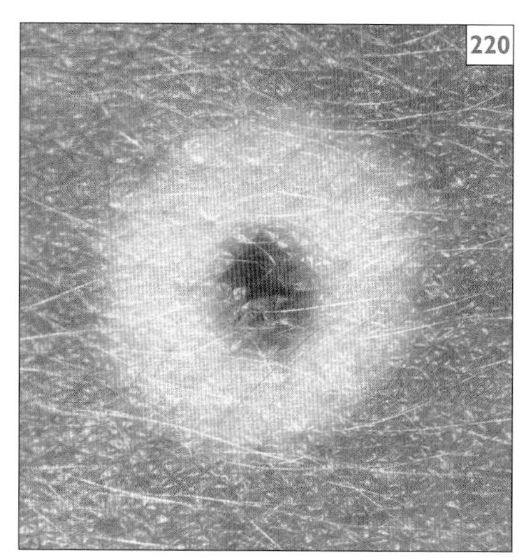

220 Halo naevus.

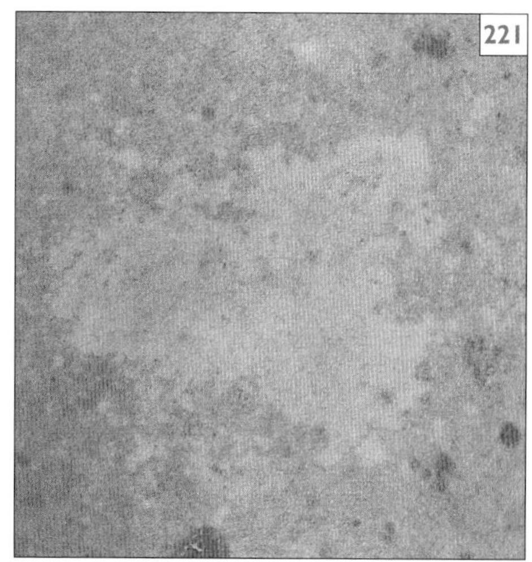

221 Naevus depigmentosus.

Halo naevus

DEFINITION AND CLINICAL FEATURES

An acquired halo of depigmentation around a melanocytic or neuronal naevus. Most halo naevi are benign melanocytic naevi (**220**), but this phenomenon may also occur around malignant melanomas and neurofibromas. Lesions are commonest on the trunk and may be multiple. The naevus tends to flatten and may disappear completely. The phenomenon is common in children and young adults and is associated with vitiligo and other autoimmune diseases.

DIFFERENTIAL DIAGNOSIS

Eczema and postinflammatory hypopigmentation around naevi, malignant melanoma.

INVESTIGATIONS

Excision biopsy if diagnostic doubt.

TREATMENT

None usually necessary.

Naevus depigmentosus

DEFINITION AND CLINICAL FEATURES

A circumscribed area of depigmentation also known as hypochromic naevus presenting at birth. The naevus may be unilateral, circular, or rectangular in shape and is most commonly found on the trunk (**221**). Microscopy of the skin reveals normal numbers of melanocytes, with sometimes rather stubby dendrites, containing autophagosomes with aggregates of melanosomes.

DIFFERENTIAL DIAGNOSIS

Ash leaf macules of tuberose sclerosis.

INVESTIGATIONS

None necessary.

TREATMENT

None necessary.

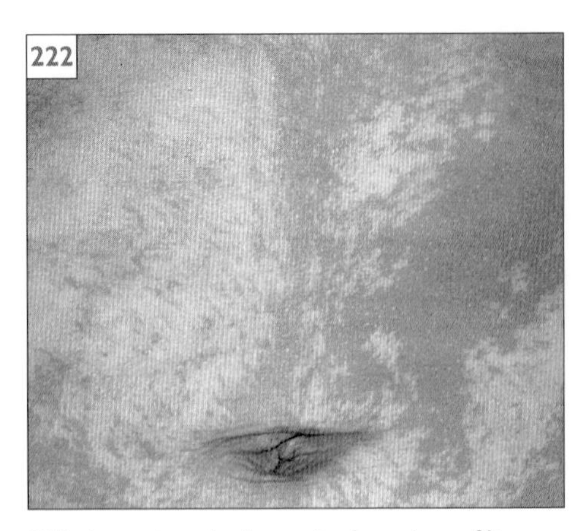

222 Incontinentia pigmenti achromians of Ito.

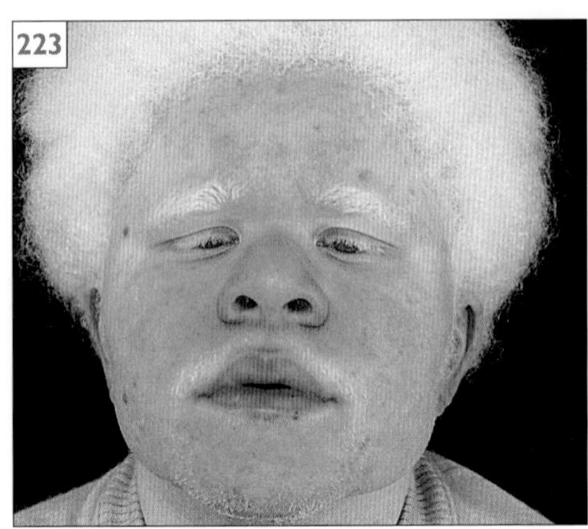

223 Oculocutaneous albinism.

Incontinentia pigmenti achromians of Ito

DEFINITION AND CLINICAL FEATURES

This is a distinct neurocutaneous syndrome where hypomelanosis is associated with neurological and muskuloskeletal abnormalities. Skin changes are usually present at birth, with symmetrical, bizarre whorls and streaks of hypomelanosis (**222**) on the trunk, extremities, or face. Associated ectodermal and CNS abnormalities include seizures, mental retardation, hypertelorism, scoliosis, strabismus, and myopia. Females are more commonly affected than males and familial cases have been reported.

DIFFERENTIAL DIAGNOSIS

Naevus depigmentosus, focal dermal hypoplasia, late stage incontinentia pigmenti.

INVESTIGATIONS

Histology to exclude other disorders as above.

TREATMENT

None available, but affected families should be offered genetic counselling.

Oculocutaneous albinism (OCA)

DEFINITION AND CLINICAL FEATURES

A heterogeneous group of inherited disorders characterized by a partial or complete failure to produce melanin in the skin and eyes. In tyrosinase-negative albinism the skin is pink, the hair is white, and the iris translucent resulting in a prominent red reflex. Most patients have horizontal or rotatory nystagmus and photophobia. The commoner tyrosinase-positive OCA has marked but incomplete dilution of pigment of the skin, hair, and eyes and, with increasing age, some pigment formation and the development of flaxen-yellow hair. In Afro-Caribbeans, the skin is a yellowish-brown colour that with age develops dark-brown freckles, resembling PUVA lentigines, in sun-exposed areas (**223**). In temperate climates, the visual defects cause the greatest disability. In hot climates, sun-damaged skin and early development of skin cancers is the main problem.

DIFFERENTIAL DIAGNOSIS

Other very rare genetic disorders associated with albinism, e.g. Chediak–Higashi syndrome.

INVESTIGATION

None usually necessary.

TREATMENT

Strict sun protection and regular examinations of the skin for premalignant and malignant lesions.

Piebaldism

DEFINITION AND CLINICAL FEATURES

Piebaldism is a rare autosomal dominant condition characterized by stable vitiligo-like areas of skin which are present at birth and associated with a white forelock (**224**). The distribution is characteristic with frontal or paramedian patches and asymmetrical involvement of the upper chest, abdomen, and limbs, sparing the hands, feet, and back. Islands of normal or hypermelanotic skin occur within the white areas (**225**).

DIFFERENTIAL DIAGNOSIS

Waardenburg's syndrome where the interpupillary distance is increased and 20% of patients are deaf, naevus depigmentosus.

INVESTIGATIONS

The absence of melanocytes and melanosomes on microscopy differentiates piebaldism from naevus depigmentosus.

TREATMENT

Cosmetic camouflage and photoprotection.

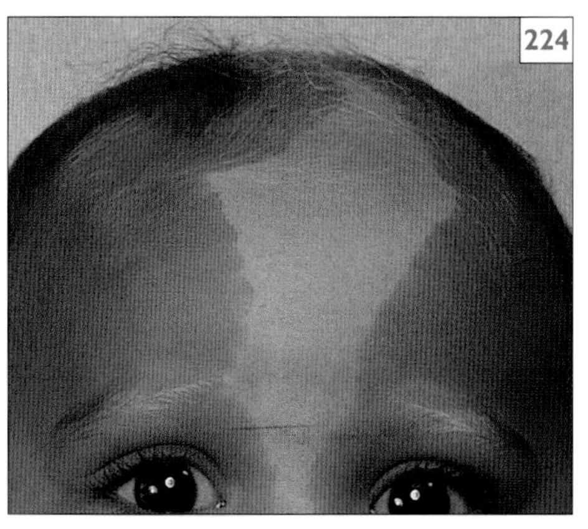

224 Piebaldism.

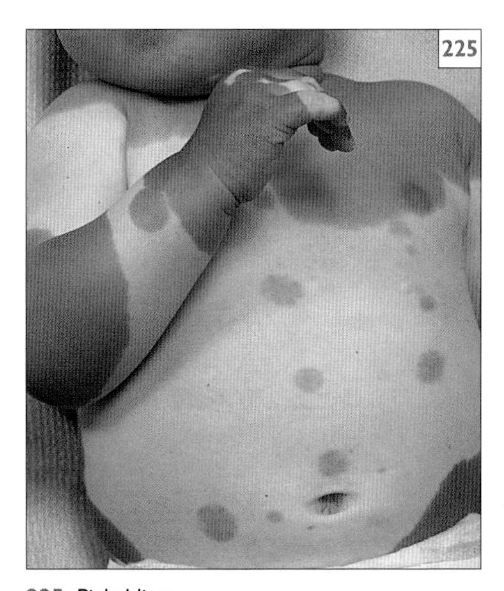

225 Piebaldism.

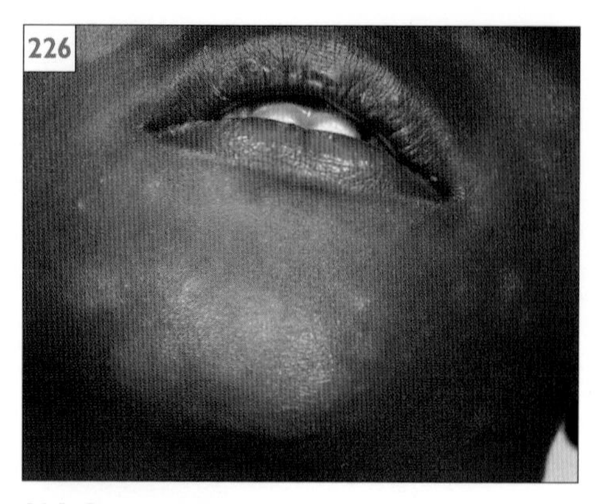

226 Pityriasis alba.

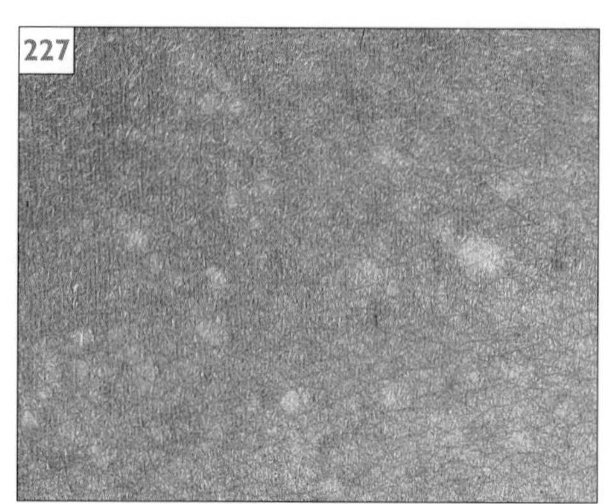

227 Idiopathic guttate hypomelanosis.

Pityriasis alba

DEFINITION AND CLINICAL FEATURES

Pityriasis alba is a common, acquired hypomelanosis characterized by poorly circumscribed, fine, scaly macules on the face of children (**226**). There may be mild inflammation. It is thought to represent a low-grade form of eczema. It may also occur on the limbs and is more noticeable in dark skinned races. There is a slow improvement and most cases resolve by puberty.

DIFFERENTIAL DIAGNOSIS

Vitiligo, tinea, hypopigmented mycosis fungoides.

INVESTIGATIONS

None usually necessary. Skin scrapings to exclude tinea. Biopsy if diagnostic doubt.

TREATMENT

Bland emollients and mild potency topical corticosteroids or topical calcineurin inhibitors (tacrolimus/pimecrolimus).

Idiopathic guttate hypomelanosis

DEFINITION AND CLINICAL FEATURES

A common condition of acquired hypomelanosis presenting as small, sharply defined, white macules. These range from 2–6 mm in diameter with sharply defined, angular, or irregular borders (**227**). In Caucasian skin they typically occur on sun-exposed areas of the limbs. Sun damage is thought to be an important factor. Non-actinic lesions are seen in Afro-Caribbeans and may be found in unexposed areas on the trunk.

DIFFERENTIAL DIAGNOSIS

Vitiligo.

INVESTIGATIONS

Histology shows a decrease in pigment granules and a reduction in the number of melanocytes.

TREATMENT

None necessary. Fair skinned individuals should use sun protection as this is usually a sign of chronic sun damage.

MISCELLANEOUS

Other important causes of hypopigmented skin lesions such as leprosy and sarcoidosis and pityriasis versicolor are found elsewhere in this book.

Non-melanin pigmentation

DEFINITION AND CLINICAL FEATURES

Alteration in skin colour due to excess or abnormal forms of normal body constituents or exogenous substances such as metals (see below). Jaundice is a common yellow discolouration of the skin and sclera caused by staining of the skin with bilirubin when circulating levels are raised. Yellow pigmentation also occurs in carotenaemia, due to excessive carotene levels (p.116), and with mepacrine therapy.

INVESTIGATIONS

Histology with special stains and spectroscopy may help identify the nature of non-melanin pigment. Metal deposits can be demonstrated by histology with dark field illumination and electron microscopy.

TREATMENT

Withdrawl of the offending exogenous agent. However, pigmentation may be permanent.

Haemosiderosis

Haemosiderosis is caused by deposition of the iron-containing pigment haemosiderin within the skin. This commonly results from the local destruction of red blood cells, but also occurs in haemochromatosis (bronze diabetes). Haemosiderin deposition stimulates melanogenesis, so that varying degrees of hypermelanosis are usually associated. It is seen most commonly on the lower legs in venous hypertension (hypostatic haemosiderosis); involved areas initially show grouped specks of orange-red pigment (**228**) but, with increasing hypermelanosis, later produce a more uniform deep-brown pigmentation that persists even if the venous hypertension is corrected. In capillaritis (e.g. Schamberg's disease) (p. 141) , cayenne pepper-like haemosiderosis without detectable hypermelanosis is seen especially on the lower legs and thighs (**229**).

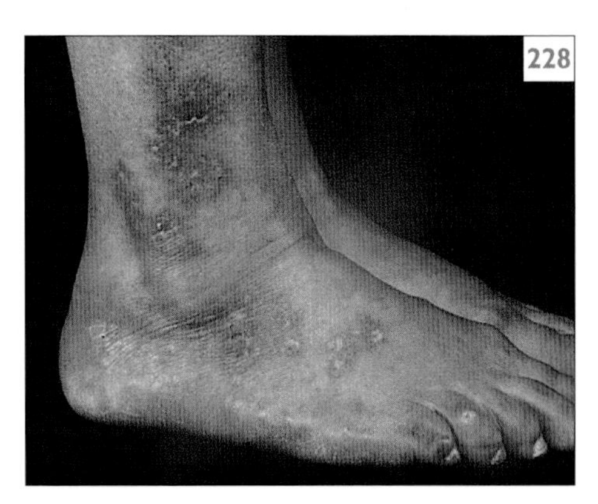

228 Hypostatic haemosiderosis.

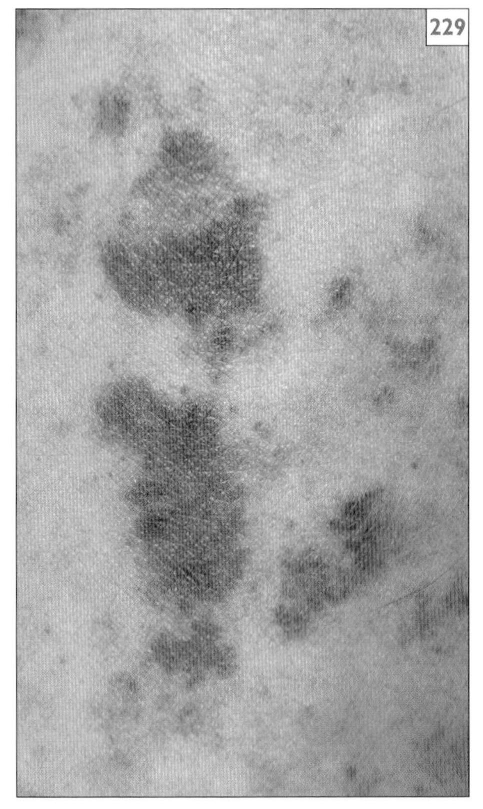

229 Capillaritis.

Carotenaemia

Carotenaemia is a yellow discolouration of the skin and palate due to excessive blood carotene levels. This yellow discolouration is most marked in areas of hyperkeratosis, especially the palms and the soles (**230**), or where subcutaneous fat is plentiful. It is seen in patients taking *β*-carotene or in food faddists who eat excessive amounts of carotene-containing foods such as carrots or oranges. Diagnosis is confirmed by measuring blood carotene levels. Rarely, carotenaemia is due to an inborn error of metabolism. It may be associated with hyperlipidaemia, diabetes, nephritis, or hypothyroidism.

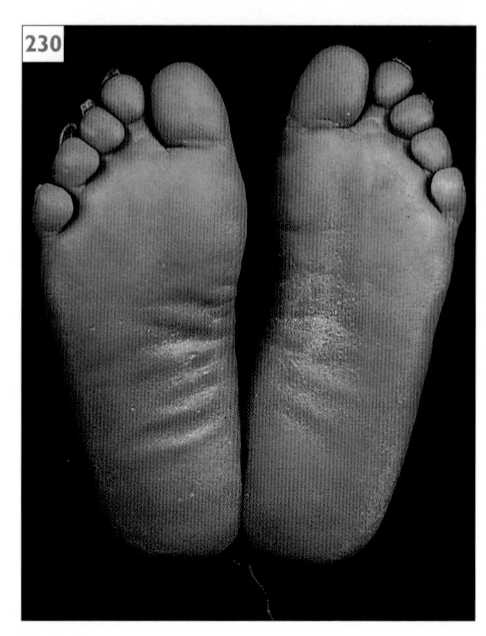

230 Carotenaemia.

Ochronosis

Ochronosis is the deposition of a melanin-like, brownish-black pigment derived from polymerized homogentisic acid. Exogenous ochronosis usually arises due to the long-term application of hydroquinone-containing skin-lightening creams. A dusky, cutaneous pigmentation is usually most marked over the cheeks and forehead. Ochronosis may also occur due to an inborn error of metabolism (alkaptonuria) with widespread pigmentation of the connective tissue, ear cartilages, and eyes.

Argyria

Argyria is the deposition of silver within the skin, either from industrial exposure or from medication. A slate blue-grey pigmentation slowly accumulates over many years until clinically apparent, especially in sun-exposed areas of skin. Sclerae, nails, and mucous membranes may also become pigmented, the pigmentation being permanent.

Lead poisoning may result in a blue-black line at the gingival margin with grey discolouration of the skin.

Chrysiasis

Chrysiasis is a permanent pigmentation of the skin due to parenteral treatment with gold salts.

Drug-induced pigmentation

DEFINITION AND CLINICAL FEATURES

A drug-induced alteration in skin colour resulting from a number of mechanisms, including increased melanin synthesis, postinflammatory hyper-pigmentation (see fixed drug eruption, p.170), and cutaneous deposition of drug-related material. Withdrawal or a reduction in the dose of the offending drug is usually appropriate unless other alternatives are not available.

The clinical picture varies according to the drug in question. The oral contraceptive pill, for instance, may induce melasma. Long-term antimalarial therapy may result in brown or blue-black pigmentation on the shin, face, and hard palate. Amiodarone or long-term high-dose chlorpromazine can both cause a blue-grey pigmentation of sun-exposed areas (**231**). Minocycline-induced pigmentation is not uncommon following prolonged high-dose courses and may present as a diffuse or generalized hyperpigmentation or as a blue-black pigment at sites of previous inflammation such as acne scars (**232**). Skin biopsy shows brown-black granules in the upper dermis that stain for iron.

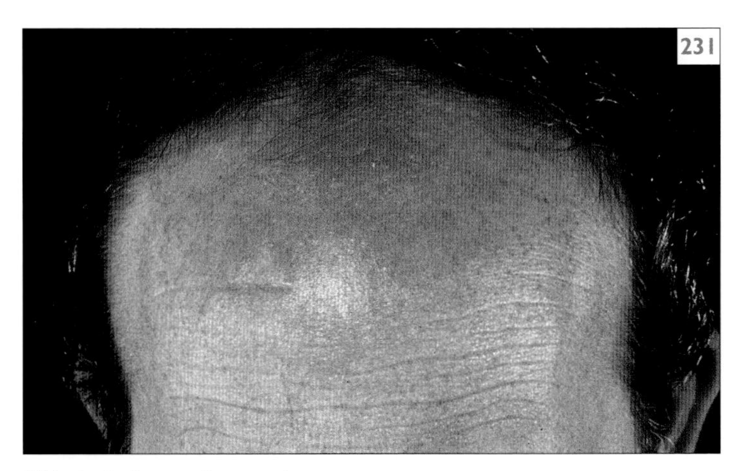

231 Amiodarone pigmentation.

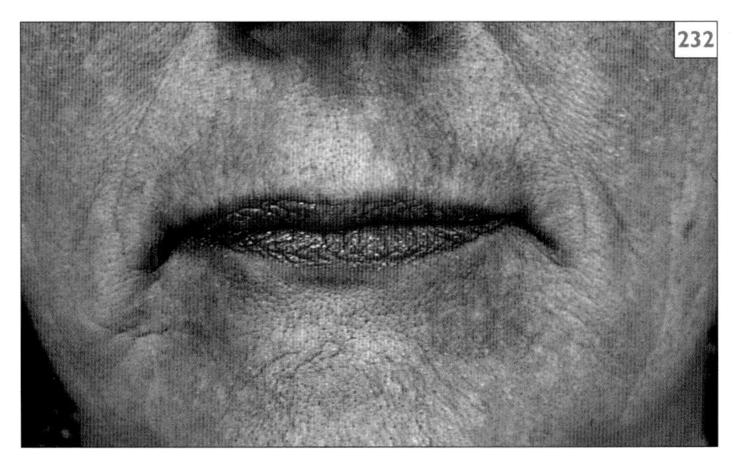

232 Minocycline-induced pigmentation.

PHOTOSENSITIVITY DISORDERS

Ultraviolet irradiation (UVR) has early and late effects on the skin. Early effects include inflammation (sunburn), tanning, hyperplasia, vitamin D synthesis, and down-regulated skin immunity. Late effects include photoageing and photocarcinogenesis.

The erythema, pain, heat, swelling and, in severe cases, blistering of sunburn develops over hours (maximal effects 24–72 hours) and settles over days (**233**). Photoageing effects include wrinkling, dryness, coarseness, laxity, loss of tensile strength, telangiectasia (**234**), mottled pigmentation and comedones (**235**). Histologically, changes of solar elastosis are seen. Colloid milium is a degenerative change with yellowish, translucent papules on light-exposed skin (**236**).

Acquired idiopathic photodermatoses

Acquired idiopathic photodermatoses include polymorphic light eruption (the commonest of all photodermatoses), actinic prurigo, chronic actinic dermatitis, and solar urticaria. They all appear to be immunologically mediated. The history and examination are distinctive in each case.

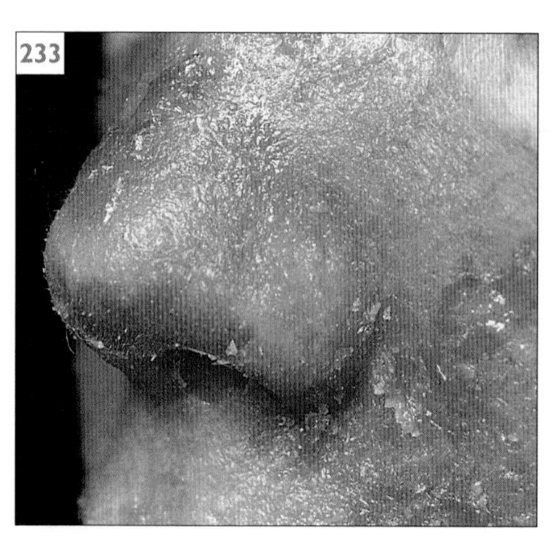

233 Sunburn.

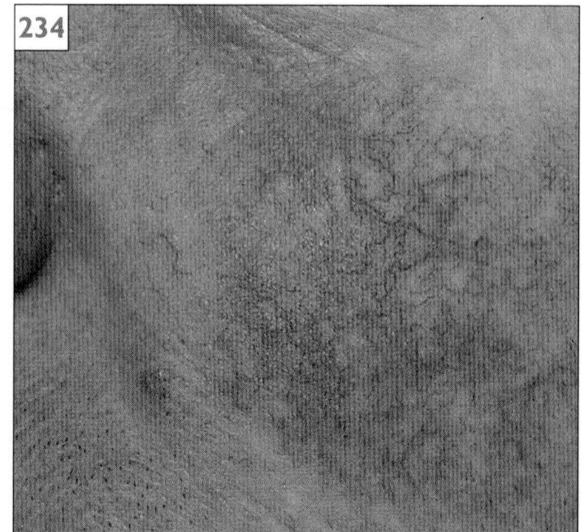

234 Telangiectasia.

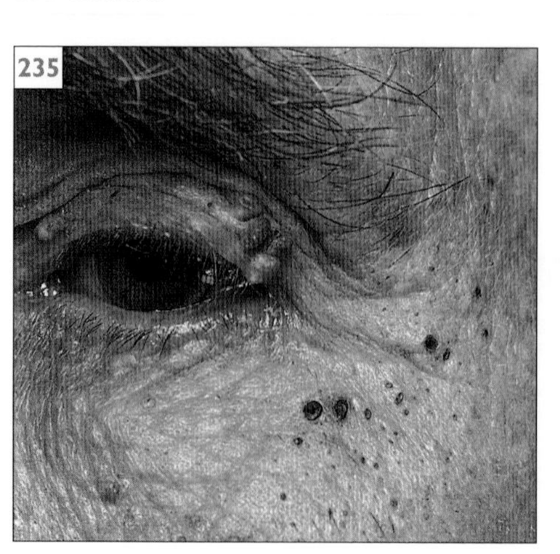

235 Comedones.

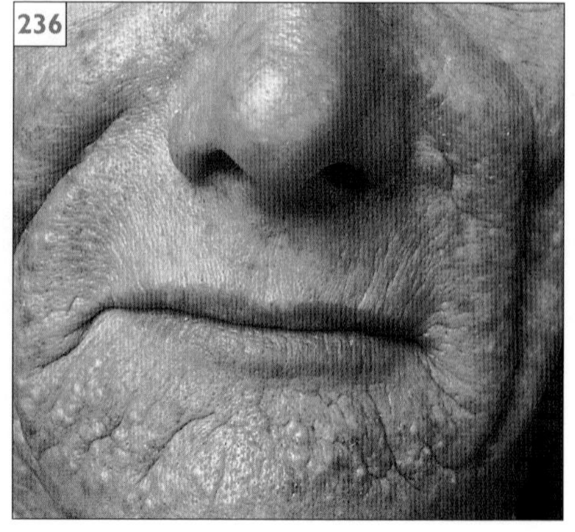

236 Colloid milium.

Polymorphic light eruption (PLE)

DEFINITION AND CLINICAL FEATURES

This is a common intermittent skin reaction to UV exposure, which may represent a delayed-type hypersensitivity response to UV-induced cutaneous antigens. It affects up to 20% of the population in temperate areas, particularly women under 30 years of age. PLE presents with an itchy, non-scarring, symmetrical papular rash on light-exposed sites (**237**) within hours or days of significant sun exposure. Large and small papules, papulopustules, and vesicles can occur, sometimes coalescing into oedematous plaques. The eruption is transient, and resolves within several days, but it may persist if exposure continues. Chronically exposed sites such as the face are often spared. The eruption is usually restricted to the spring and early summer and often improves (i.e. tolerance develops) as the summer progresses. Juvenile spring eruption is probably a variant of PLE and typically presents as itchy blisters on the light-exposed helices of young boys following sun exposure (**238**). Tolerance to UV exposure usually develops, so the complaint is commonest in the spring months.

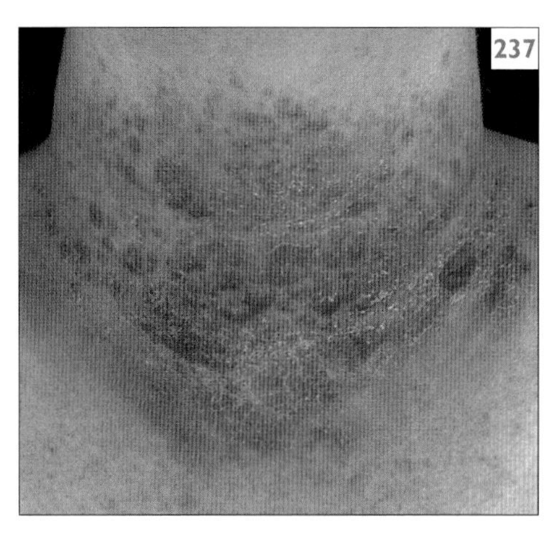

237 Polymorphic light eruption.

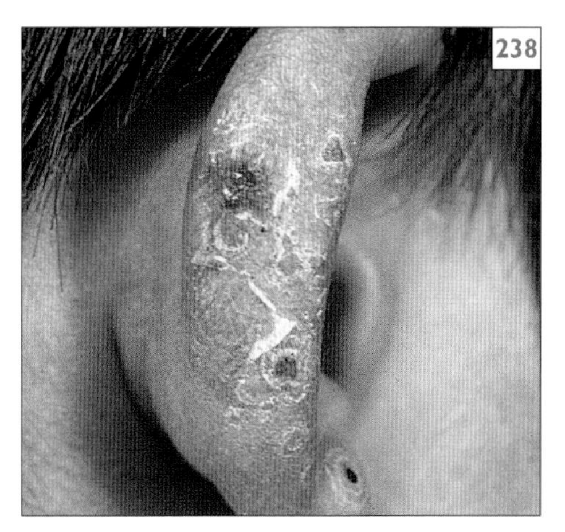

238 Juvenile spring eruption.

DIFFERENTIAL DIAGNOSIS

The history and clinical features of PLE will usually distinguish it from other photodermatoses. Photoallergic contact dermatitis may be difficult to exclude where there is a history of sunscreen use, and patch/photopatch testing considered. Cutaneous lupus should be considered, and a minority of patients with PLE may subsequently develop lupus after several years.

INVESTIGATIONS

Circulating antinuclear antibodies and extractable nuclear antibodies should be measured to exclude cutaneous lupus. Lesional histology may support the diagnosis. If diagnostic uncertainty persists, phototesting with monochromator irradiation or a solar simulator can be performed.

SPECIAL POINTS

PLE is often provoked by longer wavelength UVA, or UVA and UVB, and so may be induced through window glass (e.g. when driving) or through thin clothing.

TREATMENT

Most patients can control their rash by sensible sun exposure and regular applications of highly protective combined UVA/UVB sunscreens. More severely affected patients may need prophylactic treatment with UVB or PUVA therapy. For treatment of an acute attack, potent topical corticosteroids or a short course of oral corticosteroids is usually effective.

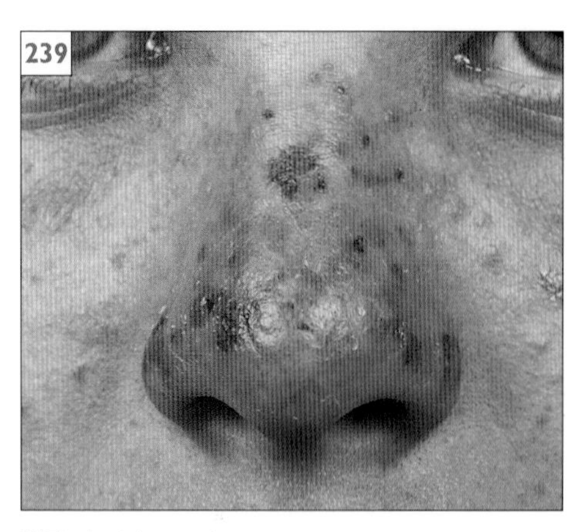

239 Actinic prurigo.

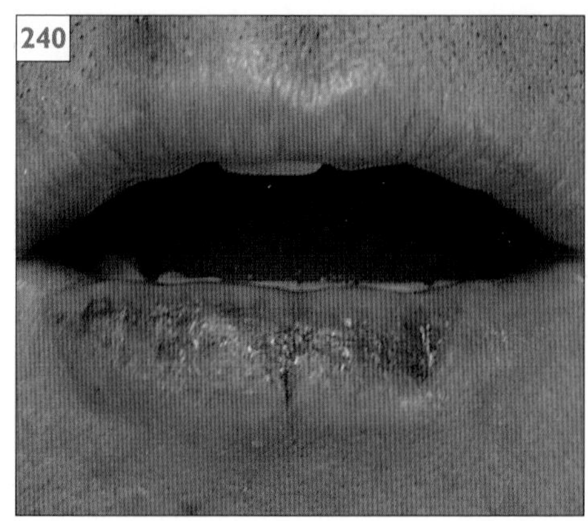

240 Associated cheilitis.

Actinic prurigo

DEFINITION AND CLINICAL FEATURES

Also known as Hutchinson's summer prurigo, this rare and chronic photodermatosis is likely to have an immunological basis. Actinic prurigo (AP) is sometimes regarded as a persistent variant of PLE, but its clinical features are quite distinct. Actinic prurigo is extremely itchy and lesions are therefore excoriated. It affects light-exposed and, to a lesser extent, non-exposed sites (**239**). The rash consists of excoriated nodules and papules, which may be crusted if secondarily infected. Unlike PLE, the eruption usually starts in childhood and may improve following puberty. Lesions persist into winter, often failing to clear completely and, when severe, the eruption often extends to involve the covered skin of the limbs and buttocks. Characteristically all light-exposed sites are affected, the lesions leaving pitted scars on resolution. Cheilitis (**240**) and conjunctivitis are recognized associations. AP is more common in females and has an association with HLA DR4 in Caucasoid populations. It has different HLA associations in the American Indians where it is a relatively common and frequently severe dermatosis.

INVESTIGATIONS

Two-thirds of patients are abnormally sensitive to monochromatic irradiation, most commonly within the UVA wavelengths.

TREATMENT

Appropriate clothing and UVA protective sunscreens should be used. Intermittent courses of low-dose thalidomide are effective in severe cases. PUVA or UVB phototherapy may be helpful (as for PLE).

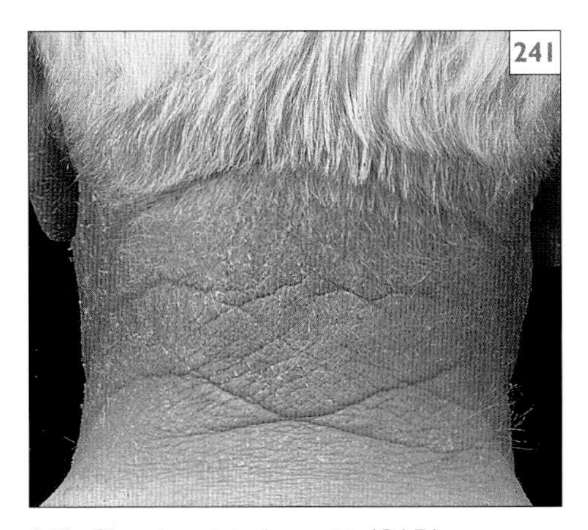

241 Chronic actinic dermatitis (CAD).

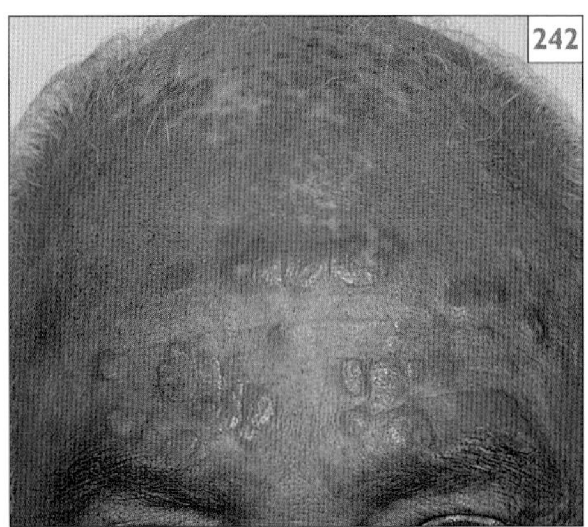

242 Severe CAD mimicking lymphomatous infiltration.

Chronic actinic dermatitis

DEFINITION AND CLINICAL FEATURES

Chronic actinic dermatitis (CAD), also known as photosensitivity dermatitis (PD) or actinic reticuloid syndrome (AR), is a disabling eczematous photodermatosis mostly affecting light-exposed sites. It is probably immunologically based, possibly a delayed-type hypersensitivity reaction to an UV-induced neoantigen. Older men are most commonly affected with persistent eczematous papules and plaques on photo-exposed sites (**241**). CAD may, when severe, mimic lymphomatous infiltration both clinically (**242**) and histologically. Some patients have had a preceding photoallergic or airborne contact dermatitis, others a history of endogenous eczema. CAD is worse in summer and after sun exposure but patients may fail to recognize this, particularly if affected all year round. Any skin type may be affected although it is seen most commonly in fair-skinned individuals with an occupational or recreational history of many years of outdoor existence.

DIFFERENTIAL DIAGNOSIS AND INVESTIGATIONS

Photosensitive eczema and photoallergic contact dermatitis may present similarly and, indeed, may co-exist. Patch and photopatch tests will establish any associated contact sensitivities.

INVESTIGATIONS

Abnormal phototesting results in CAD characteristically show a low erythemal threshold to UVB, often to UVA and, occasionally, also to visible irradiation.

TREATMENT

Rigorous avoidance of UV and other known allergens and regular use of high protection factor sunscreens is important but is rarely sufficient. Topical or intermittent oral corticosteroids are often needed, and for recalcitrant disease intermittent courses of azathioprine or ciclosporin may be required. Topical tacrolimus may be helpful.

Solar urticaria

DEFINITION AND CLINICAL FEATURES

Solar urticaria (SU) is an uncommon photodermatosis and form of physical urticaria in which sun exposure leads to wheals on exposed skin. SU appears to be an immediate (Type I) hypersensitivity response involving a circulating photoallergen, which is generated on absorption of UV radiation or visible light by a precursor. Within 5–10 minutes of exposure to sunlight, patients develop an itching or burning sensation that is rapidly followed by erythema and patchy or confluent whealing (**243**). With sun avoidance the rash resolves completely within 12 hours (unlike PLE). If severe, there may be accompanying systemic symptoms or even syncope. When severe this is an extremely incapacitating condition.

DIFFERENTIAL DIAGNOSIS

The history of an immediate reaction resolving rapidly should distinguish SU from PLE. Artificial irradiation testing may be able to induce typical lesions and demonstrate the wavelengths responsible.

INVESTIGATIONS

Phototesting should confirm the diagnosis with immediate whealing using monochromator or broad band UV sources.

TREATMENT

Sunscreens are seldom sufficient. Non-sedative antihistamines in high doses may give reasonable protection. Regular exposure to the inducing wavelengths occasionally helps, and PUVA, given with fractionated doses under specialist supervision, may provide useful remissions.

Hydroa vacciniforme

DEFINITION AND CLINICAL FEATURES

Hydroa vacciniforme (HV) is an exceedingly rare photodermatosis usually confined to childhood. HV is characterized by recurrent crops of vesicles on sun-exposed skin with subsequent vacciniform scarring. The aetiology is unknown.

Within hours of sun exposure, clusters of 2–3 mm erythematous macules appear on light-exposed sites, especially the face and the backs of the hands, often associated with a severe burning sensation. These rapidly progress to papules and then vesicles which umbilicate over a day or so; they then dry, form a crust (**244**) and heal into pitted, varioliform scars (**245**). Occasionally there are associated systemic features such as headache, fever, or malaise. Remission often occurs during adolescence. The diagnosis is made clinically. Repetitive broad spectrum UVA and UVB will often induce typical lesions.

TREATMENT

Broad spectrum sunscreens with UVA protection should be prescribed.

Phytophotodermatitis

DEFINITION AND CLINICAL FEATURES

This is a distinctive linear blistering eruption on exposed sites caused by skin contact with the sap of psoralen (furocoumarin)-containing plants and exposure to sunlight. Plants of the Umbelliferae and Rutaceae families are common culprits. It represents a phototoxic reaction. Painful erythema and blistering occur 24 hour or later after exposure and are often followed by long-lasting post-inflammatory hyperpigmentation (**246**).

DIFFERENTIAL DIAGNOSIS

Allergic contact dermatitis from plants predominantly affects the hands and fingertips, although other exposed sites including the face may be involved from airborne exposure.

INVESTIGATIONS

The history and clinical features are characteristic. If contact with a known phototoxic plant can be confirmed, patch tests are not necessary. The causative plant should be identified so that further inadvertent contact can be avoided.

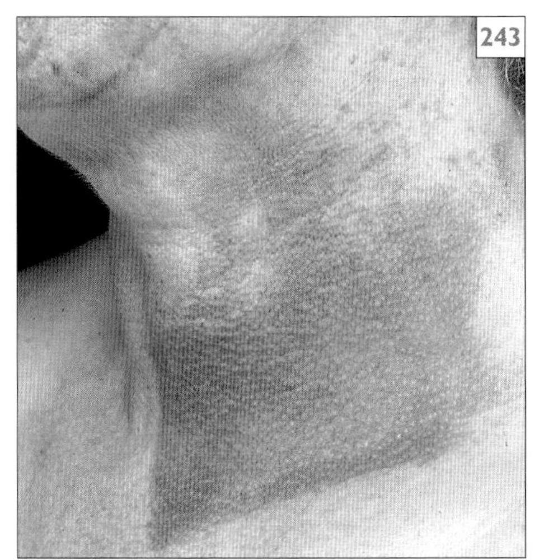

243 Solar urticaria.

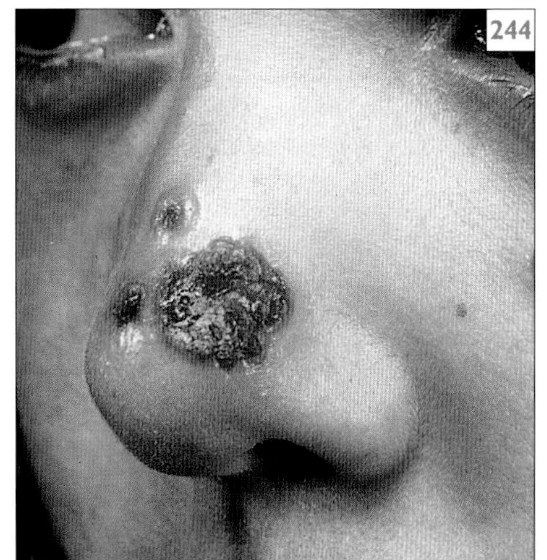

244 Hydroa vacciniforme.

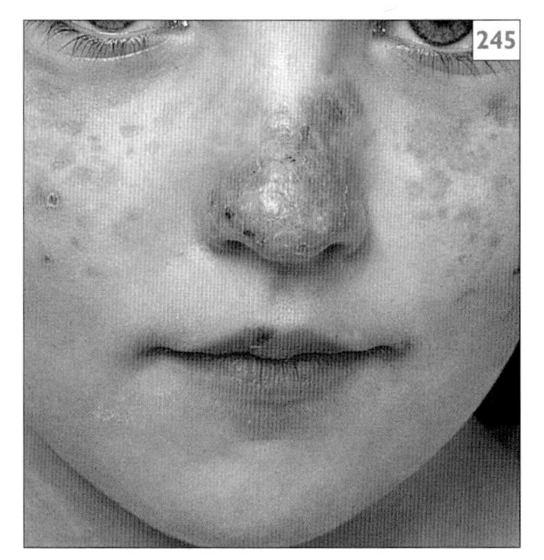

245 Varioliform scars.

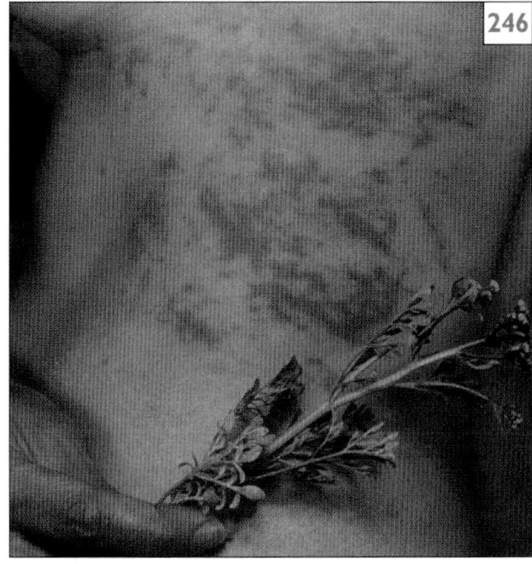

246 Phytophotodermatitis.

Genetic and metabolic photodermatoses

Cutaneous porphyrias

The cutaneous porphyrias are disorders of haem synthesis in which excessive formation of porphyrins, secondary to partial enzyme deficiencies, produce photosensitization. There are five main types. For the clinician, the important distinction is between those that can cause acute attacks and those that only cause skin disease.

Cutaneous disease only:
- Porphyria cutanea tarda (PCT).
- Erythropoietic protoporphyria (EPP).
- Congenital erythropoietic protoporphyria (CEP).

Cutaneous disease and acute attacks:
- Variegate porphyria.
- Hereditary coproporphyria.

All the cutaneous porphyrias except EPP present with fragility and blistering on light exposed skin, and biochemical analysis is necessary to differentiate reliably between them.

Porphyria cutanea tarda

DEFINITION AND CLINICAL FEATURES

Porphyria cutanea tarda (PCT) is the commonest porphyria, presenting with blisters and skin fragility of light-exposed sites. It is due to uroporphyrinogen decarboxylase deficiency and has a complex inheritance, with iron-dependent inactivation of the enzyme contributing to one of four different types of familial predisposition. The onset of symptoms requires interaction between several acquired and inherited factors, so clinical manifestations of PCT usually only occur in association with other disorders such as alcoholic liver disease or oestrogen ingestion. Hepatic siderosis, associated with high alcohol intake, may progressively inactivate hepatic uroporphyrinogen decarboxylase activity to a level where cutaneous disease develops.

The only consistent feature of PCT are lesions on exposed skin. These include hypertrichosis (**247**), pigmentation, erosions and subepidermal bullae (**248**). Fragility is common on the dorsal hands and blisters tend to heal with scarring and milia. Acute photosensitivity is uncommon.

DIFFERENTIAL DIAGNOSIS

Other porphyrias, especially variegate porphyria, need to be excluded by porphyrin analysis. Skin fragility, blistering, and milia also occur in the rare immunobullous disease, epidermolysis bullosa acquisita, but these changes are not restricted to sun-exposed sites and porphyrin levels are normal. Porphyrin levels are also normal in pseudoporphyria, which may be induced by a range of drugs especially NSAIDS.

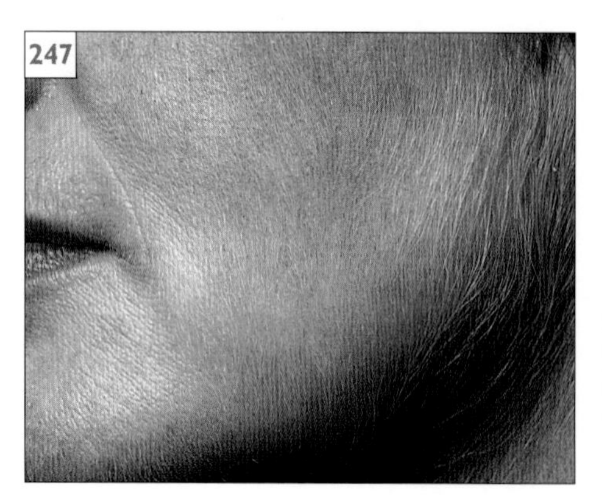

247 Hypertrichosis in porphyria cutanea tarda.

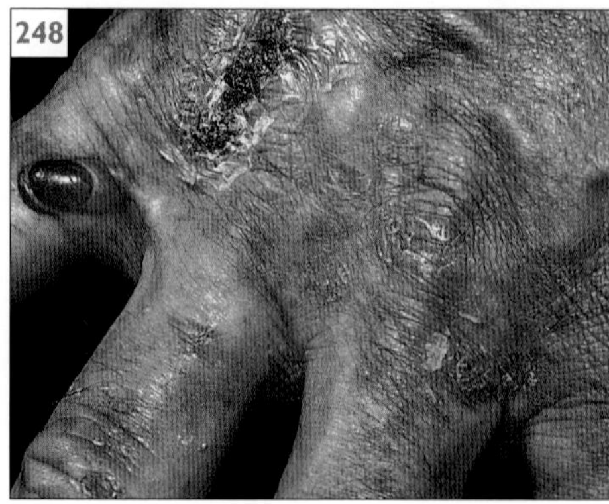

248 Subepidermal bullae.

INVESTIGATIONS

Diagnosis of PCT is confirmed by finding elevated levels of predominantly Type I uro- and coproporphyrin isomers in the urine and stools. Screen for haemochromatosis and viral hepatitis.

TREATMENT

Apart from avoidance of alcohol and oestrogens, PCT will generally respond to either depletion of body iron stores by venesection or low-dose hydroxychloroquine.

Erythropoietic protoporphyria

DEFINITION AND CLINICAL FEATURES

Erythropoietic protoporphyria (EPP) is a rare photosensitizing porphyria resulting from the accumulation of protoporphyrin secondary to decreased ferrochetalase activity. Patients present with acute photosensitivity starting in early childhood. An intense pricking, itching, burning sensation usually occurs within 5–30 minutes of sun exposure, although occasionally this is delayed for several hours. The patient experiences burning pain often with no visible signs although severe attacks produce erythema, oedema and occasionally later crusting, petechiae, or small vesicles (**249**). Acute photo-onycholysis may occur and after repeated attacks the skin characteristically becomes thickened, waxy, and pitted with small circular or linear scars, especially on the nose, around the mouth, and over the knuckles (**250**). Liver damage from accumulated protoporphyrin crystals in hepatocytes commonly gives abnormal liver biochemistry. Progressive hepatic failure and porphyrin gallstones are rare.

INVESTIGATIONS

Diagnosis of EPP is established by demonstrating increased free protoporphyrin in erythrocytes. It may be necessary to distinguish this from increased zinc protoporphyrin found in iron deficiency, lead poisoning, and some anaemias, which may coexist fortuitously with photosensitivity.

TREATMENT

Sunlight avoidance is the only effective treatment. High factor UVA-protecting sunscreens and oral *β*-carotene help marginally.

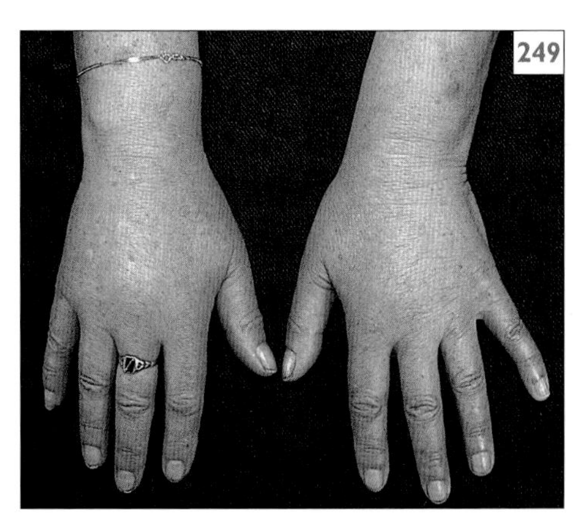

249 Erythropoietic protoporphyria (EPP).

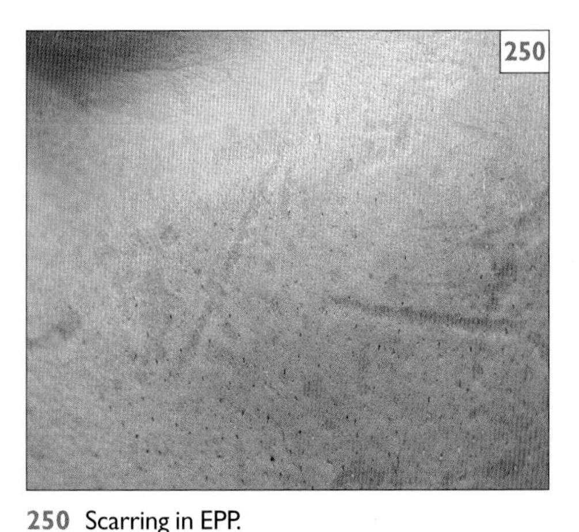

250 Scarring in EPP.

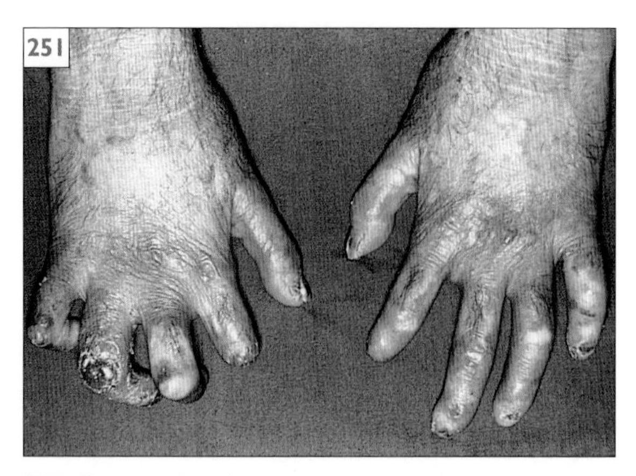

251 Congenital erythropoietic protoporphyria.

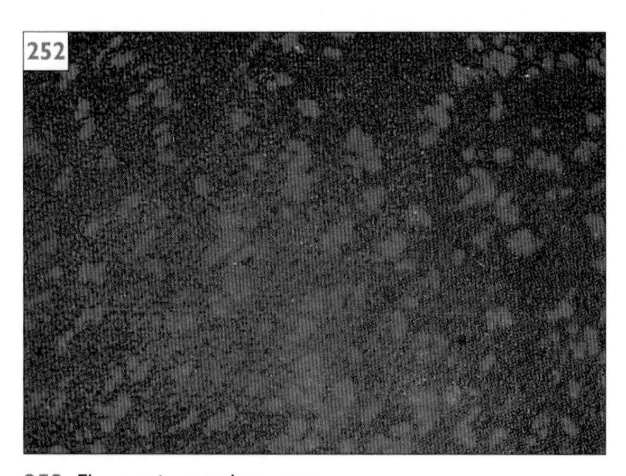

252 Fluorescing erythrocytes.

Congenital erythropoietic protoporphyria

DEFINITION AND CLINICAL FEATURES

Congenital erythropoietic protoporphyria (CED), also known as Gunther's disease, is a rare autosomal recessive disorder with severe photosensitivity, scarring, and deformity resulting from uroporphyrinogen III synthase deficiency and consequent accumulation of Type I uro- and coproporphyrin isomers in the blood and tissues. Classic CEP presents in early childhood with acute painful erythema, swelling, and blistering after sunlight exposure. Severe photosensitivity leads to extensive scarring and photomutilation (**251**). The urine is pink from the excessive amounts of porphyrin, and the teeth stain brown and show red fluorescence (erythrodontia). Erythrocytes also fluoresce (**252**) and haemolytic anaemia with splenomegaly is common, probably caused by photodamage of porphyrin-laden erythrocytes. Chronic changes include face and hand deformities, eye damage, and hypertrichosis. A fatal outcome from hepatic cirrhosis or haemolytic anaemia is not unusual. There is also a late onset form of CEP which is much less severe and may be mistaken for PCT.

INVESTIGATIONS

Diagnosis is established by finding increased levels of uro- and coproporphyrin in urine, faeces, and erythrocytes (RBCs). There are increased levels of both free and zinc-protoporphyrin in RBCs.

DNA repair-deficient photodermatoses

DEFINITION AND CLINICAL FEATURES

This is a very rare group of photosensitivity dermatoses associated with established defects in the repair of UV-induced DNA damage. They include xeroderma pigmentosum, Cockayne's syndrome, trichothiodystrophy, and Bloom's syndrome. These autosomal recessive genodermatoses have a variable association with cancer.

Xeroderma pigmentosum

Xeroderma pigmentosum (XP) is a heterogeneous disorder which can affect all races. It is characterized by extreme photosensitivity, accelerated photo-ageing, and early death from cutaneous malignancy. The cutaneous features usually begin in late childhood with exaggerated blistering sunburn, and exposed skin ages prematurely with dryness, freckling, and telangiectasia (**253**). Patients with XP are prone to a variety of benign and malignant skin tumours with at least a thousand-fold increased risk of melanoma and non-melanoma skin cancer. XP variants with milder clinical manifestations may occur.

INVESTIGATIONS

Diagnosis is by clinical assessment, by irradiation skin tests, which show enhanced delayed erythemal responses to UVB, and by demonstration of reduced DNA repair in cultured fibroblasts.

TREATMENT

Patients must minimize UV exposure with highly protective clothing, sunglasses, and sunscreens.

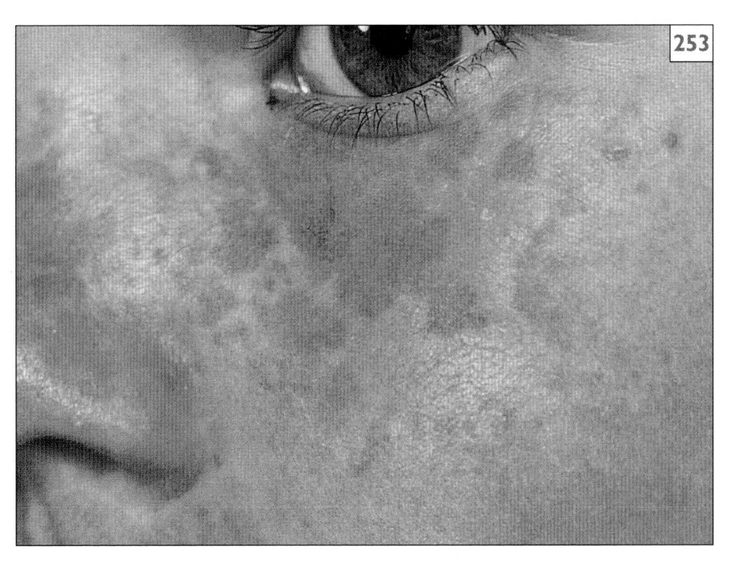

253 Xeroderma pigmentosum.

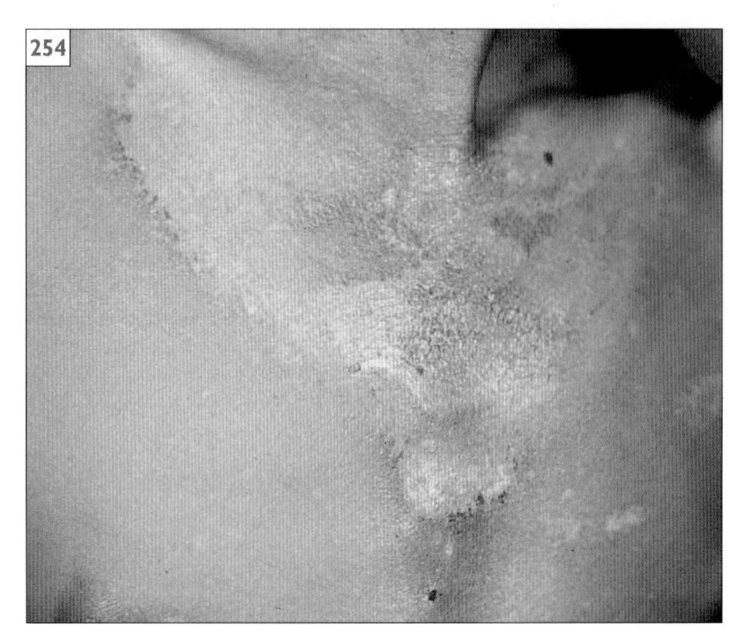

254 Casal's necklace in pellagra.

Other metabolic dermatoses

Some metabolic and nutritional disorders are associated with photodermatitis. The most important of these is pellagra.

Pellagra

DEFINITION AND CLINICAL FEATURES

Pellagra is caused by deficiency of niacin resulting from a dietary deficiency or, in the Western world, from an unbalanced diet due to alcoholism, gastrointestinal disease, or psychiatric disturbance. Rare causes include carcinoid tumours, Hartnup disease, and therapy with isoniazid or 6-mercaptopurine.

Pellagra produces the classic triad of dermatitis, diarrhoea, and dementia. The dermatitis is typically photosensitive with redness, scaling and, subsequently, hypermelanosis of light-exposed areas. A symmetrical butterfly rash on the face and a well-marginated eruption on the anterior chest (Casal's necklace) are characteristic (**254**). Mild associated mental disturbance such as depression or apathy may go unnoticed.

DIFFERENTIAL DIAGNOSIS

The main differential diagnoses are a phototoxic drug eruption, porphyria, or chronic actinic dermatitis. Zinc deficiency or other vitamin B deficiencies may co-exist.

TREATMENT

High dose oral nicainamide should be given and improvement expected within days.

DISORDERS OF THE BLOOD VESSELS

Structural abnormalities

There is a wide variety of vascular abnormalities, both congenital and acquired. These are manifest as alterations in the distribution of blood vessels in the skin.

Lymphangioma; lymphangiectasia

DEFINITION AND CLINICAL FEATURES

Dilatation of lymphatics resulting in fluid-filled blebs. Lymphangioma circumscriptum (**255**) is a developmental abnormality which appears as clusters of small blisters or warty papules filled with a mixture of blood and lymph. Lesions can be present at birth, usually on the trunk or proximal limbs, or may appear in childhood or early adult life. There may be an extensive deeper component in the subcutaneous tissue or muscle.

Lymphangiectases (**256**) are lymphatics that are dilated because of obstruction by a wide variety of inflammatory and neoplastic processes.

DIFFERENTIAL DIAGNOSIS

Keratotic lesions can be confused with angiokeratomata and verrucous haemangiomata.

TREATMENT

If surgical treatment of lymphangioma circumscriptum is to be curative, the underlying deeper lymphatic defect must be treated. If this is not possible, injection of a sclerosant may help.

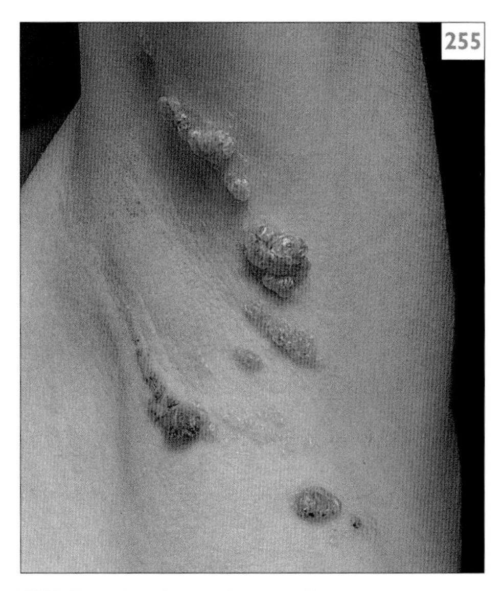

255 Lymphangioma circumscriptum.

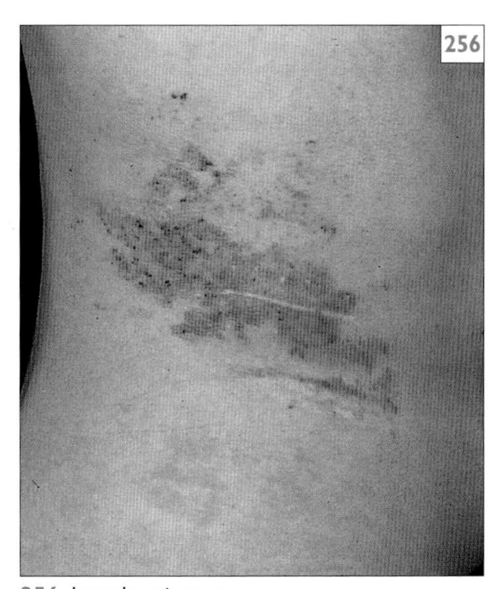

256 Lymphangiectases.

Telangiectasia

DEFINITION AND CLINICAL FEATURES

This is a permanent dilatation of capillaries and small venules. The visible vessels, on both the skin and mucosae, appear as red lines and dots that fade on pressure. Telangiectases can be isolated or grouped, giving rise to differing clinical patterns. They are classified as primary, of unknown origin, or secondary, when other dermatological conditions or external factors such as UV exposure or ionizing radiation have damaged the vessels.

Primary telangiectasia can be present at birth as part of a vascular naevus (**257**) or may appear in childhood or adult life (angioma serpiginosum [**258**], essential telangiectasia [**259**]). Vascular abnormalities may be a sign of systemic diseases such as ataxia telangiectasia and Osler–Rendu–Weber syndrome (hereditary haemorrhagic telangiectasia) (**260**).

Spider naevi (**261**) are telangiectases formed from a central feeding vessel, with a star of surrounding vessels. They are a common finding in childhood and pregnancy and may regress spontaneously. Spider naevi may be numerous in patients with liver disease.

Venous lakes (**262**) are flat or papular, blanchable, blue–red lesions seen in the elderly, often on the lips. Telangiectasia may also be a feature of several dermatoses, e.g. rosacea, connective tissue disorders, mastocytosis, and venous stasis.

DIFFERENTIAL DIAGNOSIS

Purpura can be distinguished because it is not blanched by pressure.

INVESTIGATIONS

Depends on the type of lesion and focuses on finding the underlying cause and extent of the abnormality.

TREATMENT

Spider naevi may be treated with fine point electrocautery. Larger or more widespread telangiectasia can be cleared by pulsed-dye laser therapy.

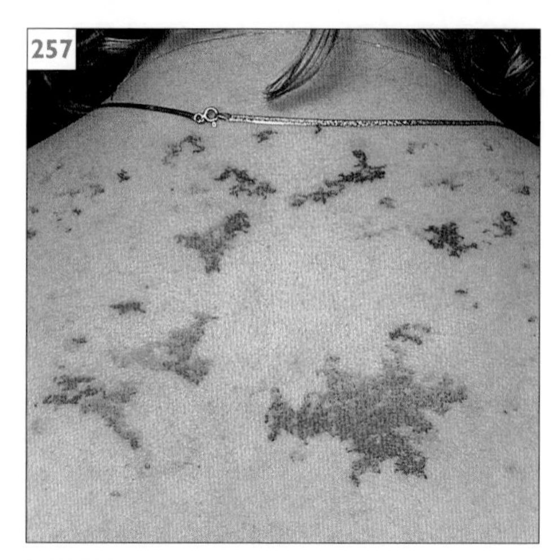

257 Telangiectatic naevus.

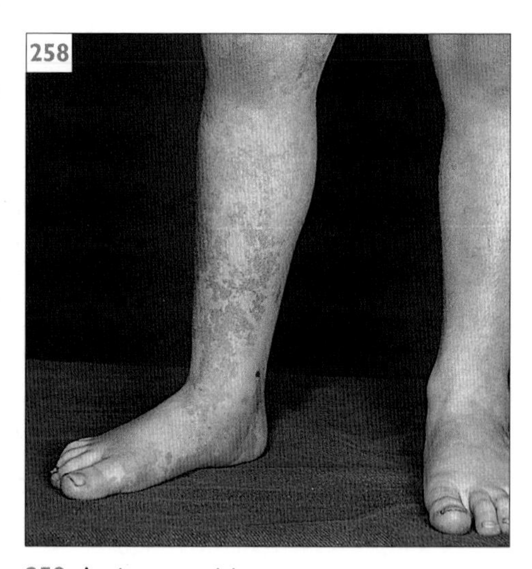

258 Angioma serpiginosum.

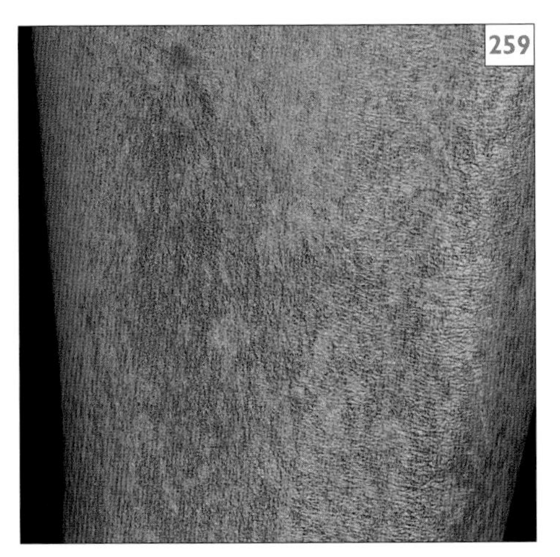

259 Essential telangiectasia.

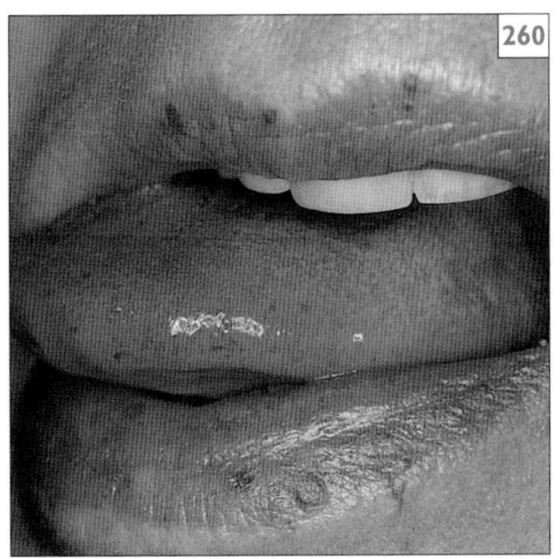

260 Haemorrhagic telangiectasia.

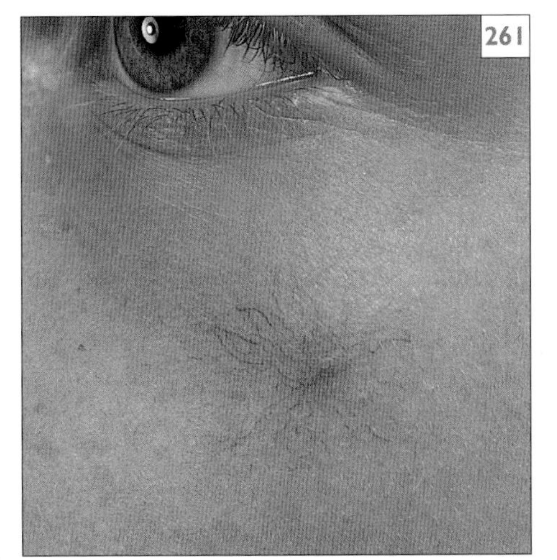

261 Spider naevus.

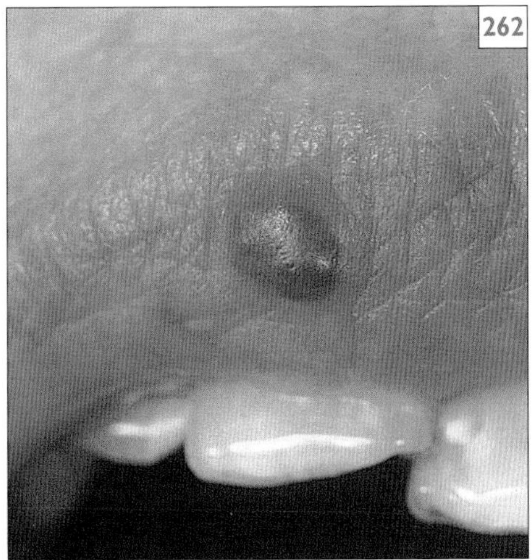

262 Venous lake.

Angiokeratomata

DEFINITION AND CLINICAL FEATURES

Dilated and distorted vessels with overlying hyperkeratosis. They occur as solitary lesions, plaques, or may be part of multi-system disease. Solitary angiokeratomata are dark-red, warty lesions. The common Campbell de Morgan or cherry spot (**263**) is a brighter red and shows less keratosis but is similar histologically. Angiokeratoma circumscriptum (**26**) are warty vascular plaques present at birth or in early childhood. Angiokeratoma of Mibelli (**265**) usually occur on the fingers and toes of girls in later childhood. Scrotal angiokeratomata (**266**) are multiple, small dark-red papules (see also p. 82). Angiokeratoma corporis diffusum occur in association with underlying disorders of lysosomal enzymes such as Anderson–Fabry's disease. Scattered cutaneous lesions (**267**) are associated with hypertension, renal failure, ocular changes, and digital pain.

DIFFERENTIAL DIAGNOSIS

Solitary lesions can, when very dark, be mistaken for malignant melanoma. Multiple lesions can be confused with vasculitis.

INVESTIGATIONS

Histology. A decreased level of galactosidase A in plasma and cultured skin fibroblasts is diagnostic of Anderson–Fabry's disease.

TREATMENT

Small lesions may be curetted and cauterized, excised, or laser ablated. Treatment is seldom requested for Campbell de Morgan spots once their benign nature is explained. Enzyme replacement therapy is available for Anderson–Fabry's disease.

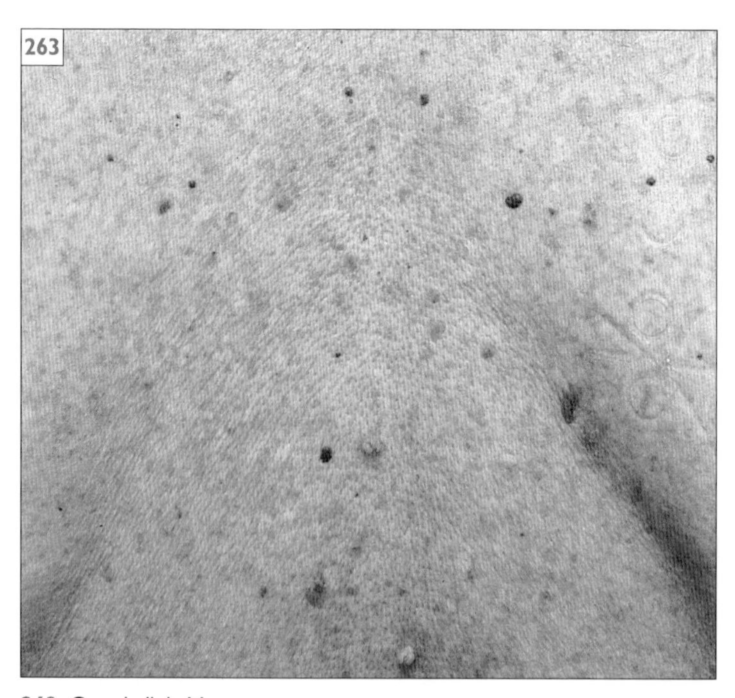

263 Campbell de Morgan spots.

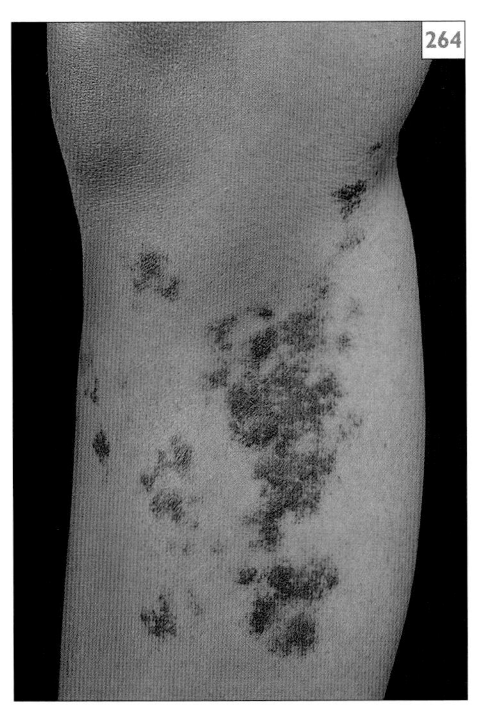

264 Angiokeratoma circumscriptum.

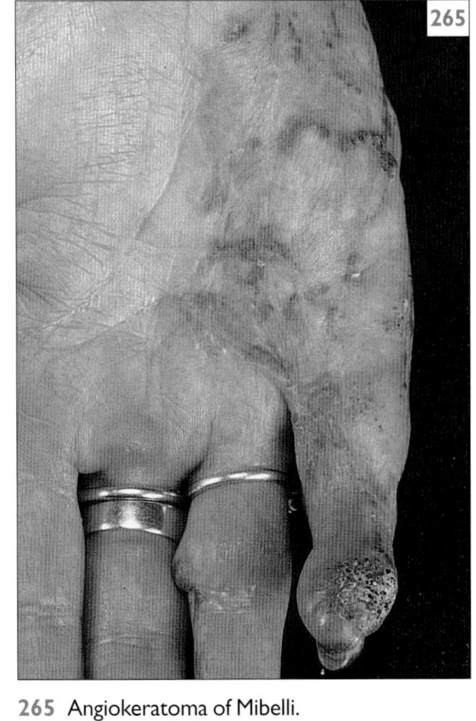

265 Angiokeratoma of Mibelli.

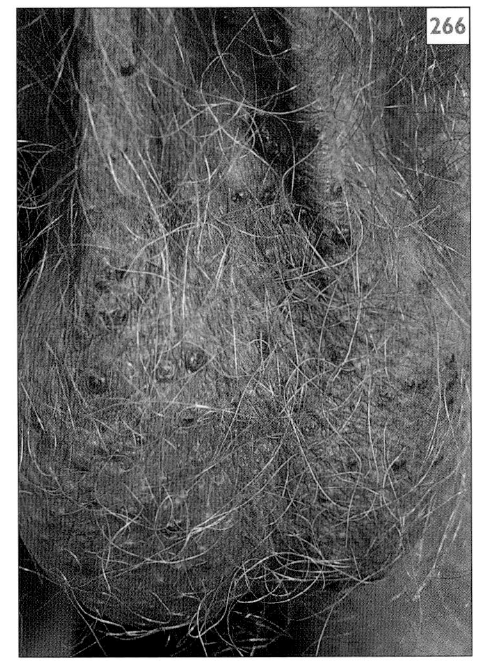

266 Scrotal angiokeratomata.

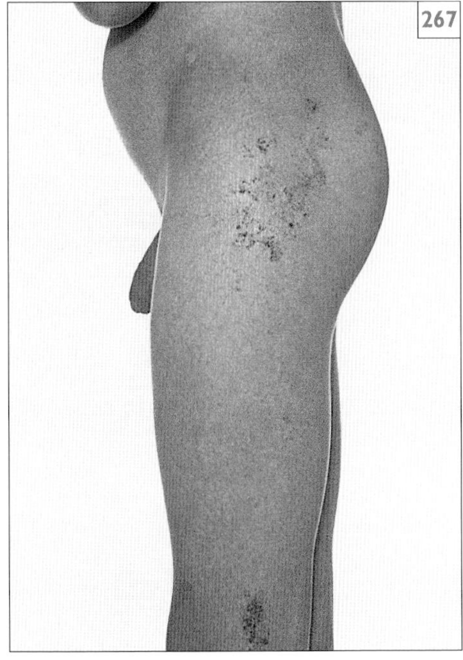

267 Angiokeratoma corporis diffusum (Anderson–Fabry's disease).

Portwine stain
(naevus flammeus)

DEFINITION AND CLINICAL FEATURES

A vascular birth mark characterized by persistent macular erythema and dilation of superficial dermal capillaries. It is less common than a salmon patch (p. 135) but more significant because of the potential for associated abnormalities. Underlying eye and brain lesions occur in up to 15% of patients with facial portwine stains, e.g. Sturge–Weber syndrome, where there is an underlying ipsilateral leptomeningeal vascular malformation. Portwine stains are usually unilateral and often affect the face and neck (**268**). Lesions are present but flat at birth, and thicken and darken with age (**269**).

A variety of lymphatic and venous abnormalities may be associated with portwine stains, particularly on the trunk and limbs. The Klippel–Trenaunay syndrome is a combination of a portwine stain on a limb and soft tissue swelling, with or without bony overgrowth (**270**).

DIFFERENTIAL DIAGNOSIS

Salmon patch. In the much rarer Parkes–Weber syndrome, limb hypertrophy is caused by multiple arteriovenous fistulae, and any associated vascular stain is paler.

INVESTIGATIONS

Uncomplicated lesions do not need investigation. CT or MRI scanning in patients with portwine stains of the upper face, to detect leptomeningeal vascular malformations (Sturge–Weber syndrome).

TREATMENT

Portwine stains on the face and neck can cause great distress to the sufferer and social disability. Cosmetic camouflage was once the main treatment. Early laser therapy carried a high risk of scarring, but modern pulsed-dye laser therapy may give great cosmetic benefit, and fade or clear lesions, especially if treated in early childhood. Patients with lesions close to the eyes should be seen regularly by an ophthalmologist to screen for glaucoma.

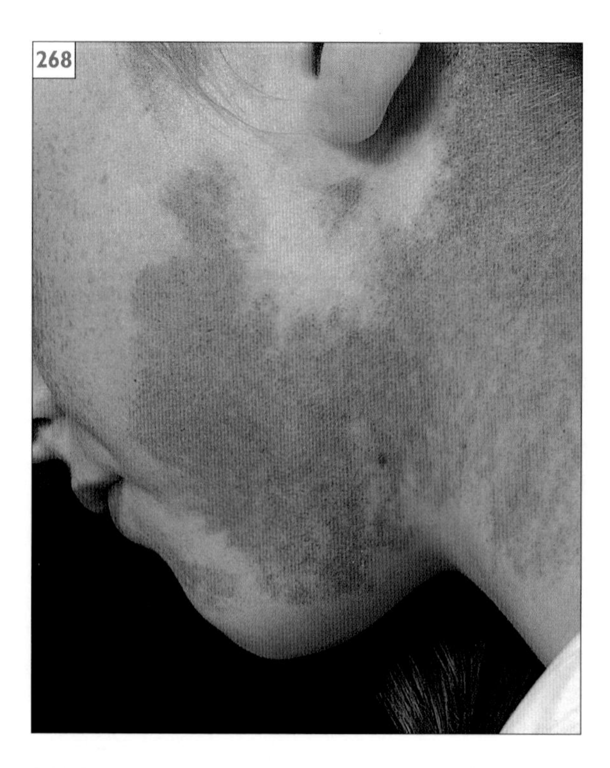

268 Portwine stain.

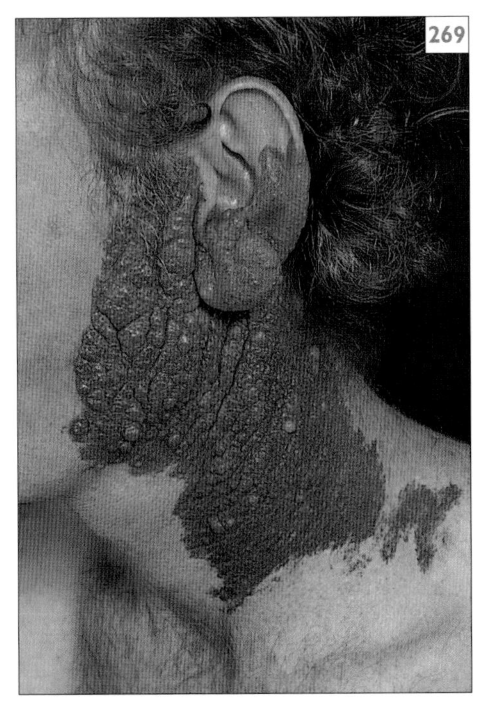

269 Thickened and darkened portwine stain.

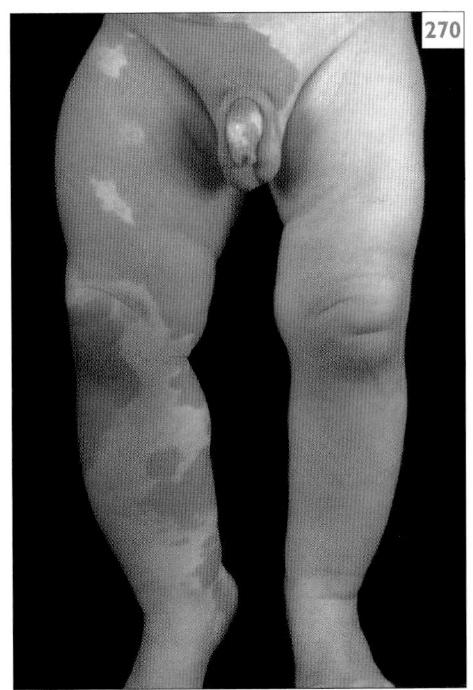

270 Klippel–Trenaunay syndrome.

Salmon patch
(stork mark; erythema nuchae)

DEFINITION AND CLINICAL FEATURES
These lesions, the most common of the vascular birth marks, are sometimes called telangiectatic naevi and affect up to 50% of newborns. The cause is unknown. They appear at birth as a pink or red patch of dilated vessels, affecting the forehead, eyelids, upper lip, and/or the back of the neck (**271**). With time the lesions on the face fade. The nuchal lesion is hidden by hair but can often be found in adults who are usually unaware of its existence. Sacral lesions may be associated with spinal dysraphism, especially when associated with a second abnormality such as a pit or hypertrichosis.

DIFFERENTIAL DIAGNOSIS
Portwine stains are usually unilateral.

INVESTIGATIONS
None usually necessary.

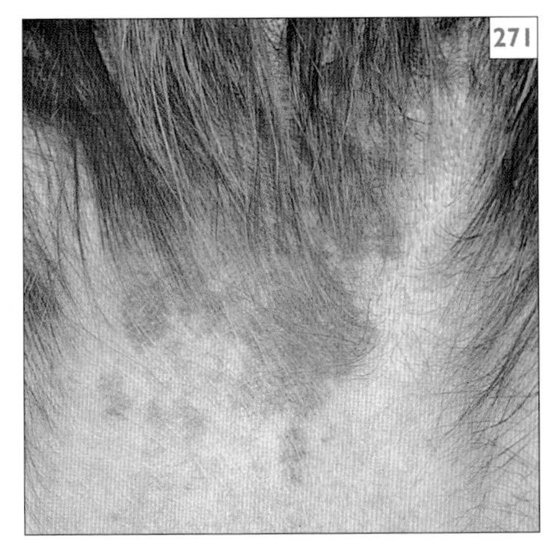

271 Salmon patch.

TREATMENT
None usually needed as facial lesions usually fade rapidly.

Naevus anaemicus

DEFINITION AND CLINICAL FEATURES

A congenital abnormality of the skin presenting as a circumscribed macular area of pallor due to reduced blood flow, with normal texture and melanin pigmentation (**272**). The lesion may reflect a locally increased vascular reactivity to catecholamines, and is more a pharmacological anomaly that an anatomical one.

Naevus anaemicus occurs most commonly on the trunk. Lesions may be single or multiple, rounded, oval or linear; small pale blotches may be irregularly grouped. Under diascopic pressure, the naevus becomes indistinguishable from the blanched surrounding normal skin. Rubbing the skin causes reactive hyperaemia in the surrounding normal skin but not within the naevus.

DIFFERENTIAL DIAGNOSIS

Naevus depigmentosus or vitiligo.

INVESTIGATIONS

Diascopy can reliably distinguish naevus anaemicus from other lesions of circumscribed pallor as above.

TREATMENT

None usually required. Cosmetic camouflage may be used if requested.

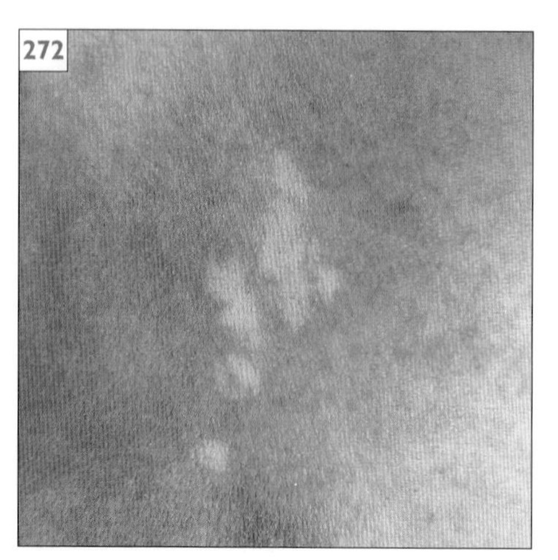

272 Naevus anaemicus.

Haemangiomas

DEFINITION AND CLINICAL FEATURES

Benign proliferative tumours of blood vessels, occurring usually in infancy, and often resolving spontaneously. The most common type is known as strawberry or capillary naevus (**273**). Strawberry naevi affect up to 10% of babies, with an increased incidence in premature infants. Seen as an area of pallor at birth, the bright red swelling develops in the first few months of life, often enlarging with alarming rapidity; lesions usually reach maximum size by 6–12 months. Thereafter the surface becomes grey and the lesion shrinks (**274**). Regression is complete by the fifth birthday in 50% of children but further improvement is unlikely after the age of 7 years. Deeper lesions, sometimes termed cavernous haemangioma (**275**), are seen as bluish subcutaneous swellings, often with a superficial strawberry component. The deeper areas often fail to regress completely. They may be complicated by ulceration and recurrent, especially from lesions in the nappy area and obstruction of orifices or vision. In eruptive neonatal haemangiomatosis multiple lesions affect the skin, liver, lungs, and sometimes other organs (**276**). Shunting may result in heart failure. Blue rubber bleb naevus syndrome (**277**) is an autosomal dominant condition. Multiple deep painful haemangiomata appear in later childhood, affecting the skin and the gastrointestinal tract. Verrucous naevus (**278**) is a warty, nonregressing haemangioma usually on the legs.

DIFFERENTIAL DIAGNOSIS

Portwine stains can be confused, particularly if there is a concomitant arteriovenous malformation.

INVESTIGATIONS

None needed in isolated lesions.

TREATMENT

The majority of strawberry naevi resolve without therapy. Complicated lesions have been treated with corticosteroids, interferon, laser therapy, and pressure garments. Verrucous haemangiomata are best excised as they continue to enlarge.

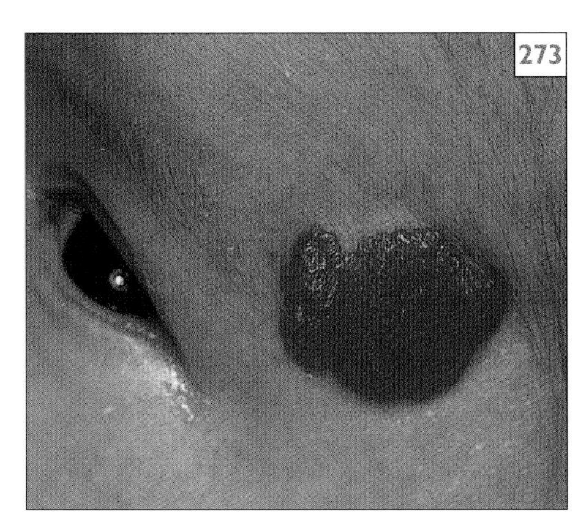

273 Strawberry or capillary naevus.

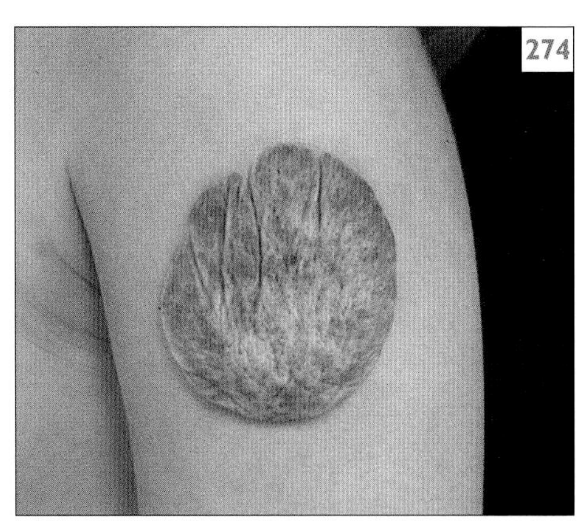

274 Regressing strawberry naevus.

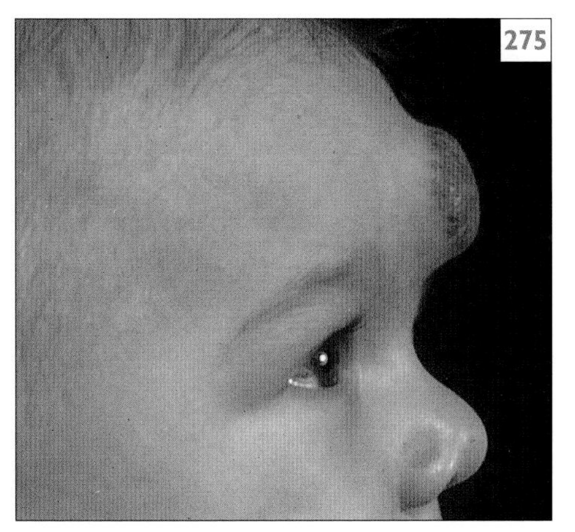

275 Cavernous haemangioma.

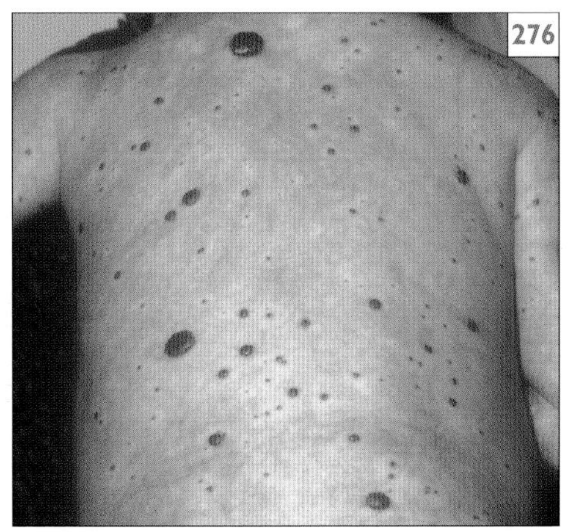

276 Neonatal haemangiomatosis.

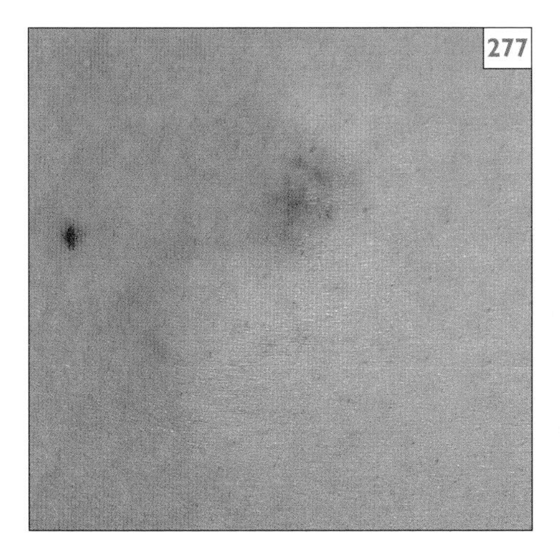

277 Blue rubber bleb naevus.

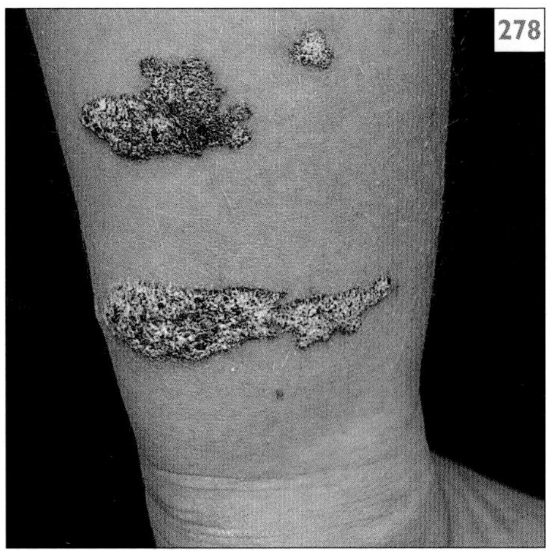

278 Verrucous naevus.

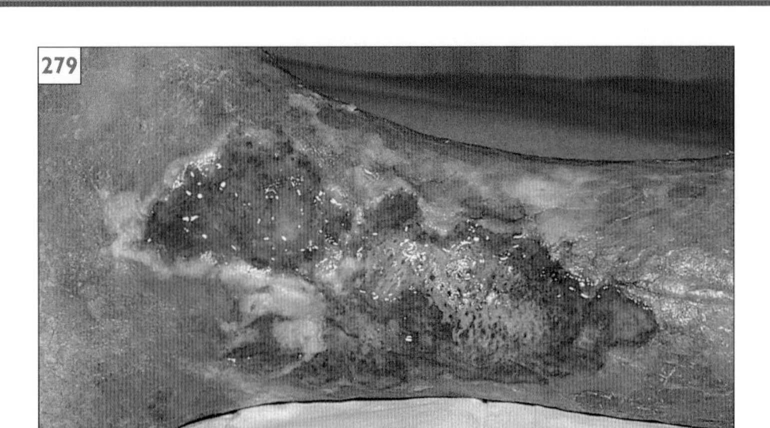

279 Varicose ulcer.

Vascular leg ulcers

DEFINITION AND CLINICAL FEATURES

There are many causes for ulceration of the lower leg. In industrialized nations the most common ulcers are those due to chronic venous insufficiency secondary to deep vein valvular incompetence or deep venous thrombosis. Arterial disease and diabetes are the other main causes. These are a major financial burden and cause of morbidity due to their chronicity.

Varicose ulcers usually affect the medial side of the lower leg (**279**) but may become circumferential. The surrounding skin will often show the changes of varicose eczema. The limb is often oedematous and there may be areas of atrophie blanche (**280**), seen as firm white plaques with telangiectasia. Lymphoedema (**281**), either congenital or acquired, can predispose to chronic ulceration. Arterial ulcers are often small but painful. They are often acral or over bony prominences. Diabetic ulcers (**282**) vary in appearance depending on the degree of large or small vessel damage, and the presence of neuropathy. Chronic ulcers on the legs are also a feature of several haematological diseases including sickle cell disease (**283**).

DIFFERENTIAL DIAGNOSIS

Distinguishing venous and arterial ulcers is essential. Ulcers are also seen in sickle cell anaemia, pyoderma gangrenosum, vasculitis, and other rarer conditions. Malignant change (**284**) can both mimic and complicate venous ulcers.

INVESTIGATIONS

Ankle or brachial Doppler pressure index to exclude significant arterial impairment. Contact dermatitis from medicaments is a common complication for which patch testing may be helpful.

TREATMENT

A wide range of dressings and topical agents are available for the treatment of ulcers. The mainstay of treatment for venous ulcers remains adequate compression bandaging. This must be applied correctly in order to be effective. Healing of arterial ulcers is usually dependent on vascular surgical intervention to improve the circulation.

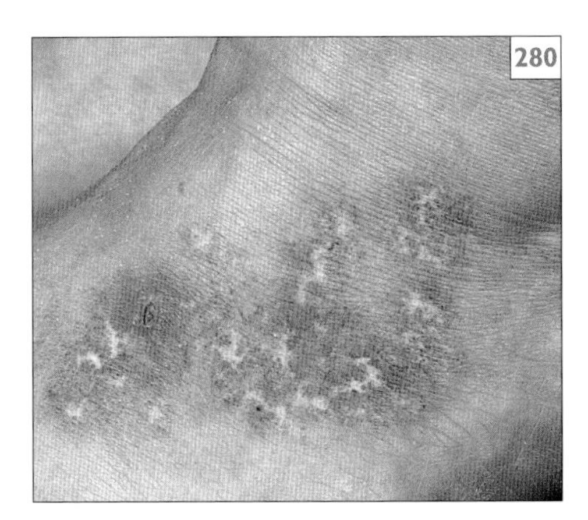

280 Atrophie blanche.

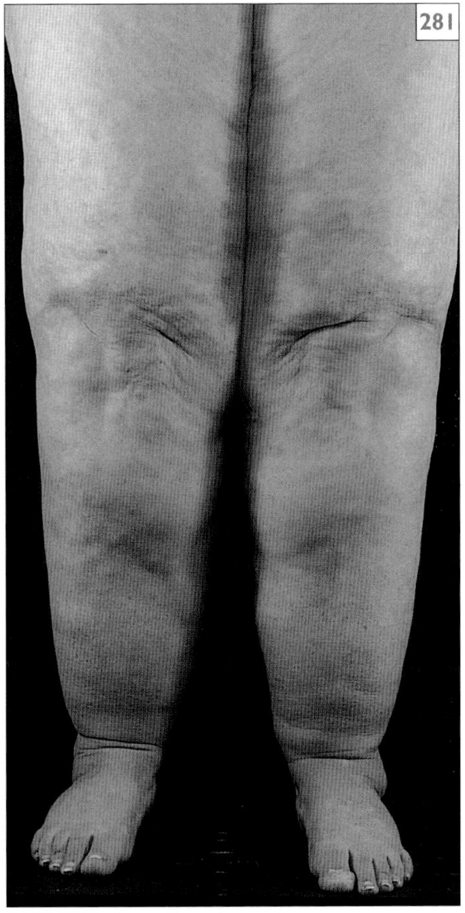

281 Lymphoedema.

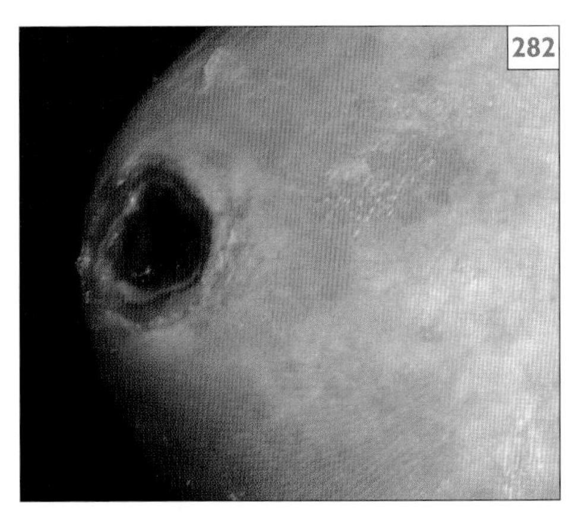

282 Diabetic ulcer on the heel.

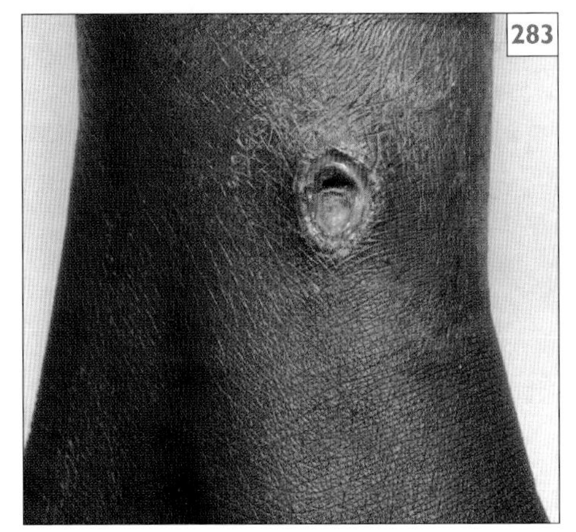

283 Leg ulcer in sickle cell disease.

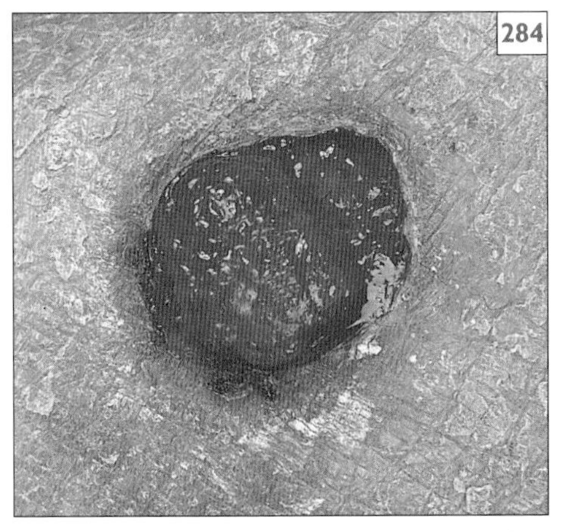

284 Malignant ulcer (squamous cell carcinoma).

Inflammatory disorders

Inflammation of blood vessels can be detected histologically in many different dermatological conditions. It may occur as a primary process, or secondary to many other processes causing microvascular occlusion such as coagulopathies and infection. The term vasculitis is applied more specifically to the combination of inflammation and necrosis of blood vessels.

Chilblains (perniosis)

DEFINITION AND CLINICAL FEATURES

A cold-related tissue injury, producing inflammatory tender lesions on the peripheries and thighs (**285**). Exposure to cold and humidity, in a susceptible individual, causes persistent constriction of large peripheral cutaneous arterioles and dilation of more superficial vessels. Chilblains usually appear in autumn or early winter when humidity is high, as this exacerbates conductive heat loss. Most cases are idiopathic but underlying causes include sepsis, dysproteinaemias, myelodysplasia, connective tissue disease, and anorexia nervosa.

DIFFERENTIAL DIAGNOSIS

Chilblain lupus erythematosus, peripheral vascular insufficiency, acrocyanosis, cryoglobulinaemia, lupus pernio.

INVESTIGATIONS

Full blood count, ESR, autoimmune profile, cryoglobulins. Histology may be useful to exclude other diseases.

TREATMENT

Lesions are usually self limiting and a warm living environment and warm clothing help. Vasodilating calcium channel blockers are an effective treatment and preventative therapy.

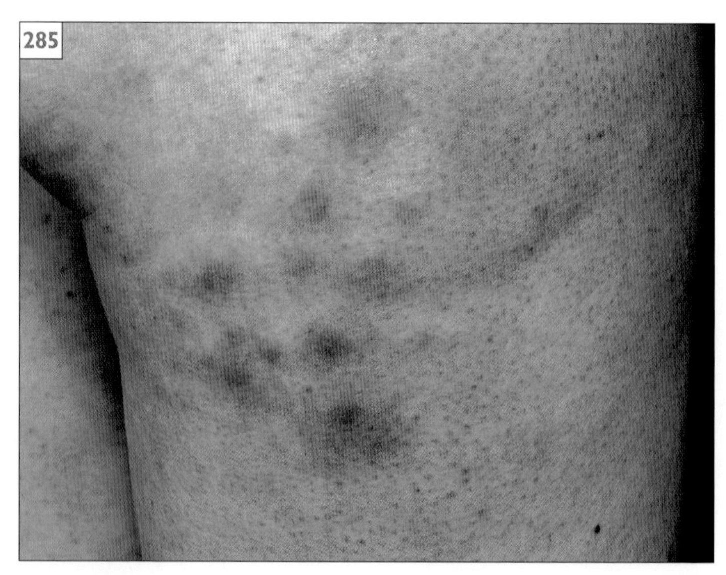

285 Chilblains.

Capillaritis
(pigmented purpuric dermatoses)

DEFINITION AND CLINICAL FEATURES
A group of chronic dermatoses characterized by a maculopapular purpuric eruption, and inflammation of capillaries. The cause is usually unknown, but capillaritis has been reported following many different drugs. It presents as mildly pruritic orange-red 'cayenne pepper' papules and plaques (**286**) and typically affects the lower legs. Old lesions become brown as haemosiderin is deposited. Different clinical patterns have been recognized and given descriptive or eponymous names including Schamberg's disease (progressive pigmented purpuric dermatoses), Majochi's disease (purpura annularis telangiectoides), itching purpura, lichen aureus (**287**) and pigmented purpuric lichenoid dermatoses of Gougerot and Blum.

DIFFERENTIAL DIAGNOSIS
Stasis dermatitis, contact dermatitis, purpura secondary to haematological disorders.

INVESTIGATIONS
Histology is usually supportive. No further investigations are usually necessary.

TREATMENT
Lesions may clear spontaneously, although slowly. Itching usually responds to topical corticosteroids or antihistamines, but the skin changes are usually resistant to treatment.

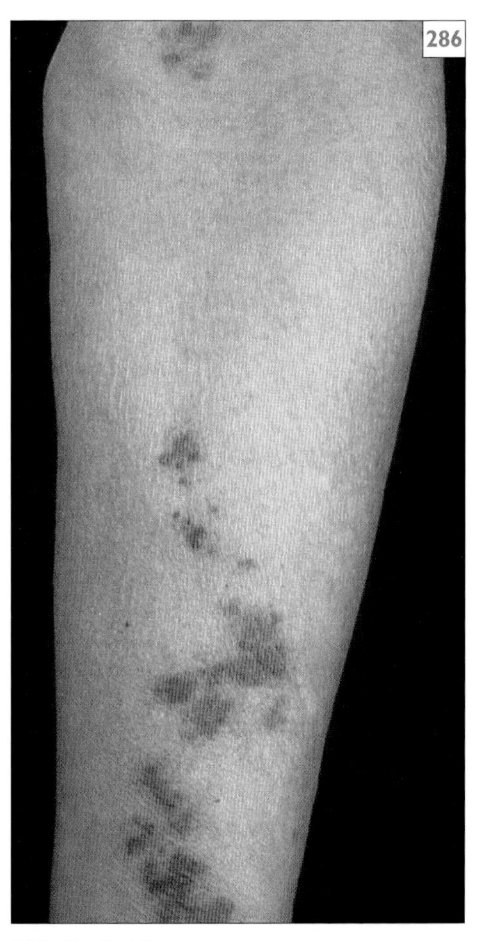

286 Capillaritis.

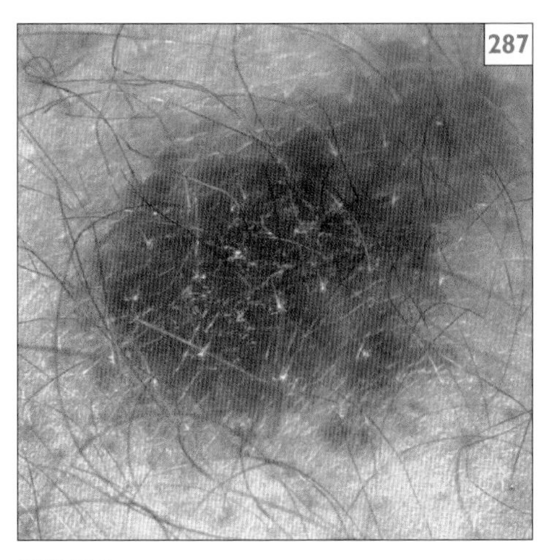

287 Lichen aureus.

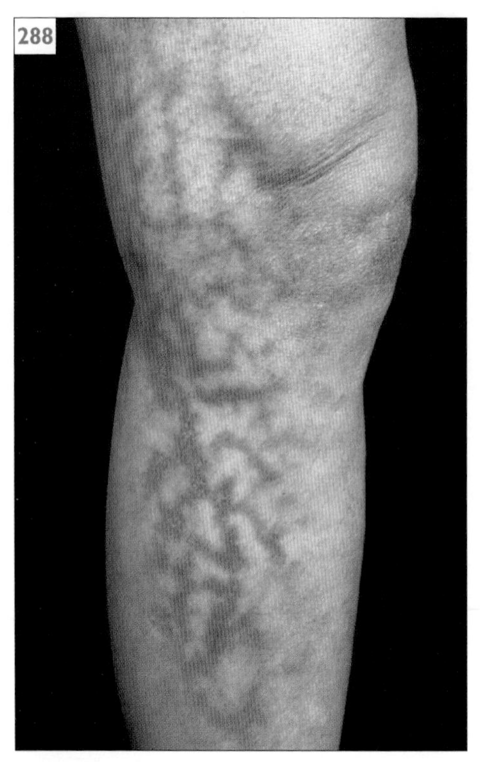

288 Livedo reticularis.

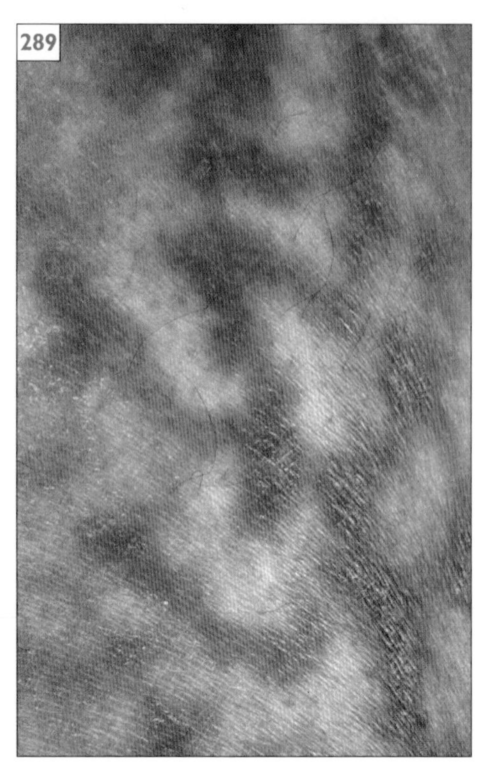

289 Erythema ab igne.

Livedo reticularis

DEFINITION AND CLINICAL FEATURES

A purple mottled discolouration of the skin, in a net-like pattern, resulting from a disturbance of dermal circulation. It is accentuated by cold and the colour changes are thought to arise due to stagnation of cyanotic blood in dilated capillaries at areas of anastamoses. Physiological livedo is common in children and young adults and usually seen over the thighs and calves (**288**). Erythema ab igne is a variant of livido reticularis caused by prolonged application of heat to the skin, usually in the elderly to relieve cold or pain. It is in effect a low-grade burn and early erythematous changes are typically followed by long-lasting hyperpigmentation (**289**).

A wide range of conditions can cause livedo reticularis. These can be grouped into: disorders of the vessel wall, including vasculitis; structural abnormalities of the vasculature; increased viscosity of the blood; microemboli; and unknown.

DIFFERENTIAL DIAGNOSIS

Livedoid drug rash, angioma serpiginosum.

INVESTIGATIONS

Physiological livedo does not require any further investigations. Patchy asymmetrical livedo requires may be secondary to vasculitis or haematological disease, which should be investigated accordingly.

TREATMENT

Uncomplicated livedo does not require treatment.

Vasculitis

DEFINITION AND CLINICAL FEATURES

Vasculitis is inflammation and damage of the blood vessels. The pathogenesis of vasculitis is a complex subject as there are likely to be many different causes. It may occur as a local or systemic process and can be a primary disorder or secondary to another disease process. The clinical features depend on the size and site of affected vessels. The skin is often involved in vasculitides so dermatologists can play an important role in the diagnosis and evaluation of patients. Classification of vasculitis is confusing but is broadly based on the size of the damaged vessels and the nature and degree of damage. In most forms of vasculitis, gravitational effects result in the lower legs being most severely affected.

Cutaneous small vessel vasculitis (leukocytoclastic vasculitis) is the most common type of vasculitis in dermatology. It is characterized by palpable purpura ranging in size from 1 mm to several centimetres and often occurring in crops (**290**). These may evolve into blisters or pustules and subsequently ulcerate (**291**). Other forms include erythematous swelling known as urticarial vasculitis (**292**) and livedo reticularis (see **288**). Cutaneous small vessel vasculitis may be triggered by infection or drugs. It is usually a self-limiting disease, without extra-cutaneous features, but patients should be thoroughly evaluated to exclude infection, connective tissue disease, drug hypersensitivity, and cancer.

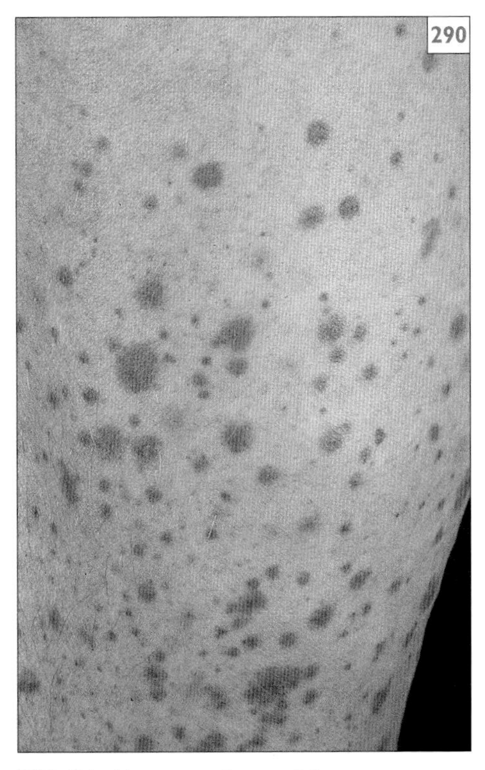

290 Palpable purpura in vasculitis.

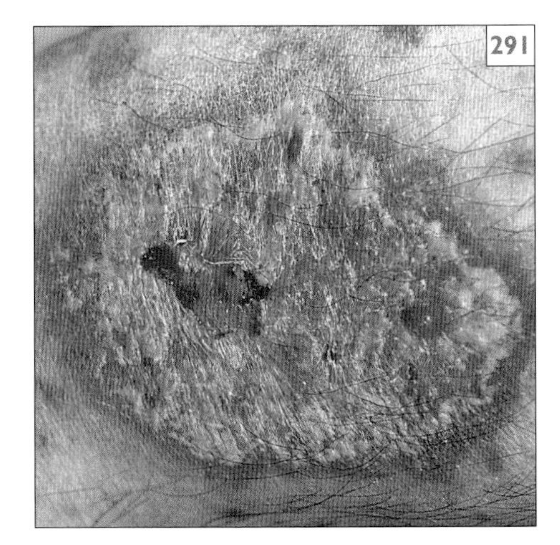

291 Vasculitic ulceration of the skin.

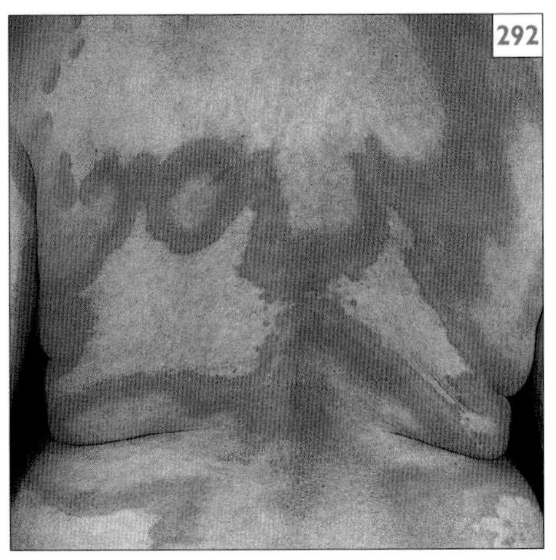

292 Urticarial vasculitis.

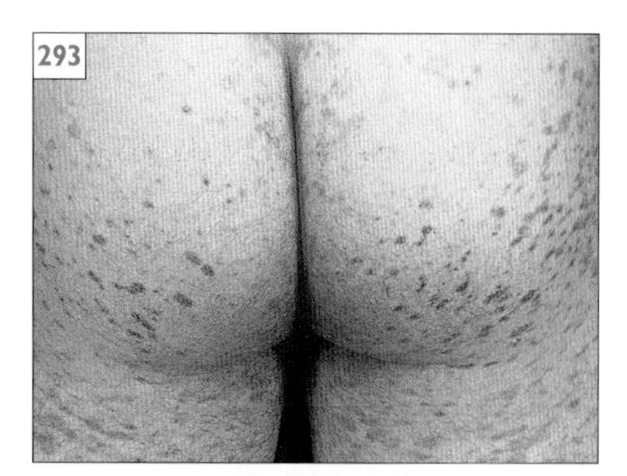

293 Henoch–Schönlein purpura.

Henoch–Schönlein purpura is a small vessel vasculitis with deposition of IgA complexes that involves the skin, gastrointestinal system, and kidneys. There may be an associated arthritis. It is commonest in young children and the classical symptoms are a rash, arthritis, and abdominal pain. The eruption typcially affects the extensor aspects of the limbs and buttocks (**293**).

Nodular vasculitis (erythema induratum of Bazin) results from the involvement of deeper vessels in the subcutaneous tissue, leading to inflammation of the adipose tissue (panniculitis). It is characterized by painful red or bruise-like lumps (**294**) on the calves which may ulcerate and suppurate, healing with discoloured areas or depressed scars. It may be associated with streptococcal infections or tuberculosis.

Polyarteritis nodosa (**295**) affects small and medium-sized arteries, resulting in nodules in the skin and livedo reticularis, often with multisystem involvement. Wegener's granulomatosis (**296**) is a form of vasculitis in which granulomas are seen histologically. It affects the upper and lower respiratory tracts and the kidneys, but can affect other systems. In the skin it produces a range of signs, from purpura to pyoderma-like ulceration.

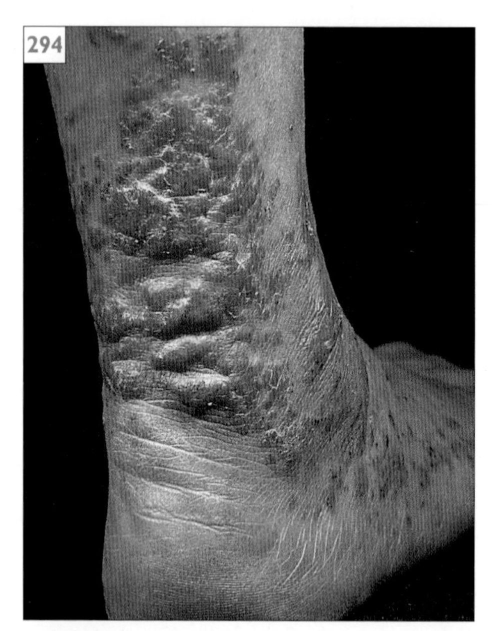

294 Nodular vasculitis.

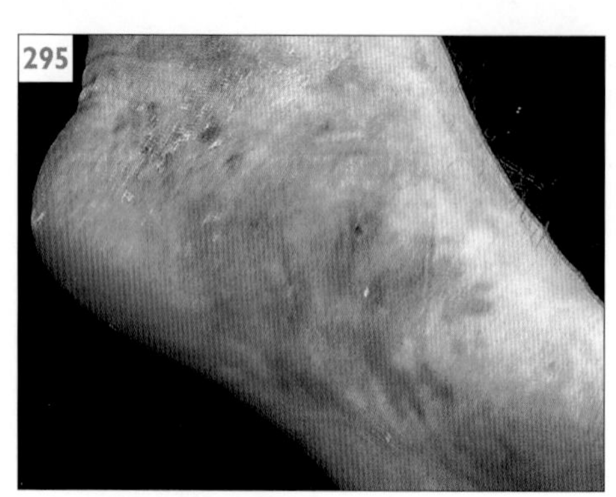

295 Polyarteritis nodosa.

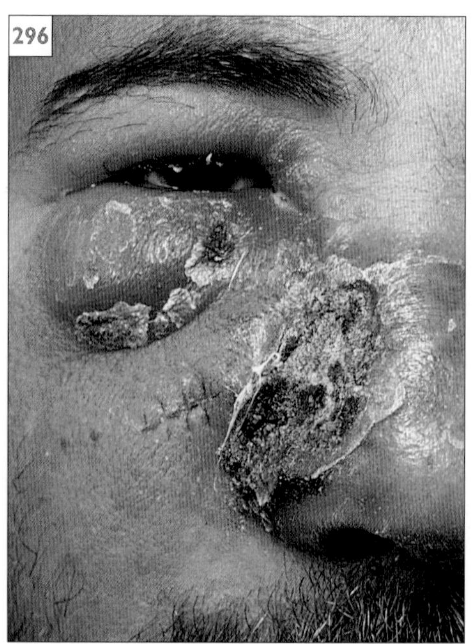

296 Wegener's granulomatosis.

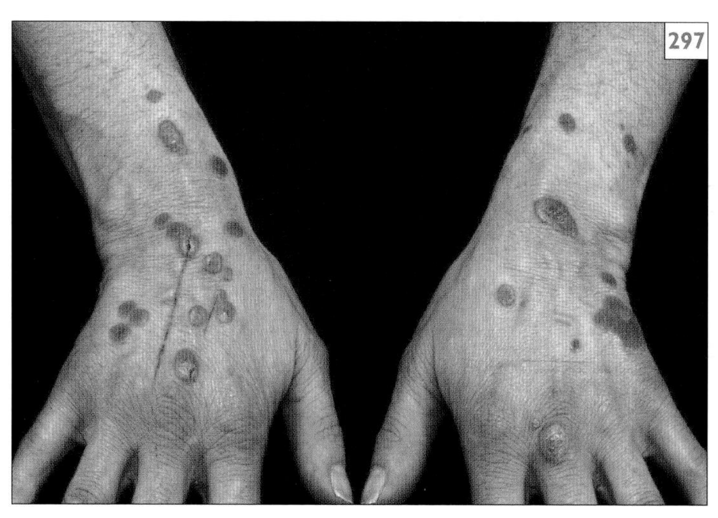

297 Erythema elevatum diutinum.

DIFFERENTIAL DIAGNOSIS

Causes of purpura such as coagulopathies. Nodular vasculitis and panniculitis can be confused with atypical infections.

INVESTIGATIONS

Histology should confirm the diagnosis, identify the size of blood vessel affected and the nature of the inflammatory infiltrate. Further investigations aim to determine the extent of systemic involvement and the underlying cause. A full blood count, ESR, renal and liver blood tests, and autoantibody screen should be tested. Urinalysis by dip testing and microscopy is important in the early detection of renal involvement.

TREATMENT

Treatment depends on the severity of skin eruption, involvement of other organs, and the underlying cause. Any triggering infection or drug should be treated or discontinued. Leg elevation and NSAIDs may help. Oral corticosteroids are usually given for more severe cutaneous disease or systemic involvement, followed by steroid-sparing drugs such as dapsone or colchicine and immunosuppressants.

Erythema elevatum diutinum

DEFINITION AND CLINICAL FEATURES

This rare chronic eruption is characterized by fibrosing plaques on the dorsal hands, knees, buttocks, and Achilles tendons, with histological evidence of leukocytoclastic vasculitis (**297**). Lesions are red-violaceous-brown initially and may be painful. They last for several years and fibrose to leave atrophic scars.

DIFFERENTIAL DIAGNOSIS

Other cutaneous small vessel vasculitis, Sweet's syndrome.

TREATMENT

The disease usually shows an excellent response to dapsone, but may relapse on discontinuation.

Pyoderma gangrenosum

DEFINITION AND CLINICAL FEATURES

A rare non-infectious disorder of the skin characterized by a dense inflammatory neutrophil-rich infiltrate and a variable degree of vascular damage. It may be idiopathic or associated with a variety of systemic diseases, particularly inflammatory bowel disease, arthritis, haematological malignancies, and monoclonal gammopathies. The lower legs and trunk are most frequently affected but the lesions can affect any site. Painful red–blue nodules develop central ulceration, spreading rapidly with ragged blue–black undermined edges (**298**). Variants include superficial lesions, pustular, vegetative and bullous forms (**299**). Patients are often unwell with general malaise and fever. Healing usually occurs with atrophic cribriform scars. A delay in the diagnosis and treatment of pyoderma gangrenosum or inappropriate surgical intervention can lead to rapidly progressive skin ulceration.

DIFFERENTIAL DIAGNOSIS

Venous leg ulcers, post-operative wound infections, syphylis and other infections, vasculitis, and disorder of coagulation.

INVESTIGATIONS

Histology is variable and often non-specific, but helps to exclude other diagnoses. Special stains and culture of skin may be needed to exclude infective causes of ulceration.

TREATMENT

Systemic corticosteroids are usually needed for rapidly advancing or widespread disease.

Immunosuppressants such as ciclosporin and mycofenolate mofetil may be used as an adjunct in unresponsive cases or as steroid-sparing drugs. Successful use of biologic TNF-alpha inhibitors has also been reported. Aggressive surgical debridement is contraindicated as it may exacerbate pyoderma gangrenosum. However, split-skin grafts and cultured keratinocyte autografts may aid wound healing if used with concurrent immunosuppressants.

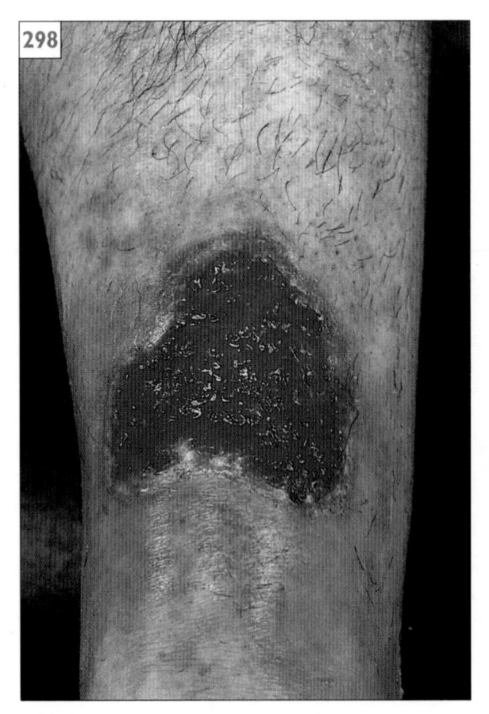

298 Pyoderma gangrenosum – ulceration.

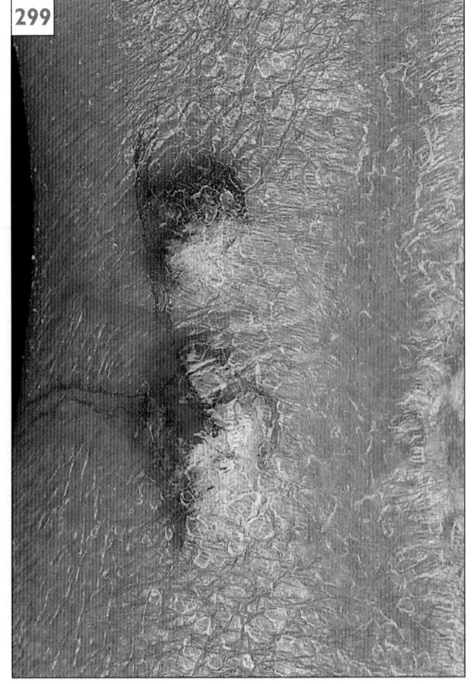

299 Pyoderma gangrenosum – bullae.

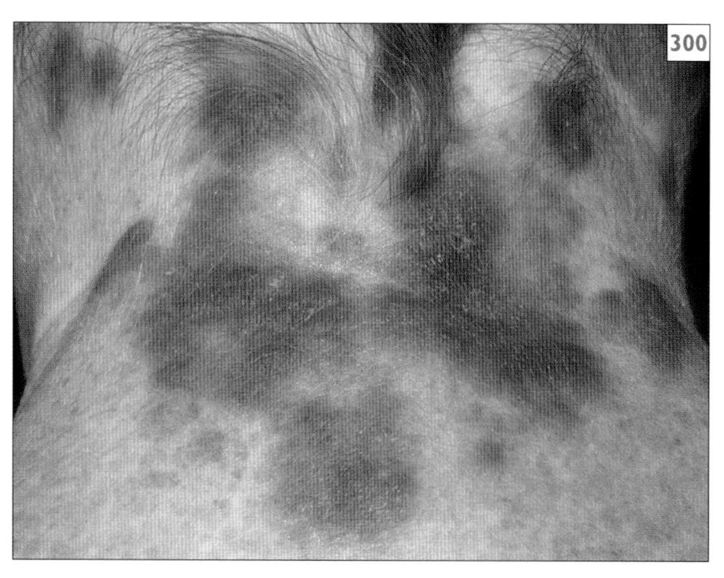

300 Sweet's syndrome.

Sweet's syndrome
(acute febrile neutrophilic dermatosis)

DEFINITION AND CLINICAL FEATURES

A neutrophil-rich dermatosis characterized by the acute onset of painful inflammatory plaques and nodules (**300**) in association with a fever and peripheral neutrophilia. Sweet's syndrome may be idiopathic, drug-induced, or associated with an underlying disease, especially haematological malignancies such as acute myeloid leukaemia. An underlying cause can be identified in about 50% of cases. The skin lesions of Sweet's syndrome may be the initial manifestation of malignancy and may preceed the diagnosis by many months. The patient is usually acutely unwell with a persistent high fever and malaise, and lesions typically affect the face and upper body.

DIFFERENTIAL DIAGNOSIS

Pyoderma gangrenosum, vasculitis.

INVESTIGATIONS

Histology shows a dense neutrophil-rich inflammatory infiltrate in the upper dermis. There may be features of vasculitis, but this is thought to arise secondarily to the inflammatory process. Full blood count shows leukocytosis and neutrophilia; ESR, and CRP are raised.

TREATMENT

There is usually a good response to a 4–6 week course of oral corticosteroids. Occasionally longer-term treatment is needed to prevent relapse. Potassium iodide, colchicine, and indomethacin are also effective.

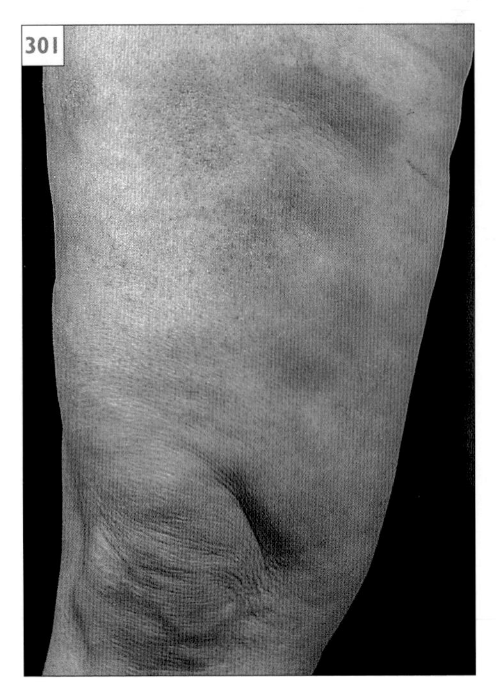

301 Panniculitis.

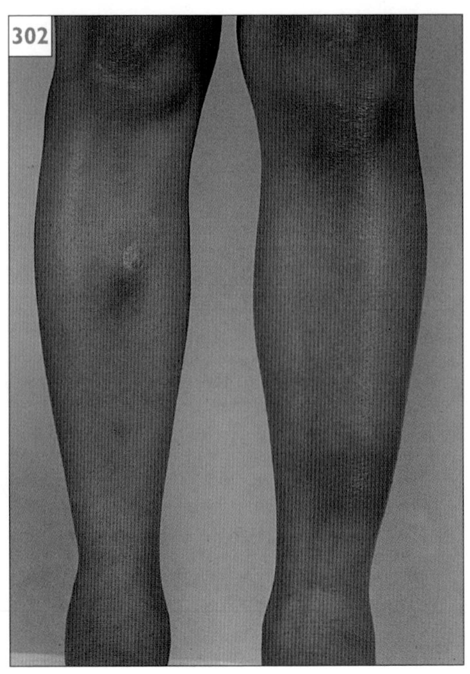

302 Erythema nodosum.

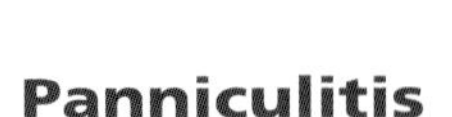

Panniculitis

DEFINITION AND CLINICAL FEATURES

Inflammation of the subcutaneous fat. Most lesions are chronic, lasting for weeks or months, and present as erythematous, tender, indurated deep nodules or plaques (**301**), which may be followed later by extensive fibrosis or fat atrophy. Like vasculitis, panniculitis may occur as a primary disorder or secondary to a range of diseases including connective tissue diseases, infections, sarcoidosis, pancreatic enzymatic deficiencies, alpha-1 antitrypsin deficiency, lymphoma, cold injury, and physical trauma. Four main histological patterns of panniculitis are recognized: septal, lobular, mixed, and panniculitis with vasculitis. Erythema nodosum is the classic example of a septal panniculitis. It is thought to be a hypersensitivity reaction triggered by infection-associated antigens and typically presents with tender bruise-like swellings on the anterior lower legs (**302**).

DIFFERENTIAL DIAGNOSIS

Lipodermatosclerosis, vasculitis, eosinophilic fasciitis.

INVESTIGATIONS

A deep biopsy of the skin and subcutaneous tissue is essential for adequate histological diagnosis. Further investigations may be necessary depending on the differential diagnosis, for example chest radiography and ASO titre in erythema nodosum. Infective panniculitis should be suspected in any patient who is immunosuppressed and extra biopsy material sent for tissue culture.

TREATMENT

Treatment is usually supportive and depends on the underlying pathology. NSAIDs may be needed for analgesia. For more severe disease, systemic corticosteroids may be effective, but underlying infections must be excluded prior to their use. Other treatment includes dapsone, colchicine, antimalarials, thalidomide, and potassium iodide.

SKIN MANIFESTATIONS OF SYSTEMIC DISEASE

Acanthosis nigricans

DEFINITION AND CLINICAL FEATURES

Hyperpigmented, velvety plaques involving neck and flexures. Acanthosis nigricans has several causes and the common mechanism is likely to be stimulation of growth factor signalling pathways in the epidermis. This may occur in insulin-resistant syndromes due to increased stimulation of insulin-like growth factor receptors. Benign forms of acanthosis nigricans are characterized by the insidious onset of brown, thickened papillomatous skin predominantly affecting the nape of the neck (**303**) and axillae (**304**); less commonly, the anogenital and groin regions are also involved. Features suggestive of underlying malignancy include rapid onset, extension to extraflexural sites, involvement of mucous membranes and/or vermilion border, presence of deeply pigmented, verrucous plaques, associated palmar keratoderma, and nail changes. The disorder is divided into five main subgroups according to their underlying aetiology:

- Hereditary – benign autosomal dominant.
- Benign – caused by endocrine disorders, including acromegaly, Addison's disease, Cushing's disease, diabetes mellitus.
- Pseudoacanthosis nigricans – obese, Asian, or Hispanic adults.
- Drug induced – nicotinic acid, stilboestrol.
- Malignant – especially adenocarcinoma of the gastrointestinal tract, ovary, and uterus.

DIFFERENTIAL DIAGNOSIS

Chronic, lichenified eczema, confluent and reticulate papillomatosis, lichen amyloidosis.

INVESTIGATIONS

Clinical differentiation between benign and malignant forms of the disorder should indicate appropriate investigation to elucidate underlying cause.

TREATMENT

Treatment is of the underlying cause. Removal of malignant tumours may lead to improvement.

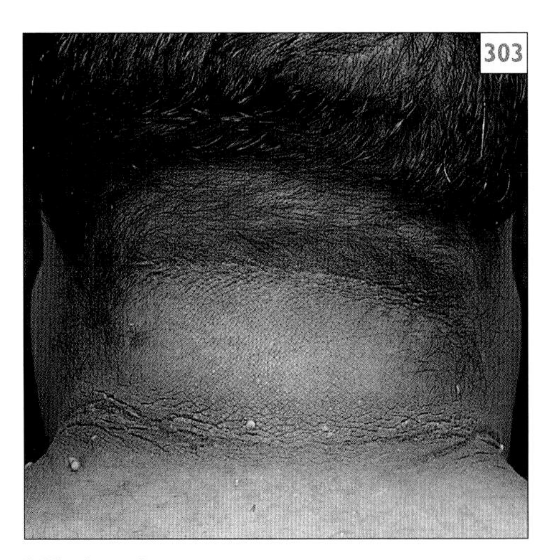

303 Acanthosis nigricans.

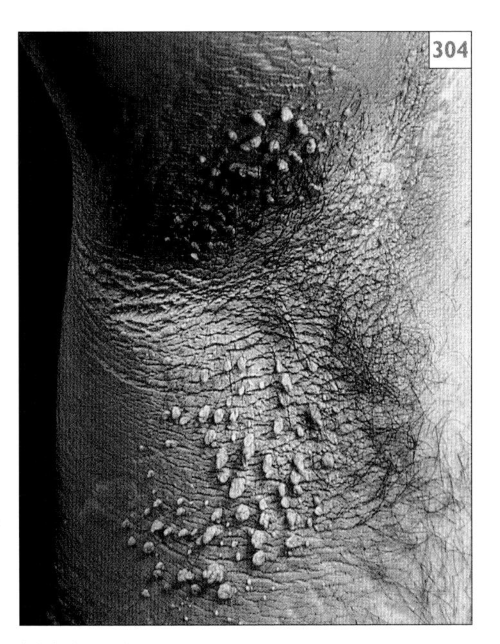

304 Acanthosis nigricans.

Porokeratoses

DEFINITION AND CLINICAL FEATURES

Porokeratoses are a group of disorders characterized by scaling lesions with a distinctive margin and a distinct histological abnormality of the epidermis, the cornoid lamella. Lesions are thought to arise from abberant clones of keratinocytes and may be inherited, usually as an autosomal dominant trait, or acquired following chronic sun exposure. Keratinocytes demonstrate variable degrees of dysplasia and may progress to overt malignancy. Lesions appear as a discrete, annular plaque with a peripheral hyperkeratotic ridge, often with a characteristic central groove (**305**), surrounding anhidrotic, hairless, atrophic epidermis. All forms of porokeratosis, with the exception of disseminated superficial actinic porokeratosis (DSAP), are rare. Five clinical subtypes are recognized:

- Porokeratosis of Mibelli refers to one (or a few) isolated plaque(s), most commonly distributed on the limbs (**306**). These begin as small papules in childhood which slowly spread centrifugally over years to reach several centimetres in diameter.
- DSAP occurs during middle age and comprises multiple, small (less than 1 cm in diameter), monomorphic, flat plaques on the lower legs (**307**) and other chronically sun-exposed sites, especially in fair-skinned individuals.
- Disseminated superficial porokeratosis (also called porokeratosis plantaris, palmaris et disseminata) may be distinguished from DSAP by the presence of lesions on non-sun-exposed sites and onset in childhood. A disseminated form has also been reported following organ transplantation.
- Linear porokeratosis is always confined to one limb or side, and may occur in a zosteriform or linear configuration (**308**).
- Punctate porokeratoses are confined to the palms and soles and comprise minute, hyperkeratotic, seed-like plaques. They may be associated with porokeratosis of Mibelli or linear porokeratosis.

DIFFERENTIAL DIAGNOSIS

DSAP must be distinguished from multiple actinic, stucco, or seborrhoeic keratoses. Linear porokeratosis may resemble linear verrucous epidermal naevus though is easily distinguishable on histopathological examination.

INVESTIGATIONS

Biopsy to demonstrate the presence of the cornoid lamella – a thin column of parakeratotic cells extending through the stratum corneum, bending away from the centre of the lesion.

TREATMENT

Cryotherapy, topical 5-fluorouracil and carbon dioxide laser therapy may be used.

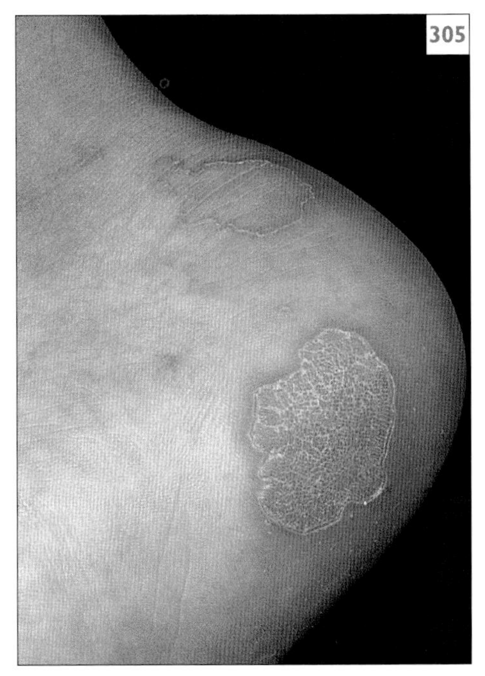

305 Porokeratosis.

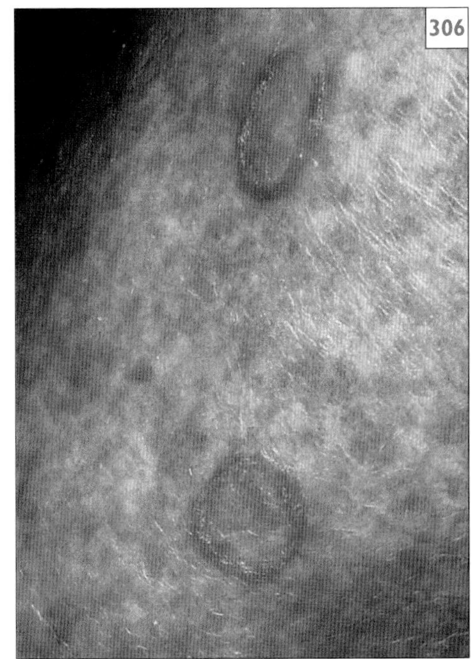

306 Porokeratosis of Mibelli.

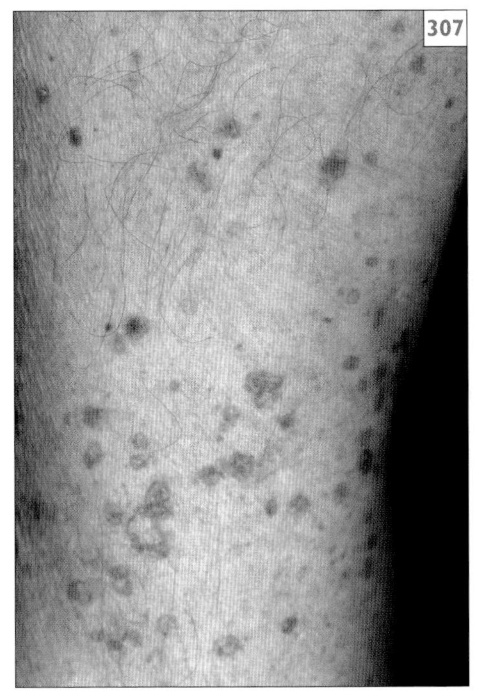

307 Disseminated superficial actinic porokeratosis (DSAP).

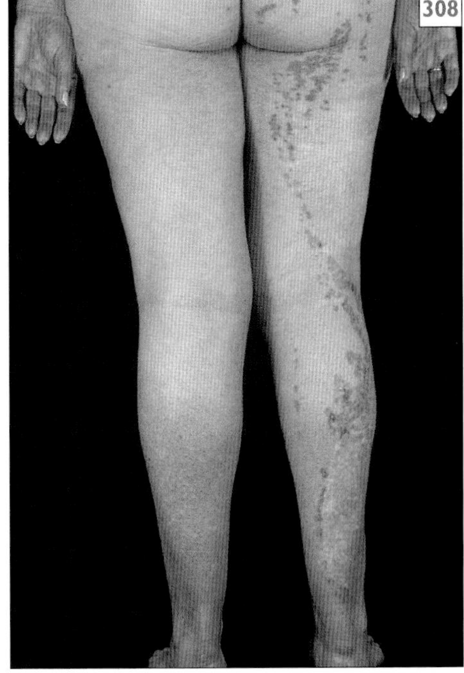

308 Linear porokeratosis.

Granuloma annulare

DEFINITION AND CLINICAL FEATURES

Granuloma annulare is relatively common disease characterized by the degeneration of dermal collagen and an associated lymphohistiocytic infiltrate (necrobiotic granuloma). The most frequent presentation of granuloma annulare is of asymmetrical anular lesions made up of individual flesh-coloured or mildly erythematous dermal papules (**309**). These lesions are most commonly found on the dorsum of the hands and feet in children and young adults and are usually asymptomatic. They enlarge centrifugally and often persist for months or years before resolving without scarring. Generalized or disseminated variants of granuloma annulare present with numerous small papules and macules which may be widespread on the trunk and limbs (**310**). There is conflicting evidence of a link between granuloma annulare and diabetes.

DIFFERENTIAL DIAGNOSIS

The clinical appearance is usually distinctive. On occasions other annular disorders, such as erythema annulare centrifugum, annular sarcoidosis, and annular lichen planus may be considered. The more diffuse form of granuloma annulare may be confused with sarcoidosis, mastocytosis, and reticulate erythematous mucinosis. Histology should be diagnostic.

INVESTIGATIONS

If there is diagnostic doubt a skin biopsy should be taken. Urine should be tested for glycosuria.

TREATMENT

Granuloma annulare tends to remit spontaneously and, in some patients, particularly children, simple reassurance may suffice. Potent topical or intralesional corticosteroids may be successful in clearing localized lesions. Generalized disease may respond to PUVA, oral retinoids, or ciclosporin.

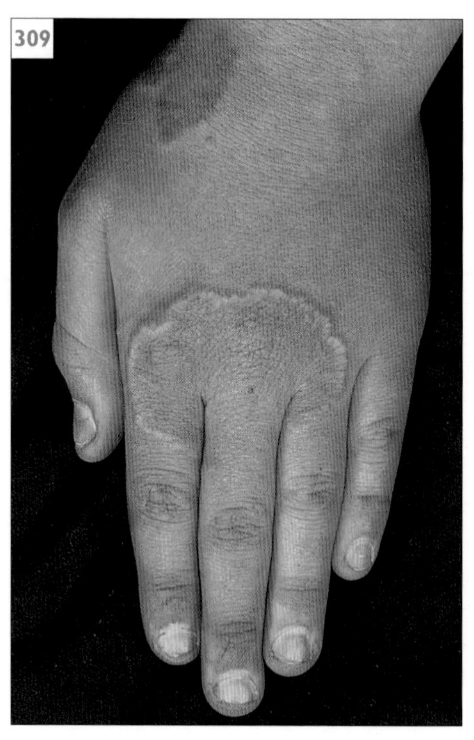

309 Granuloma annulare.

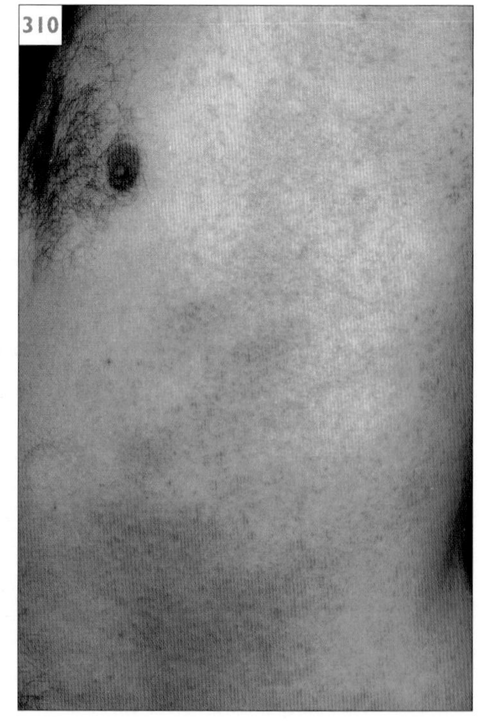

310 Diffuse granuloma annulare.

Necrobiosis lipoidica

DEFINITION AND CLINICAL FEATURES

Necrobiosis lipoidica consists of well-demarcated plaques of cutaneous atrophy with a yellowish discolouration associated with degeneration of collagen and a deep granulomatous infiltrate in the dermis and subcutis. It usually affects young and middle-aged adults and occurs on the pretibial area (**311**). Erythematous plaques enlarge by peripheral extension and the centres become glazed and atrophic with telangiectasis. Lesions tend to persist and may ulcerate (**312**). Cutaneous appendages are absent within the plaques and, in some instances, sensation is reduced. Approximately two-thirds of patients with necrobiosis lipoidica have or will develop diabetes mellitus, although there is no association with glycaemic control. The condition is uncommon, occurring in less than 1% of diabetics, and is very uncommon in the non-diabetic population.

DIFFERENTIAL DIAGNOSIS

Granuloma annulare, morphoea, sarcoid, and planar xanthomata.

INVESTIGATIONS

A skin biopsy is only required in atypical cases where the signs are not characteristic. Patients should be investigated for diabetes.

TREATMENT

Potent topical corticosteroids under occlusion or intralesional corticosteroids and topical PUVA may help, but atrophy usually persists.

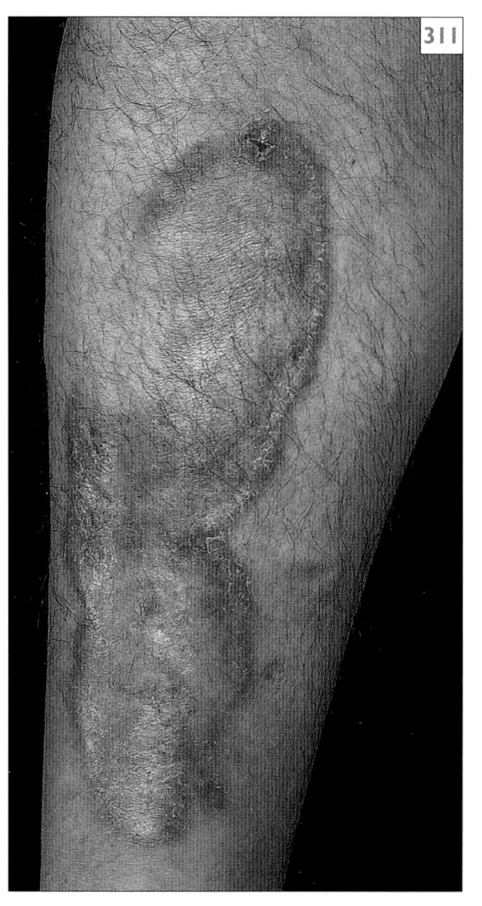

311 Necrobiosis lipoidica.

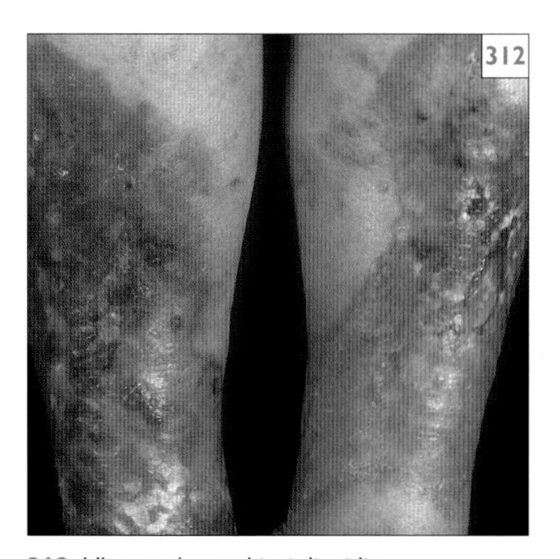

312 Ulcerated necrobiosis lipoidica.

Sarcoidosis

DEFINITION AND CLINICAL FEATURES

Sarcoidosis is a disorder characterized by the development of non-caseating, lymphocyte-poor granulomatous inflammation of unknown aetiology in multiple organs. The manifestations are protean depending on the organs involved. Cutaneous involvement is found in approximately a quarter of patients with systemic sarcoidosis. Cutaneous sarcoidosis can be found in the absence of evidence of systemic disease. The combination of erythema nodosum (a septal panniculitis) and bilateral hilar lymphadenopathy in young people is a common presentation. Other patients with a more insidious onset commonly have respiratory symptoms and one or more of the following manifestations of cutaneous sarcoidosis:

Lupus pernio is the involvement of the nasal skin with a chronic infiltrative erythema (**313**), commonly with involvement of the upper respiratory tract.

Papular and nodular sarcoidosis consist of focal dermal infiltration with naked granulomas producing discrete nodules. Papular lesions are commonly symmetrical while nodular lesions are often asymmetrical. Papular lesions are commonly found around the nape of the neck (**314**) and may be symmetrically distributed on the trunk, buttocks, and limbs. They often fade spontaneously. Nodules may be found at any site but have a particular predilection for periocular skin (**315**). Scar sarcoidosis consists of similar lesions involving old scars. There is resemblance to keloids but scar sarcoid does not itch. Annular and plaque-like variants also exist (**316**).

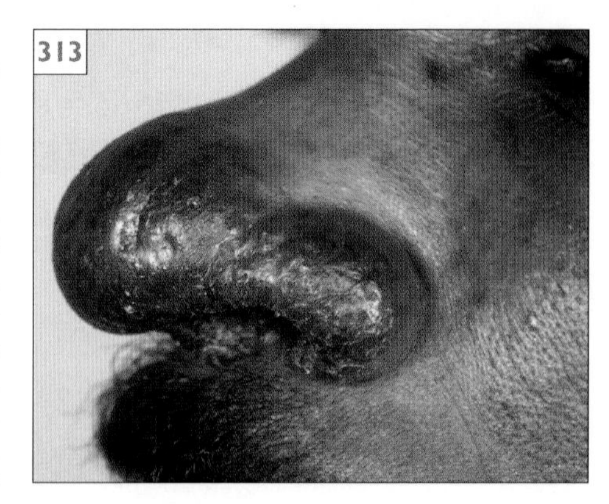

313 Lupus pernio.

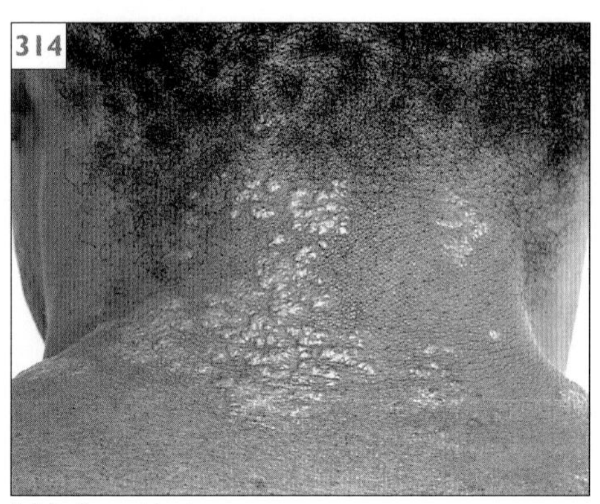

314 Sarcoidosis.

DIFFERENTIAL DIAGNOSIS

With the exception of erythema nodosum and lupus pernio, which have relatively characteristic clinical signs, sarcoidosis can be confused with granuloma annulare, necrobiosis lipoidica, infective granulomas including tuberculosis, and, sometimes, lichen planus.

INVESTIGATIONS

Histological confirmation of the diagnosis of sarcoidosis is important, so a skin biopsy should be taken. Once the diagnosis is confirmed, the patient should be investigated for systemic involvement with chest radiograph; respiratory function tests; ECG; full blood count; serum calcium; renal and liver function tests. Radiographs of the hands can be helpful if there are joint symptoms.

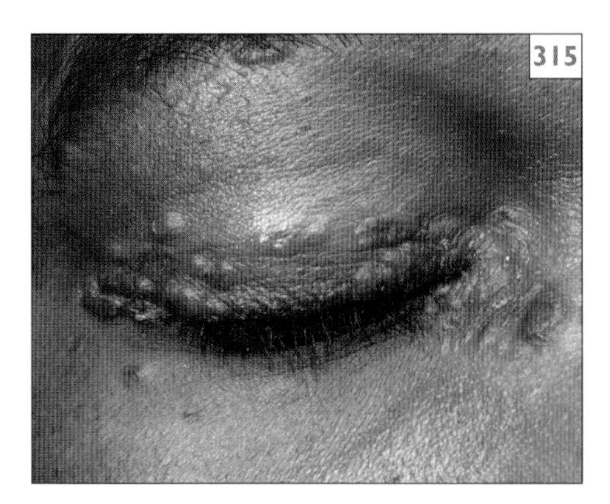

315 Papular sarcoidosis.

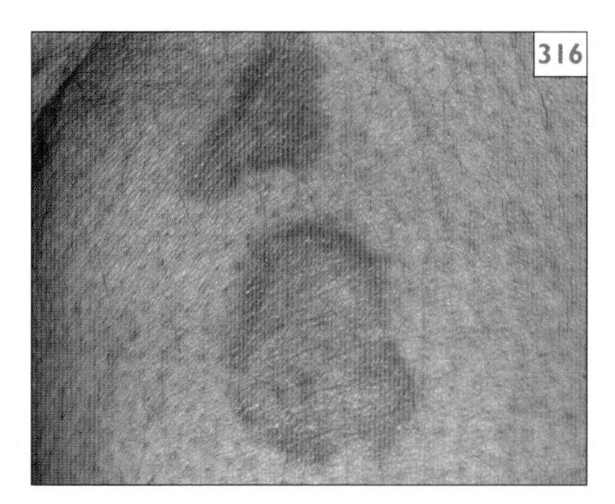

316 Annular sarcoidosis.

TREATMENT

Potent topical corticosteroids may sometimes help cutaneous lesions. A range of systemic drugs including corticosteroids, methotrexate, azathioprine, and antimalarials can be of benefit, but cutaneous lesions usually relapse quickly when they are discontinued. The decision to use these must take into account the severity of skin disease, its likely chronicity, and any associated systemic involvement.

Rheumatoid nodule

DEFINITION AND CLINICAL FEATURES

Rheumatoid nodules consist of palisaded necrobiotic granulomas in the subcutis in patients with seropositive rheumatoid arthritis. They present as non-tender, subcutaneous nodules, occurring particularly over the ulnar border of the forearm, on the dorsum of the hands, the extensor aspect of the knees, and elsewhere in patients with seropositive rheumatoid arthritis (**317**). Approximately 20% of patients with rheumatoid arthritis develop rheumatoid nodules at some stage during their disease.

DIFFERENTIAL DIAGNOSIS

In the presence of established rheumatoid arthritis the diagnosis is usually easy. Subcutaneous granuloma annulare and the nodules of rheumatic fever have similar clinical and histological appearances but are seen in a different clinical context.

INVESTIGATIONS

The diagnosis can be confirmed by serology for rheumatoid factor and histology.

TREATMENT

Symptomatic nodules may be excised or treated with intralesional corticosteroids.

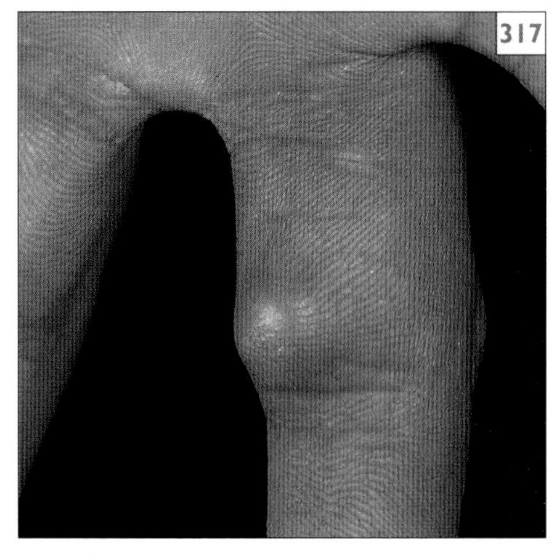

317 Rheumatoid nodule.

Granulomatous cheilitis
(Meisner's cheilitis)

DEFINITION AND CLINICAL FEATURES
This is an uncommon condition characterized by chronic granulomatous inflammation of the lips which are markedly and persistently swollen and may have a purplish discoloration (**318**). Histology reveals chronic granulomatous inflammation and in idiopathic cases there may be no evidence of granulomatous disease elsewhere. Granulomatous cheilitis may be an isolated occurrence but some patients have underlying Crohn's disease or sarcoidosis. It has also been reported as an adverse reaction to food additives including cinnamates. Granulomatous cheilitis may be associated with a fissured tongue and facial palsy (Melkersson–Rosenthal syndrome).

INVESTIGATIONS
A lip biopsy is helpful to confirm the diagnosis. Patients should be patch tested to look for evidence of allergic contact dermatitis.

DIFFERENTIAL DIAGNOSIS
In early attacks differentiation from angio-oedema may be difficult, but the swelling of granulomatous cheilitis soon becomes persistent. Many other causes of macrochelia exist including post-infectious lymphoedema and lymphoma.

TREATMENT
Treatment with intralesional corticosteroids after local anaesthesia is usually helpful but reduction cheiloplasty may be required in some cases.

Morphoea

DEFINITION AND CLINICAL FEATURES
Morphoea is a disorder of unknown aetiology in which there is localized dermal fibrosis associated with atrophy of epidermal appendages.

Morphoea can be subdivided into four main clinical types:

- Circumscribed or localized morphoea which is by far the most common and presents with a slightly erythematous plaque which, over the course of several months, becomes thickened and waxy with associated loss of hair and eccrine glands (**319**). Lesions characteristically have an inflamed lilac border and may become pigmented as they resolve.
- Linear morphoea which consists of a similar indolent process, usually affecting the limbs in childhood.
- Frontoparietal morphoea (or Parry–Romberg syndrome) which represents a similar linear process affecting half of the face, often in childhood or young adults ('coup de sabre').
- Generalized morphoea represents a similar process involving widespread involvement of the skin but without other organ involvement.

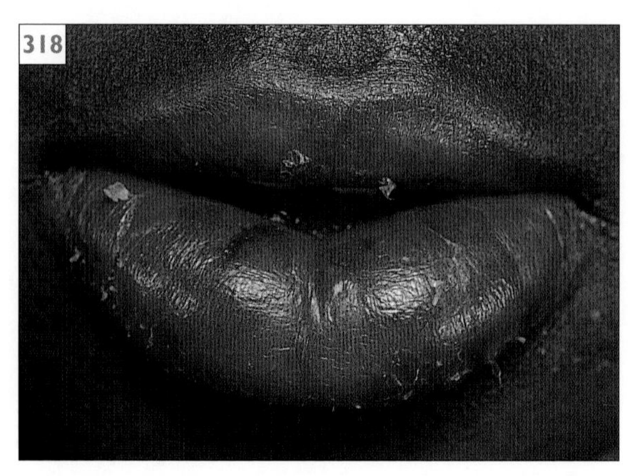

318 Granulomatous cheilitis.

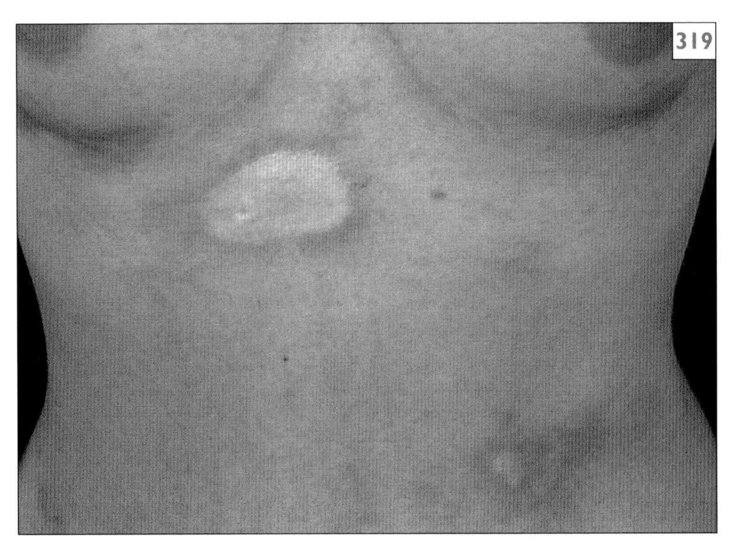

319 Morphoea.

Morphoea appears to be an immunologically mediated disease with altered circulating cytokines and fibroblast function. In some countries an association has been reported with *Borrelia burgdorferi* infection. Morphoea-like changes particularly involving the hands may occur following occupational exposure to chemicals including polyvinyl chloride, organic solvents, and pesticides.

DIFFERENTIAL DIAGNOSIS

Scleredema of Buschke usually develops more acutely and lacks the pallor of morphoea. Lichen sclerosus has a predilection for the anogenital area, generalized morphoea shares histological features with systemic sclerosis but lacks extracutanous disease. Eosinophilic fasciitis is characterized by tissue and peripheral eosinophilia and deeper fibrosis.

INVESTIGATIONS

Histological confirmation with a skin biopsy. No further investigations are needed for localized disease, but *Borrelia* serology should be checked if there is a possibility of Lyme disease. Full blood count, ESR, autoantibodies, renal and liver function tests should be tested in more widespread disease.

TREATMENT

Topical or intralesional corticosteroids and calcipotriol may help localized disease. Many systemic agents have been reported to help morphoea, including PUVA, corticosteroids, methotrexate, retinoids, and antimalarials.

Systemic sclerosis

DEFINITION AND CLINICAL FEATURES

Systemic sclerosis is a disorder of unknown aetiology which causes progressive persistent fibrosis particularly in the skin, lower respiratory tract, gut, and kidney. It frequently presents with cutaneous involvement. The earliest feature is usually Raynaud's phenomenon. Other early signs include swelling of the hands, and ulceration of the fingers which may progress to digital gangrene. Similar changes may occur on the feet. Progressive dermal fibrosis restricts movement of the fingers and gives the skin a tight waxy appearance (sclerodactyly) (**320**). There is resorption of the distal finger pulps associated with acro-osteolysis. Mat-like telangiectasia is often widespread and the face shows a beaked nose, a small mouth with restricted opening, and radial furrowing (rhagades) (**321**). Involvement of other organs includes pulmonary fibrosis, oesophageal hypomotility causing dysphagia and aspiration, malabsorption, and malignant hypertension. Women are affected more frequently than men.

DIFFERENTIAL DIAGNOSIS

Generalized morphoea. Occupational scleroderma may sometimes resemble systemic sclerosis very closely. Always ask a patient with apparently idiopathic systemic sclerosis their job!

INVESTIGATIONS

The diagnosis of systemic sclerosis is established by finding evidence of involvement of internal organs, for example with a barium swallow, renal function tests, chest radiograph, and lung function tests. Autoantibodies including ANA, ENAs such as anticentromere antibody and anti-SCL70, anti-Jo-1, and antiRo/SS-A are often raised. The ESR may be raised as an acute phase response.

TREATMENT

Symptomatic treatment is important as there is no specific therapy which alters the disease course. Patients should keep their hands warm and avoid trauma because of poor wound healing. Heated gloves help and smoking should be avoided. Vasodilators may improve peripheral blood flow and infusion of prostacyclin may be required for severe digital ischaemia. Extracorporeal photopheresis, plasmapheresis, and plasma exchange with prednisolone or cyclophosphamide have been used for severe disease.

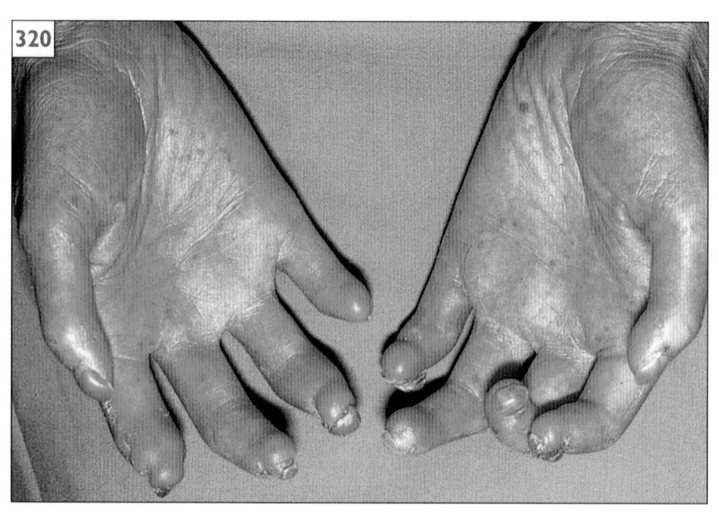

320 Systemic sclerosis.

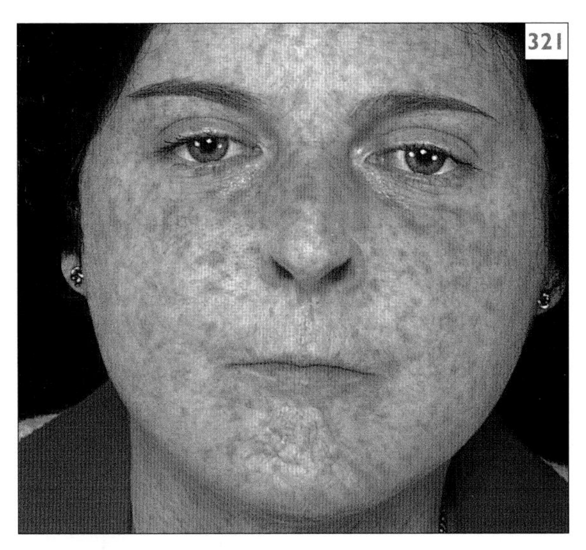

321 Systemic sclerosis.

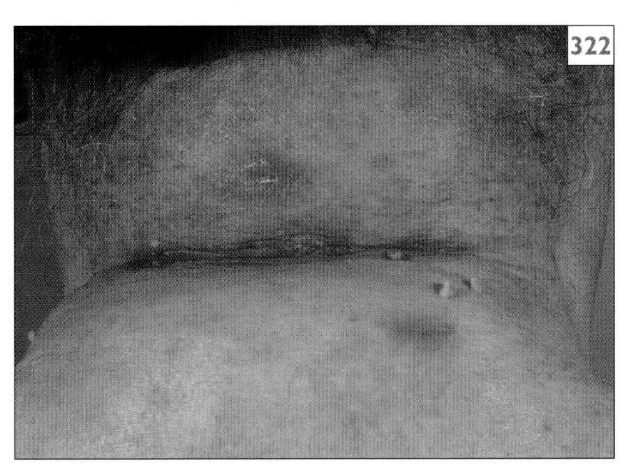

322 Sclerederma of Bushke.

Scleredema of Buschke

DEFINITION AND CLINICAL FEATURES

A rare condition in which areas of firm, indurated skin (**322**) appear spontaneously with dermal thickening due to an increase in ground substance. It may occur acutely after an upper respiratory infection, particularly in children, or develop slowly in adults with diabetes, who often have arteriopathic complications. It has also been reported with paraproteinaemia.

INVESTIGATIONS

The ASO titre may be raised in post-streptococcal cases. Fasting glucose and protein electrophoresis for paraproteinaemia in adults.

TREATMENT

No effective treatment has been established but the condition may resolve over months to years.

Dermatomyositis

DEFINITION AND CLINICAL FEATURES

Dermatomyositis is a rare disorder of skin, muscles, and blood vessels which causes a characteristic rash on the face and hands, in association with muscle weakness and inflammation. There are two distinct forms, a childhood variant which usually starts under the age of 10 and an adult variant which mainly affects the 40–60 age group. In adults the disease is commonly associated with an underlying malignancy.

The characteristic eruption of dermatomyositis is a violaceous or heliotrope rash on the face with periorbital swelling (**323**). This eruption may extend in a photosensitive distribution on to the neck and upper chest. The skin over the hands shows dilated nail fold capillaries and ragged cuticles (**324**). Gottron's papules – erythematosquamous plaques – appear over the interphalangeal and metacarpophalangeal joints in association with Dowling's lines, which are similar linear lesions on the dorsal surface of the fingers over the metacarpals.

In addition to myositis involving skeletal muscle, smooth muscle may be involved, causing dysphagia and dysphonia as well as impaired intestinal motility. Pulmonary fibrosis, myocarditis, and retinitis are well-recognized features. Cutaneous calcinosis is a late manifestation which is particularly prominent in the childhood variant. Livedo reticularis and cutaneous ulceration are rare.

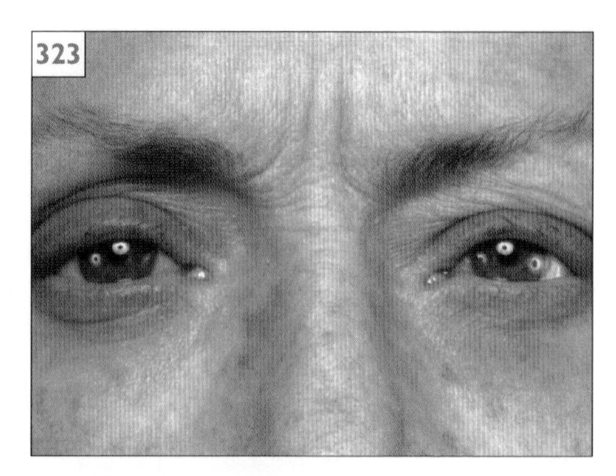

323 Dermatomyositis.

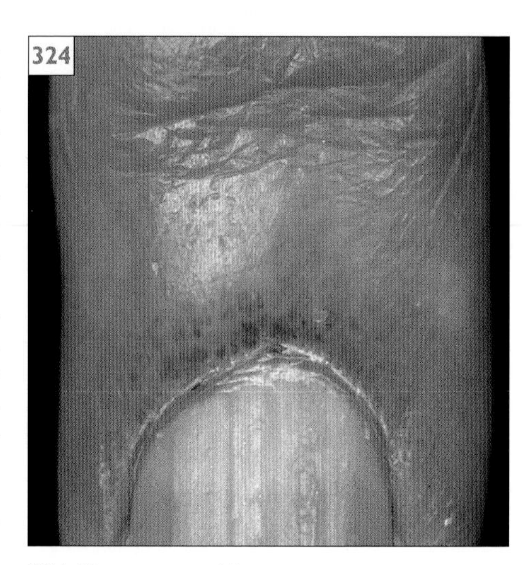

324 Dermatomyositis.

DIFFERENTIAL DIAGNOSIS

Mixed connective tissue disease, systemic sclerosis, systemic lupus erythematosus.

INVESTIGATIONS

Skin and muscle biopsies are helpful, but the histological changes may be absent or minimal. Electromyography and muscle enzymes including creatine phosphokinase (CPK) may be abnormal. Autoantibodies, including extractable nuclear antigens and anti-Jo-1, should be sought. Adults should be thoroughly examined and investigated for an occult carcinoma.

TREATMENT

High-dose oral corticosteroids are required in almost all patients with muscle involvement, the dosage depending on the degree of disease activity. A steroid-sparing drug such as azathioprine or methotrexate may be added later for long-term disease control. Calcinosis is a good prognostic factor, but responds poorly to treatment.

Discoid lupus erythematosus

DEFINITION AND CLINICAL FEATURES

Discoid lupus erythematosus is an uncommon chronic skin disorder consisting of localized erythematosquamous plaques which heal with atrophy, scarring, and pigmentary change. The plaques are commonly present on the head and neck but may also be found on the hands and occasionally in a more generalized distribution. They show erythema, scaling, follicular plugging, telangiectasia, hyper- and hypopigmentation, and scarring (**325**, **326**). Plaques may be found in the scalp and a similar process may involve the vermilion border of the lips and the oral mucosa. Chilblain-like lesions may also occur.

DIFFERENTIAL DIAGNOSIS

Granuloma faciale, lichen planus, lupus vulgaris, sarcoidosis, and other chronic granulomatous infections.

INVESTIGATIONS

Histology is characteristic with liquefaction degeneration of the basal cell layer of the epidermis, degeneration of dermal connective tissue, and a patchy lymphocytic infiltrate particularly around appendages. A full blood count, ESR, and ANA should be done to exclude the possibility of systemic involvement.

TREATMENT

Lesions may be aggravated by sunlight, so sunblocks and protective clothing should be worn. Potent or superpotent corticosteroids usually help but treatment must be supervised carefully. Oral corticosteroids, antimalarial drugs, and thalidomide can improve recalcitrant disease. Smoking may reduce the effectiveness of antimalarial therapy in cutaneous lupus erythematosus.

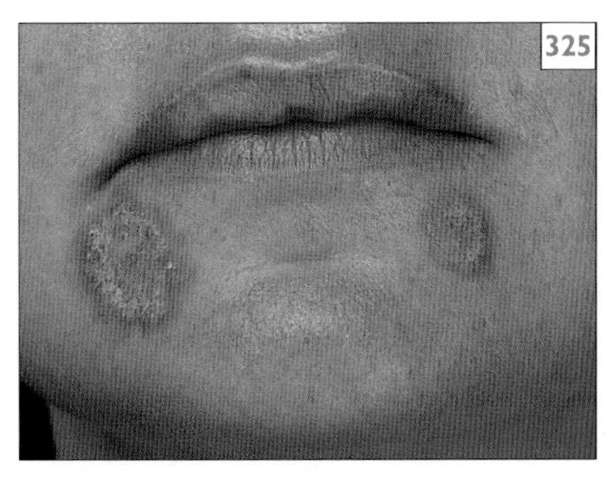

325 Discoid lupus erythematosus.

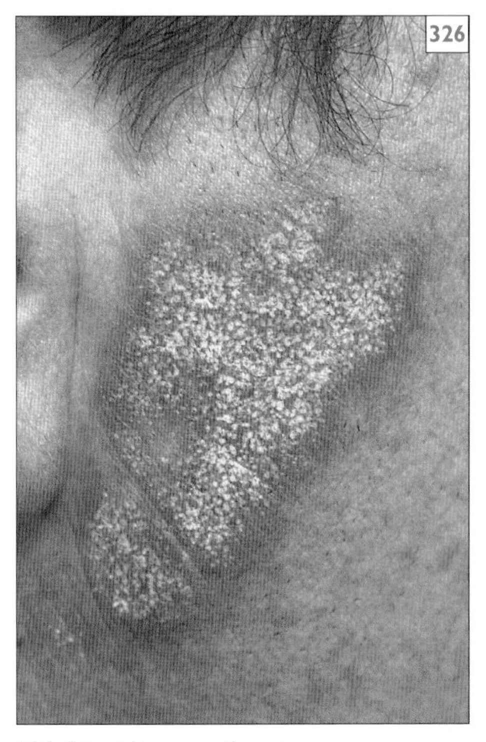

326 Discoid lupus erythematosus.

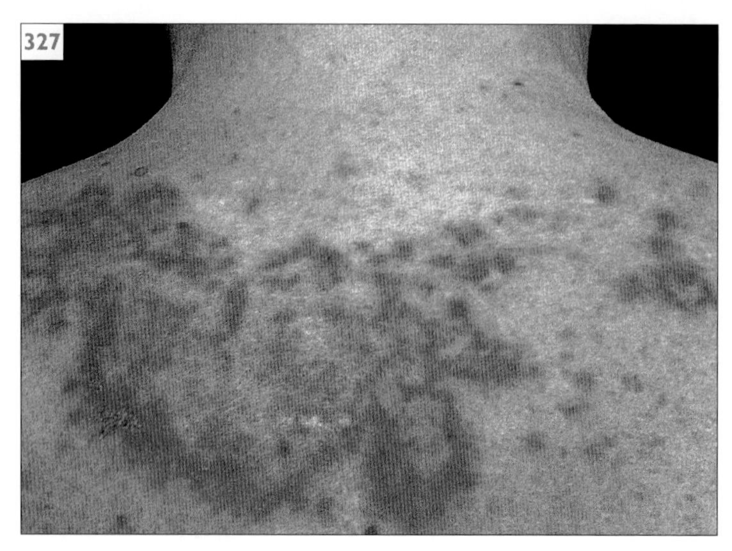

327 Subacute cutaneous lupus erythematosus.

Subacute cutaneous lupus erythematosus

DEFINITION AND CLINICAL FEATURES

This specific subset of lupus is characterized by a widespread symmetrical erythematosquamous eruption, which may be papulosquamous or annular and polycyclic (**327**). This is most prominent on the upper trunk neck and upper arms and is associated with photosensitivity and the presence of anti-Ro antibodies. Lesions resolve without scarring, in contrast to discoid lupus erythematosus. Children of mothers with subacute cutaneous lupus erythematosus are at risk of congenital heart block and neonatal lupus erythematosus. Systemic features such as arthritis are common, and patients may fulfil diagnostic criteria for SLE but their prognosis is usually good. A number of drugs have been reported to trigger SLE including thiazide diuretics, griseofulvin, terbinafine, calcium channel blockers, and etanercept.

DIFFERENTIAL DIAGNOSIS

Psoriasis, systemic lupus erythematosus, generalized discoid lupus erythematosus.

INVESTIGATIONS

Full blood count, urea, electrolytes and creatinine, liver function tests, ANA, anti-Ro, anti-La, and anti-double-stranded DNA antibodies. A thorough drug history should be taken to exclude drug-induced disease.

TREATMENT

Sun avoidance measures. Antimalarial drugs such as hydroxychloroquine and mepacrine may be used in combination. Oral corticosteroids, retinoids, and immunosuppressive agents are effective for more severe disease.

Systemic lupus erythematosus

DEFINITION AND CLINICAL FEATURES

This is a systemic multiorgan inflammatory disease most commonly affecting the skin, joints, and vasculature in association with immunological abnormalities. SLE is uncommon, and young Afro-Caribbean women are at increased risk. Non-organ specific autoantibodies are the hallmark of SLE, especially anti-double-stranded DNA antibodies and anti-Sm antibodies.

The rash of systemic lupus erythematosus consists of maculopapular erythema with fine scaling particularly on light-exposed areas (**328**, **329**). The classical butterfly facial rash is not always evident. Periungual telangiectasia is a common feature, as is oral mucosal ulceration and diffuse hair fall. Photosensitivity may be marked and cause acute lesions with blistering. Other features of acute systemic lupus erythematosus include fever, polyarthralgia, nephritis, leucopenia, serositis causing pleuritic chest pain, pericarditis, pneumonitis, and encephalopathy. The skin disease is non-scarring.

DIFFERENTIAL DIAGNOSIS

Mixed connective tissue disease, discoid LE. The facial rash may resemble dermatitis, dermatomyositis, erysipelas, or rosacea.

INVESTIGATIONS

Anti-double-stranded DNA antibodies are diagnostic. A full biochemical and haematological profile should be carried out. Haemolytic anaemia, leukopenia, lymphopenia, or thrombocytopenia and elevated ESR may occur. Renal function should be thoroughly evaluated for evidence of renal involvement. Serum complement may be reduced. Antiphospholipid antibodies including lupus anticoagulant may be positive and are associated with thrombosis and early miscarriage. Histology of lesional skin may be supportive and direct immunofluorescence can demonstrate immunoglobulin deposition at the dermo-epidermal junction in a lesional skin in both SLE and DLE ('lupus band').

TREATMENT

SLE may be precipitated or exacerbated by sunlight, stress, infection, and a range of drugs which should therefore be avoided. Corticosteroids are required in the acute phase with additional immunosuppressive drugs for unresponsive disease or as steroid-sparing agents. Antimalarial drugs are less effective than in DLE. The prognosis of SLE is very variable, with survival related to the severity of organ involvement and frequency of exacerbations.

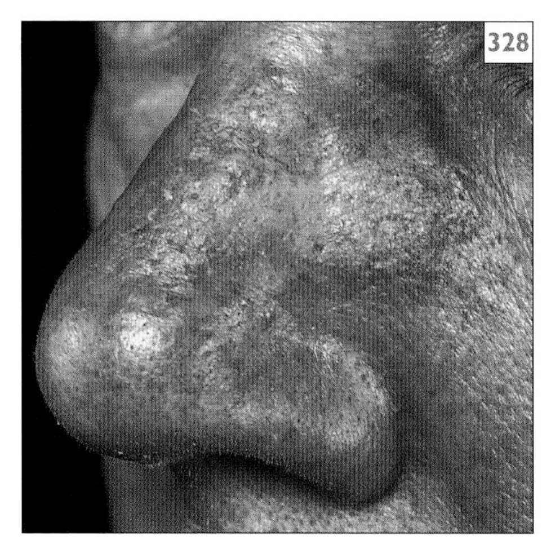

328 Systemic lupus erythematosus.

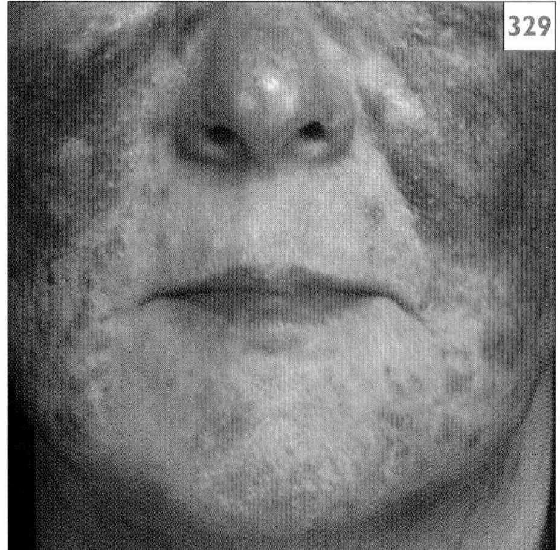

329 Systemic lupus erythematosus.

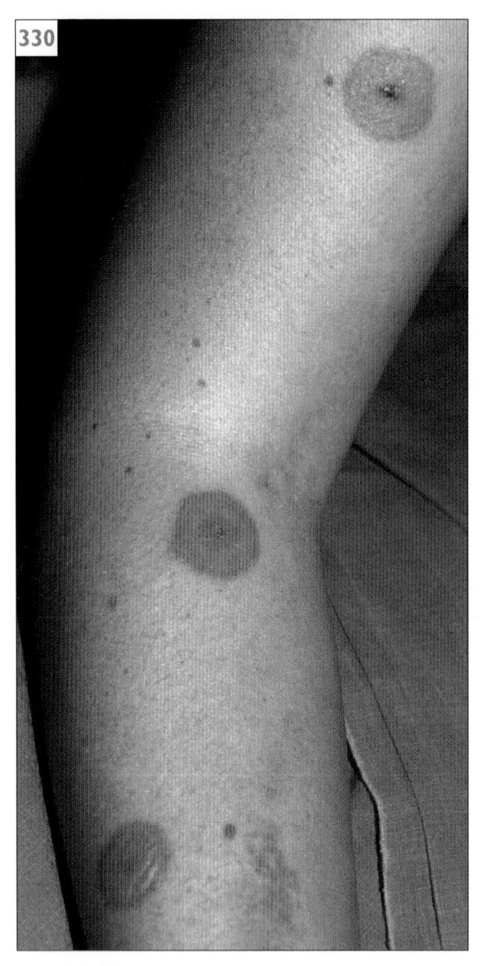

330 Erythema multiforme.

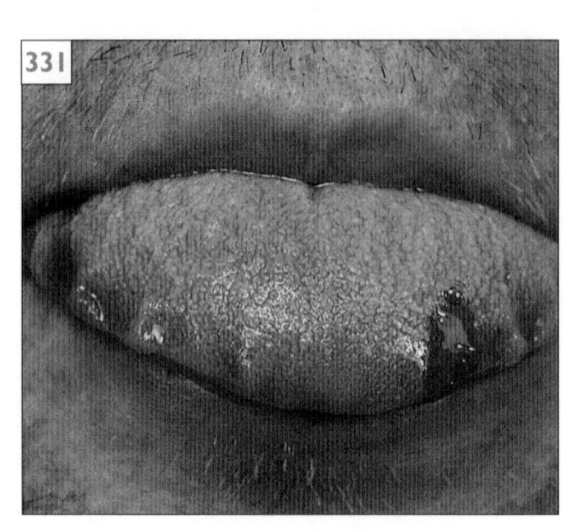

331 Erythema multiforme on the tongue.

Erythema multiforme

DEFINITION AND CLINICAL FEATURES

An acute inflammatory eruption affecting the skin and mucosa, with characteristic target or iris lesions. Potential triggering factors can be identified in about 50% of cases, most commonly herpes simplex virus or mycoplasma infection. Lesions may be macular, papular, or urticarial. The target lesion consists of an erythematous ring with dusky centre and inflammatory border (**330**). The eruption is most severe on the hands, feet, and extensor surfaces but can become widespread. Oral and genital ulcers and conjunctivitis may also occur (**331**). Attacks may be recurrent (see also bullous erythema multiforme, p. 60).

DIFFERENTIAL DIAGNOSIS

Drug eruptions, lupus erythematosus, urticarial vasculitis.

INVESTIGATIONS

Histology usually shows characteristic changes with dermal inflammation and degeneration of the lower epidermal cells.

TREATMENT

The eruption usually resolves within 2–3 weeks. Localized forms only require symptomatic treatment. Eye involvement requires the early help of an ophthalmologist. The value of systemic corticosteroids is debated, but a short reducing course tapered over a period of 1–2 weeks may be given. Adequate hydration must be maintained with intravenous fluids if there is severe oral ulceration. Long-term prophylactic use of oral antiviral drugs may help prevent relapses in patients suffering from recurrent erythema multiforme.

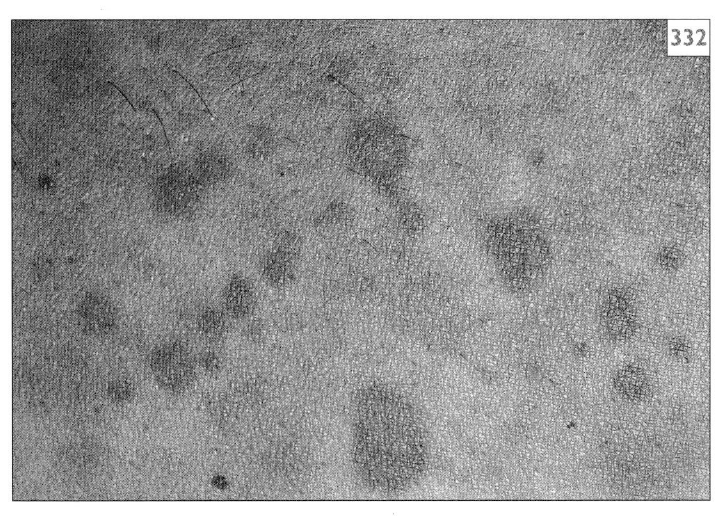

332 Still's disease.

Still's disease

DEFINITION AND CLINICAL FEATURES

Still's disease is predominantly seen in childhood. Its features include arthritis, spiking fever, sore throat, lymphadenopathy, serositis, and a transient maculopapular rash. The characteristic rash is seen in about 25% of patients and consists of non-pruritic erythematous macules with central and perilesional pallor (**332**). It occurs synchronously with a fever in the evening and is absent in the mornings. The disorder is persistent and frequently follows a sore throat.

DIFFERENTIAL DIAGNOSIS

Urticaria, reactive erythemas including erythema marginatum (rheumatic fever), lupus erythematosus.

INVESTIGATIONS

ESR is raised. Full blood count may show a neutrophilia. LFTs may show hepatitis.

TREATMENT

Non-steroidal anti-inflammatory drugs are the first line of treatment but systemic corticosteroids may be required.

DRUG ERUPTIONS

Cutaneous eruptions are one of the most frequent forms of adverse drug reaction. Their true incidence is difficult to determine because mild and transitory eruptions are often not recorded and because skin disorders may be falsely attributed to drugs. Certain patient groups are at increased risk of developing an adverse drug reaction. The ampicillin rash seen in patients with infectious mononucleosis is a classical example (**333**). The elderly and patients with acquired immunodeficiency syndrome (AIDS) appear predisposed to adverse drug reactions.

Antibiotics, non-steroidal anti-inflammatory drugs, antiepileptic drugs, and cardiac drugs such as ACE inhibitors, calcium channel-blockers, and amiodarone are commonly implicated. In patients taking multiple drugs it may be difficult to pinpoint the culprit and withdrawal of the most likely agent is usually necessary. The diagnosis may be confirmed by rechallenge, but the risks of this must be carefully considered and often outweigh the benefits. Patch testing may occasionally be diagnostic in eczematous and exanthematic eruptions.

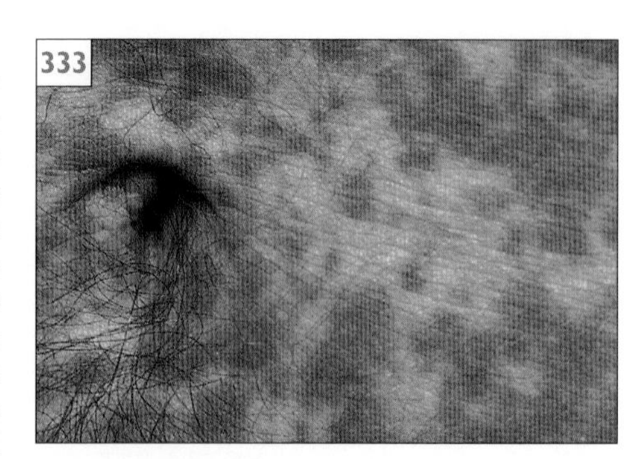

333 Ampicillin rash.

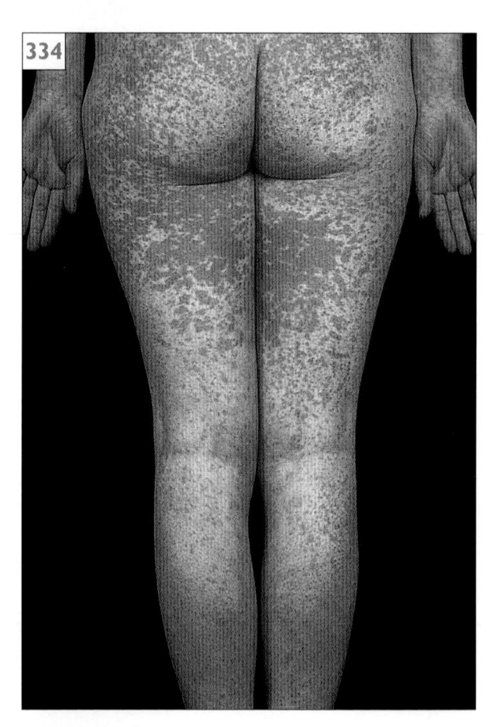

334 Exanthematic drug reaction.

Exanthematic (maculopapular) **reactions**

DEFINITION AND CLINICAL FEATURES

The commonest of all cutaneous drug eruptions, occurring in 2–3% of patients, and seen with almost any drug up to 3 weeks after administration. Typically, there is a fine erythematous morbilliform maculopapular eruption of the trunk and extremities that may become confluent (**334**). Exanthematic drug reactions often start in areas of trauma or pressure and can be very variable, with either predominantly small papules, or large macules, a reticular eruption, or polycyclic or sheet-like erythema. Intertriginous areas may be favoured, palmar and plantar involvement can occur, and the face is often spared. Purpuric lesions are common on the legs and erosive stomatitis may develop. Drug exanthem may be accompanied by fever and pruritus. These eruptions usually fade with desquamation, sometimes with postinflammatory hyperpigmentation. Viral exanthems may resemble drug exanthems but usually start on the face and spread to the trunk, and are more often accompanied by systemic upset, fever, and lymphadenopathy. Tissue and blood eosinophilia are suggestive of drug rashes.

DRUG ASSOCIATIONS

Drugs commonly causing exanthematic reactions include: ampicillin and penicillin, sulfonamides, phenylbutazone, phenytoin, carbamazepine, gold, and gentamicin.

Acute generalized exanthematous pustulosis (toxic pustuloderma)

DEFINITION, CLINICAL FEATURES AND DRUG ASSOCIATIONS

An acute pustular eruption in association with drug therapy. The main differential is pustular psoriasis. Numerous small non-follicular pustules develop in crops with a predilection for the large flexures in association with a more generalized exanthem (**335**). There may be an associated fever and eosinophilia. Most cases have been reported in association with penicillins or macrolides, but many other drugs have been implicated.

DRESS syndrome (drug rash with eosinophilia and systemic symptoms)

DEFINITION, CLINICAL FEATURES AND DRUG ASSOCIATIONS

A drug-induced delayed multi-organ hypersensitivity syndrome characterized by a rash with eosinophilia and systemic symptoms, usually starting after 3–6 weeks of drug therapy. The cutaneous features include facial oedema with infiltrated papules, and a generalized exanthematous or pustular rash which evolves into an exfoliative dermatitis. Other features are fever, lymphadenopathy, haematological abnormalities (eosinophilia, atypical lymphocytosis), hepatitis, pneumonitis, and myocarditis. Management is usually with oral corticosteroids.

A range of drugs, especially anticonvulsants and antibiotics, have been reported to cause DRESS syndrome.

Bullous drug eruptions

DEFINITION, CLINICAL FEATURES AND DRUG ASSOCIATIONS

This is a heterogeneous group involving many different clinical reactions and mechanisms. Pemphigus and pemphigoid may be drug induced (see pp. 54 and 56), as may pseudoporphyria, a porphyria-like disorder with normal porphyrin metabolism. Penicillamine-induced pemphigus is usually of the foliaceus type, while captopril causes a pemphigus vulgaris-type eruption. Cicatricial pemphigoid has been described with clonidine and previously with practolol. Fixed eruptions and drug-induced vasculitis may have a bullous component, while toxic epidermal necrolysis (TEN) (see p. 170) leads to extensive blistering. A number of drugs may induce phototoxic bullae (see p. 172). Bullae, often at pressure points, can be present in patients comatose after overdosage with barbiturates, methadone, tricyclic antidepressants, and benzodiazepines.

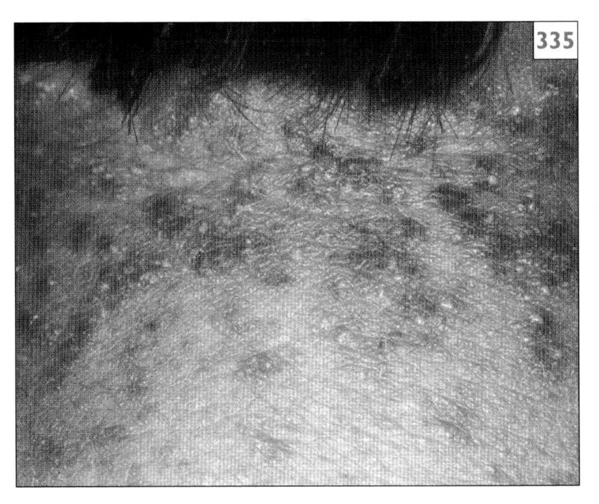

335 Acute generalized exanthematous pustulosis.

Urticaria

DEFINITION AND CLINICAL FEATURES

Urticaria is the second most common allergic cutaneous reaction to drugs. Underlying mechanisms include Type 1 (IgE antibody-mediated) hypersensitivity reaction, immune complex-mediated reactions (serum sickness), and direct liberation of histamine from mast cells. Urticarial lesions are inflamed and oedematous plaques and polycyclic wheals (**336**) which resolve without surface scaling or dryness (see p.32). Urticaria usually resolves quickly when the offending drug is withdrawn but may continue episodically for several weeks.

DRUG ASSOCIATIONS

Penicillin and salicylates are common provokers. Other commonly implicated agents include blood products, vaccines, radiocontrast agents, NSAIDs, opiates, cephalosporins, and ACE inhibitors. Chronic idiopathic urticaria may also be exacerbated by drugs including aspirin and NSAIDs, and opiates.

Vasculitis

DEFINITION, CLINICAL FEATURES

Vasculitis is a manifestation of immune complex disease with inflammation and necrosis of blood vessels (see page 143). Drug-induced vasculitis may involve the skin and/or internal organs. The pattern of the cutaneous eruption may indicate the calibre of the involved vessel. Capillaritis is characterized by cayenne pepper spots of pigmentation, venulitis by palpable purpura (**337**, and arteritis by painful nodules. All arise most commonly on the lower extremities.

DRUG ASSOCIATIONS

Many groups of drugs have been associated with vasculitis, including thiazides, sulfonamides, penicillin, fluoroquinolone antibiotics, ACE inhibitors, cimetidine, allopurinol, hydralazine, quinidine, phenylbutazone, serum products, and radiographic contrast media.

Stevens–Johnson syndrome

DEFINITION AND CLINICAL FEATURES

Stevens–Johnson syndrome is a severe variant of erythema multiforme (EM) characterized by widespread involvement of mucosal surfaces, accompanied by systemic symptoms.

A prodrome of fever and malaise is followed by eruption of mucosal bullae, with or without the widespread cutaneous target lesions of EM. Mucosal surfaces, commonly the oral mucosa, respiratory tract, and conjunctivae may be extensively involved and secondary infection is common (**338**, **339**). Morbidity is significant, with pain, ocular complications, respiratory compromise, dysuria, and difficulty maintaining adequate oral fluid intake. The value of systemic corticosteroid treatment is still debated.

DRUG ASSOCIATIONS

Erythema multiforme (see p. 164) is more commonly precipitated by various infections, but may occasionally be drug-induced, while a drug cause is likely for Stevens–Johnson syndrome. Commonly incriminated are sulfonamides/co-trimoxazole, barbiturates, phenylbutazone, phenytoin, carbamazepine, phenothiazines, chlorpropamide, thiazide diuretics, and malaria prophylaxis.

Fixed drug eruption

DEFINITION AND CLINICAL FEATURES

A cutaneous reaction that characteristically recurs in the same site(s) each time the drug is administered. Usually a single drug is involved but cross-sensitivity to related drugs may occur. Typical lesions are well-demarcated, round or oval, erythematous, dusky plaques (**340**) with subsequent postinflammatory hyperpigmentation. Bullae are quite common (**341**). Lesions arise within 8 hours of drug administration and are commoner on the extremities, genitalia, and perianal areas. Mucous membranes may be involved.

DRUG ASSOCIATIONS

A large number of drugs have been reported, but especially tetracyclines, sulfonamides, phenolphthalein, and oxyphenbutazone.

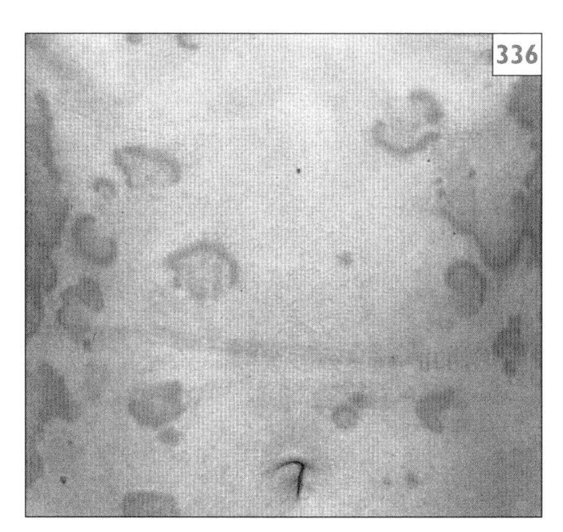

336 Urticarial drug reaction.

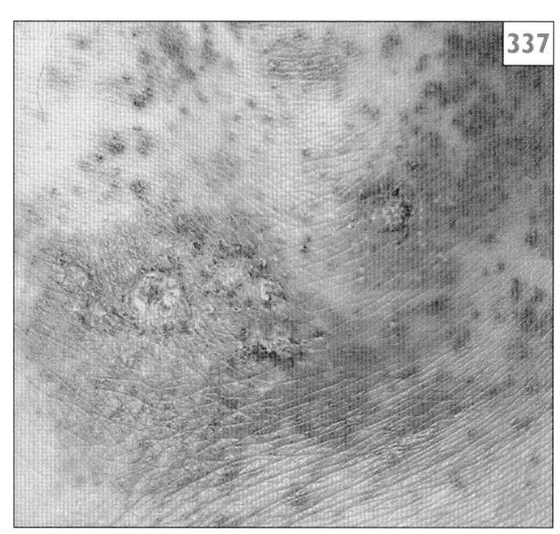

337 Drug-induced vasculitis.

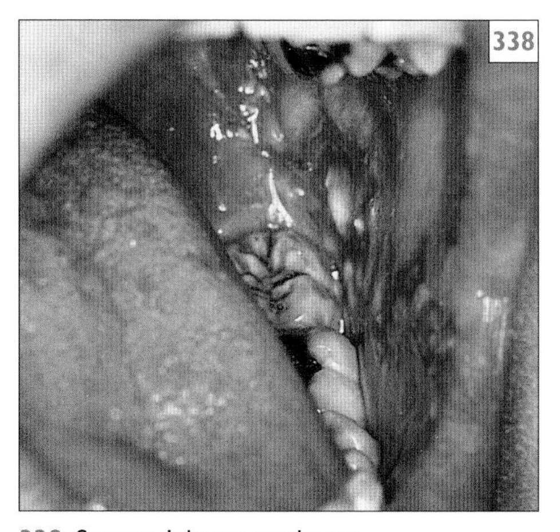

338 Stevens–Johnson syndrome.

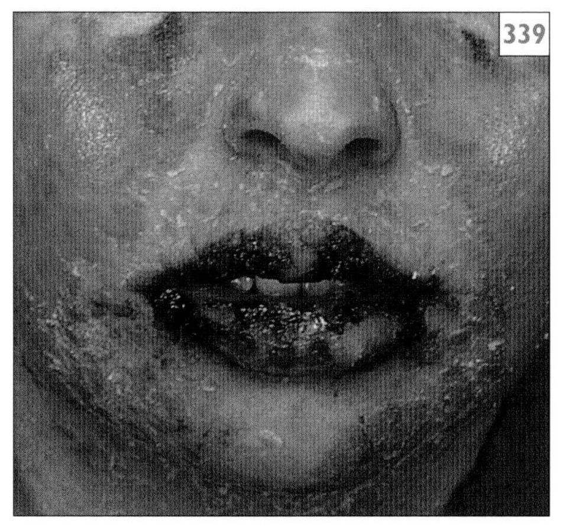

339 Stevens–Johnson syndrome.

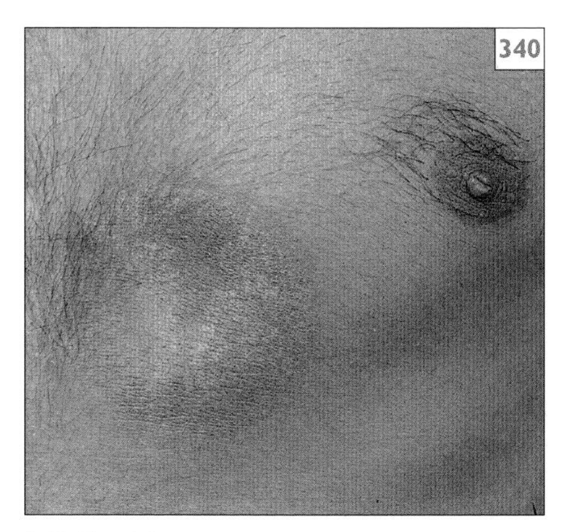

340 Fixed drug eruption.

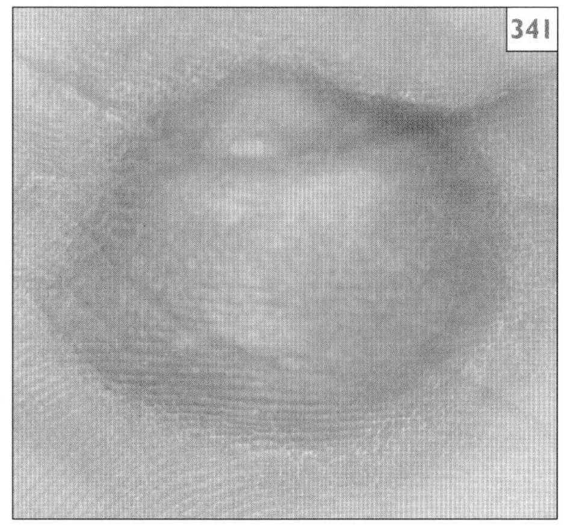

341 Fixed drug eruption.

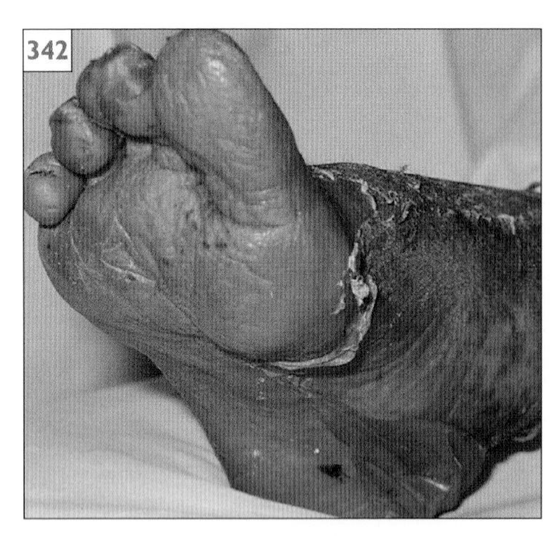

342 Toxic epidermal necrolysis.

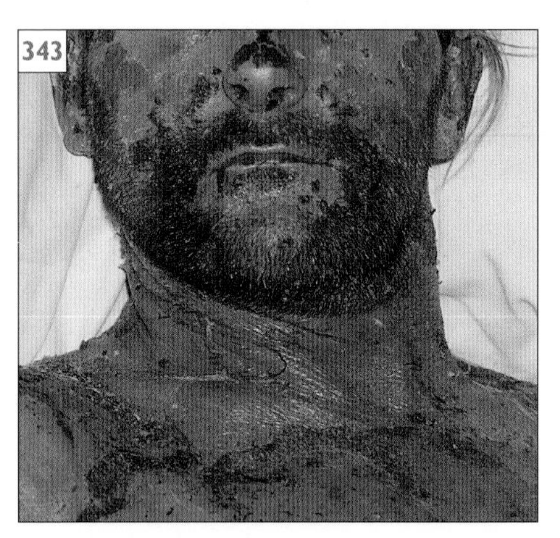

343 Toxic epidermal necrolysis.

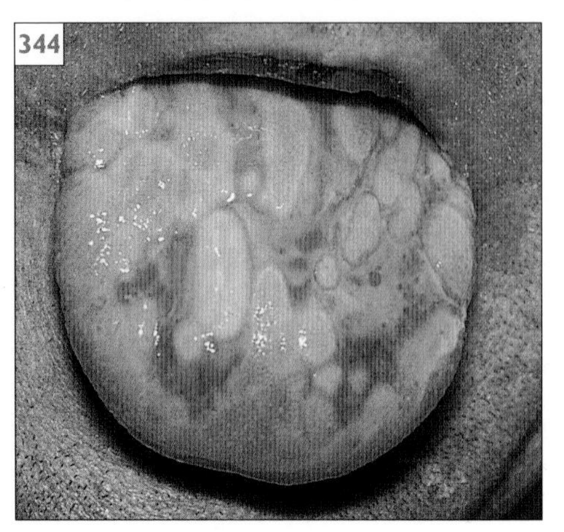

344 Toxic epidermal necrolysis.

Toxic epidermal necrolysis (TEN)

DEFINITION AND CLINICAL FEATURES

A life-threatening dermatosis characterized by full-thickness epidermal necrolysis and exfoliation, affecting more than 30% of the body surface. Often a prodrome of 1–2 days precedes a morbilliform or generalized erythema of the face and extremities. This is rapidly followed by blister formation with confluence into large, flaccid bullae that are easily ruptured, resulting in sloughing of large sheets of epidermis (**342**, **343**). Mucous membranes are usually severely affected, including the oral mucosa (**344**), conjunctivae, trachea, bronchi, and anogenital region. Nail shedding may also occur. Systemic involvement is reflected by fever, leucocytosis, electrolyte imbalance, and elevated hepatic enzymes. Complications of secondary infection and multi-organ failure are similar to those of burns victims and there is a significant mortality. Pigmentary changes and a sicca syndrome are frequent sequelae. Management is essentially supportive in an intensive care or burns unit. Other treatments such as early high-dose corticosteroids, intravenous immunoglobulin, or ciclosporin remain unproven due to the rarity of this condition.

DRUG ASSOCIATIONS

A drug aetiology is identified in up to 75% of cases. Many drugs have been associated but most frequently implicated are sulfonamides, NSAIDs, phenytoin, penicillins, allopurinol, carbamazepine, and barbiturates.

Lichenoid eruptions

DEFINITION AND CLINICAL FEATURES

A drug eruption that may closely mimic idiopathic lichen planus (see pp. 47 and 86). Histologically, there is additional focal parakeratosis and eosinophilia. Typical lesions are violaceous, flat-topped, shiny papules. Lichenoid drug eruptions tend to be extensive (**345**) and may be linked with or develop into an exfoliative dermatitis (**346**). The eruption may develop weeks or months after initiation of therapy and usually only resolves slowly with withdrawal of the inciting agent. A light-exposed distribution may occur with thiazides. Lichenoid allergic contact dermatitis may also occur after exposure to colour film developers.

DRUG ASSOCIATIONS

Lichenoid drug reactions are especially seen with gold, penicillamine, beta-blockers, captopril, thiazide diuretics, tetracyclines, antimalarials, and anti-tuberculous agents.

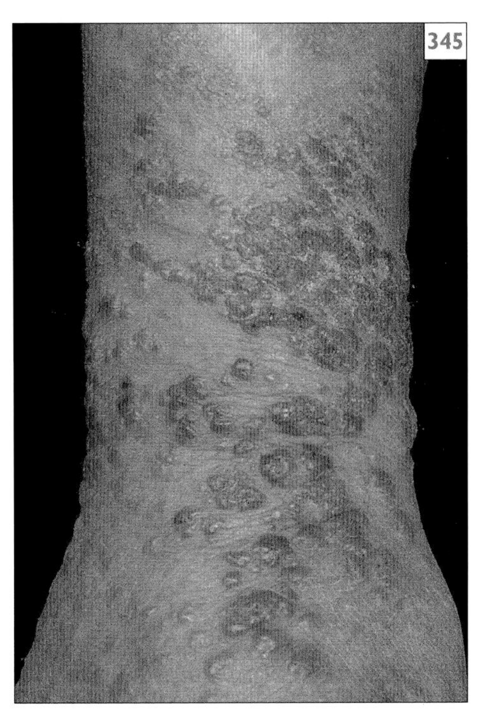

345 Lichenoid drug eruption.

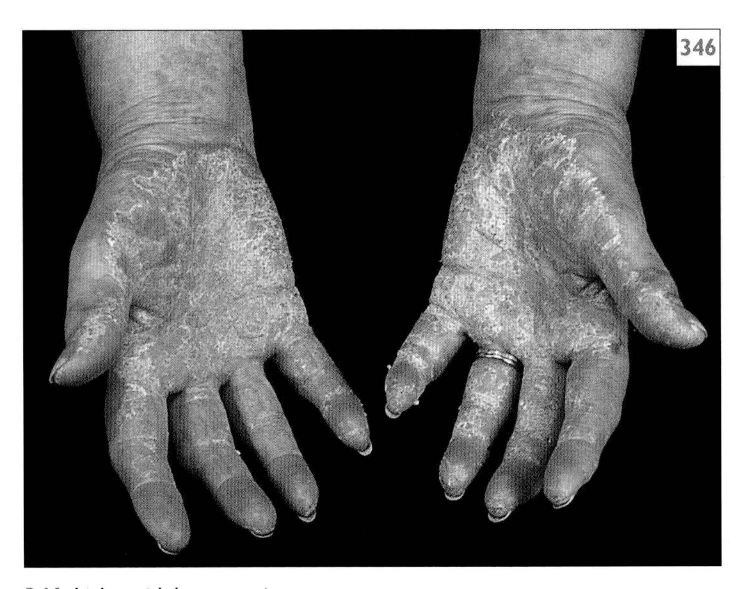

346 Lichenoid drug eruption.

Photosensitivity

DEFINITION AND CLINICAL FEATURES

Drug–light reactions may be phototoxic or photoallergic. Clinically, it may not be possible to distinguish between the two and some drugs may produce both. Phototoxic reactions are the more common and will occur in almost all individuals, given sufficient drug dosage and light exposure. Photoallergic reactions require the interaction of the drug, UV light, and the immune system.

Phototoxic reactions present as exaggerated sunburn with erythema, oedema, blistering, weeping, desquamation, and subsequent hyperpigmentation on exposed areas. Phototoxic eruptions appear within 24 hours of drug exposure and resolve within 1 week; photoallergic eruptions may take weeks or months to resolve. With photoallergic reactions the eruption is variable. Erythematous plaques, eczema, vesicles, and bullae all occur. The distribution is characteristically in sun-exposed areas, including the face and neck (**347**), and the backs of the hands and forearms. Photo-oncholysis (**348**) can occur with both phototoxic and photoallergic reactions.

DRUG ASSOCIATIONS

Common associations with photosensitivity include NSAIDs, tetracyclines (especially doxycycline), sulfonamides, thiazide diuretics, and cardiac drugs, especially ACE inhibitors and amiodarone.

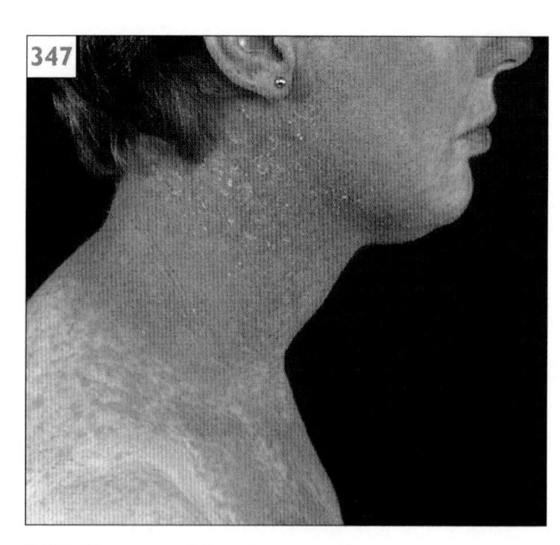

347 Photosensitive drug reaction.

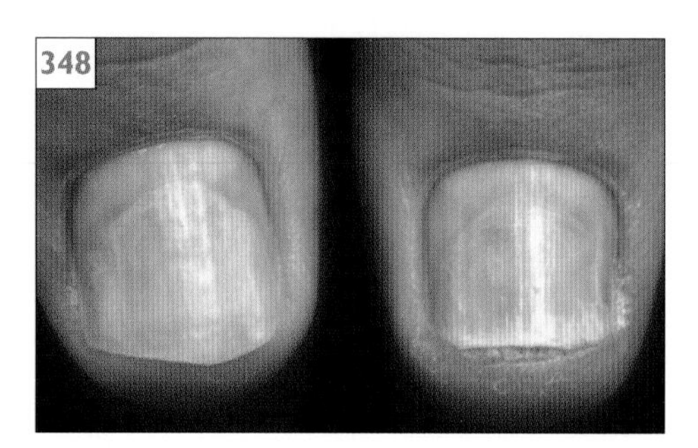

348 Photo-onycholysis.

Gingival hyperplasia

DEFINITION AND CLINICAL FEATURES

Drugs cause gingival hyperplasia by inducing neutropenia and immunosuppression or by altering fibroblast proliferation and metabolism. Ciclosporin affects both the immune system and the fibroblast.

Gingival hyperplasia related to ciclosporin is usually confined to the free gingival margin and the interdental papilla. Associated bleeding is common. Calcium-channel blockers (especially nifedipine) may cause a nodular or a diffuse gingival hyperplasia.

DRUG ASSOCIATIONS

Ciclosporin, nifedipine, and phenytoin.

Iododerma

DEFINITION AND CLINICAL FEATURES

Prolonged administration of small doses of iodide or bromide may provoke eruptions with or without mucosal or systemic symptoms. Acneiform or vegetating masses are the most distinctive. Iodine can cause urticaria, acneiform papules and pustules, tense haemorrhagic bullae arising on plaques of erythema, and hypertrophic vegetating masses. In bromism, acneiform and vegetating lesions occur more, and bullae less, frequently than with iodism. Vegetating iododermas/bromodermas may be very florid, with heaped-up masses of hypertrophic epithelium with many pustules simulating pemphigus vegetans or a granulomatous infection. Serious and even fatal reactions have been caused by radiographic contrast media in sensitized individuals.

PART 2

Tumours

- Benign tumours arising from the epidermis
- Benign tumours arising from the dermis
- Benign tumours arising from skin appendages
- Benign melanocytic lesions
- Malignant neoplasms and their precursors
- Cutaneous lymphoproliferative disorders

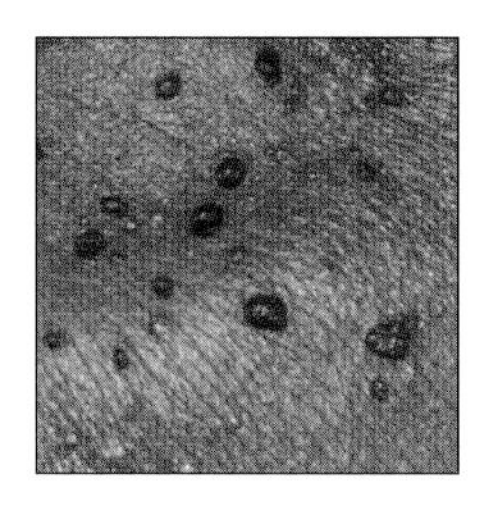
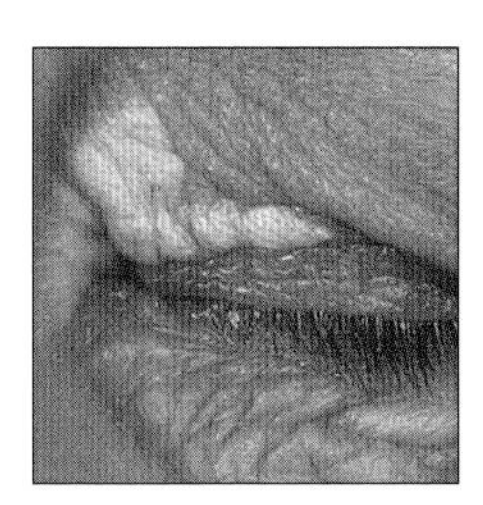
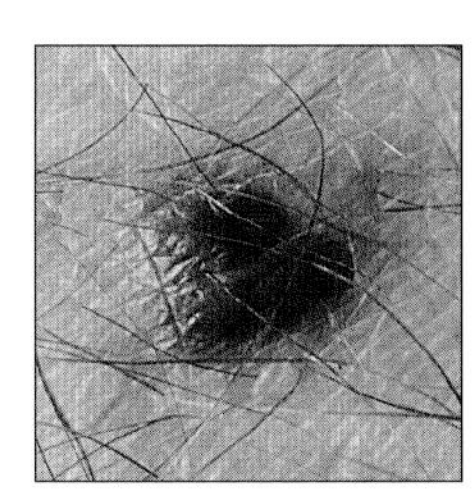
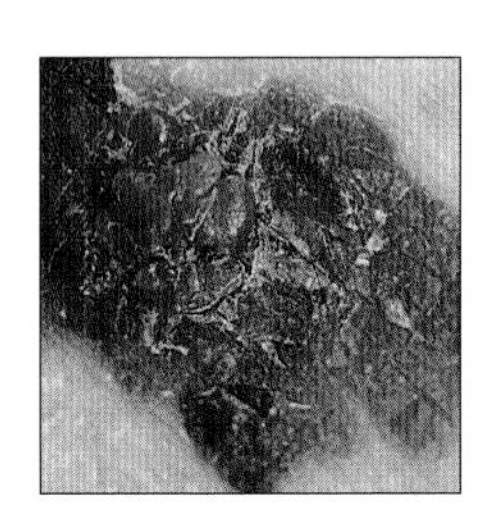

BENIGN TUMOURS ARISING FROM THE EPIDERMIS

Epidermal naevus

DEFINITION AND CLINICAL FEATURES

A naevus composed of keratinocytes which arises during development from an abnormal clone of cells. Almost all epidermal naevi follow the pattern of the lines demonstrated by Blaschko, which are thought to represent the routes of ectodermal cell migration from the neural crest during embryogenesis. Epidermal naevi are usually present at birth and affect approximately 0.1–0.5% of adults. At birth they appear as pink or slightly pigmented streaks or plaques and they darken and become more warty (verrucous) with age (**349**). A variety of developmental abnormalities may occur in association with epidermal naevi. The 'epidermal naevus syndrome' is the association of sebaceous and/or verrucous naevi with developmental abnormalities of the central nervous system, eye, and skeleton.

DIFFERENTIAL DIAGNOSIS

Linear viral warts.

INVESTIGATIONS

Histology should be performed to distinguish between epidermolytic and non-epidermolytic epidermal naevi, as individuals with the former may pass the genetic abnormality to their offspring in the form of generalized bullous ichthyosiform erythroderma (BIE) (see p. 73-).

TREATMENT

Small lesions may improve with cryotherapy or laser resurfacing. Oral retinoids may be used to reduce the hyperkeratosis of larger lesions. Patients with epidermolytic verrucous epidermal naevi should receive genetic counselling before starting a family because of the risk of parenting a child with BIE.

Sebaceous naevus

DEFINITION AND CLINICAL FEATURES

An epidermal hamartoma predominantly composed of sebaceous glands. Lesions present in neonates as smooth pink–yellow velvety plaques or patches in the scalp. At puberty they become thickened and warty (**350**) and are often unnoticed until this time. Benign appendage tumours may develop within sebaceous naevi and there is a small life-time risk of malignant transformation, the commonest tumour being basal cell carcinoma.

DIFFERENTIAL DIAGNOSIS

Seborrhoeic keratosis, syringocystadeoma papilliferum. Encephalocoele, although very rare, must be distinguished as these communicate with the brain.

INVESTIGATIONS

Biopsy.

TREATMENT

Excision in early adulthood may be required for cosmetic reasons and because of the risk of malignancy.

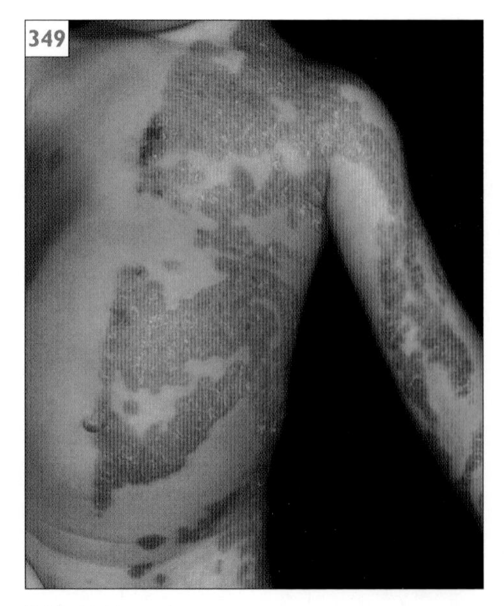

349 Epidermal naevus.

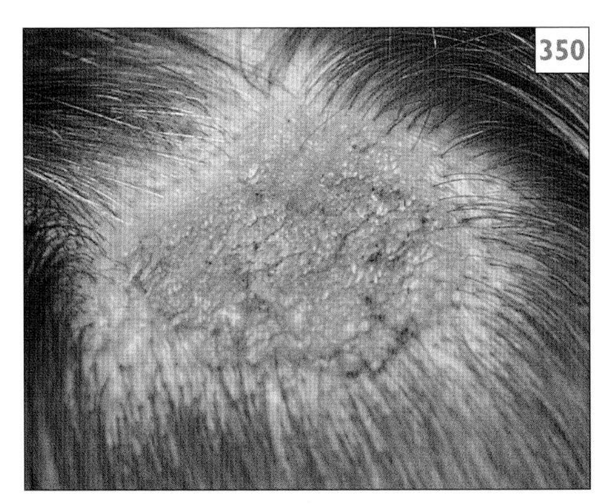

350 Sebaceous naevus.

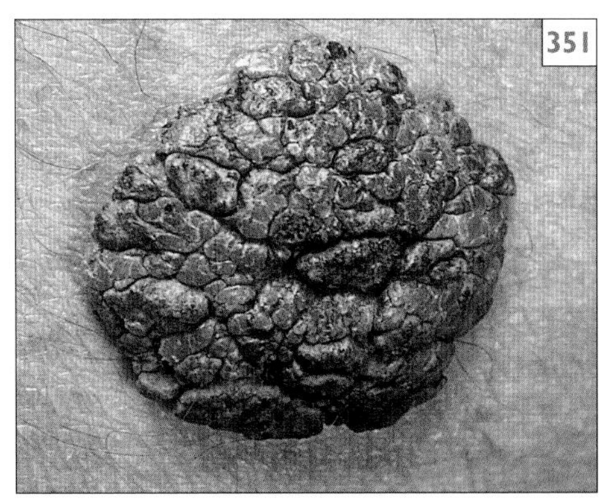

351 Verruciform seborrhoeic keratosis.

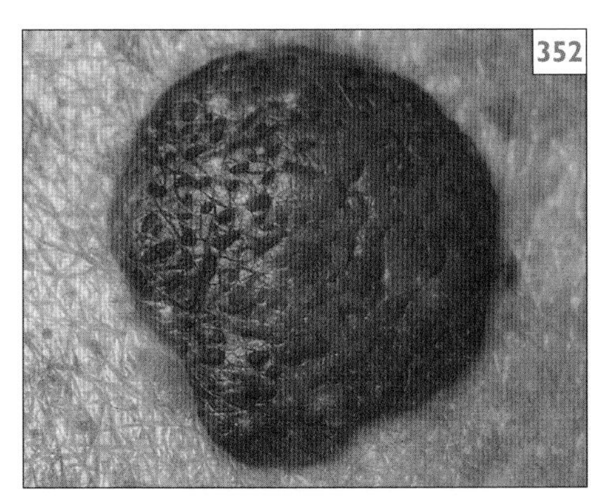

352 Dome-shaped seborrhoeic keratosis.

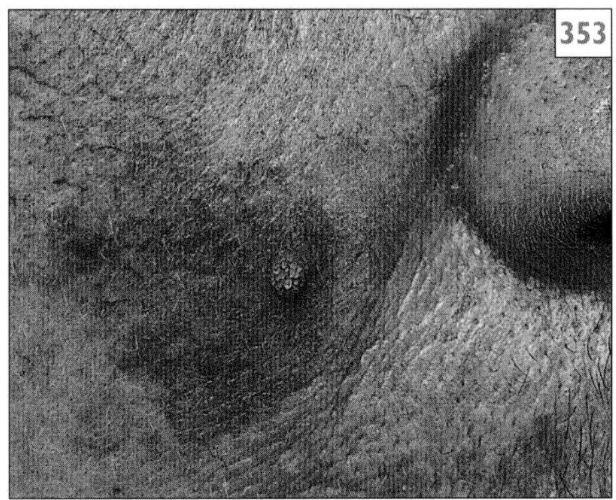

353 Irregular plaque-type seborrhoeic keratosis.

Seborrhoeic keratosis

DEFINITION AND CLINICAL FEATURES

A warty, pigmented papule or plaque due to a benign proliferation of keratinocytes. Seborrhoeic keratoses are very common in people over 40 and the number of lesions increases with age. They mostly arise on the trunk and face but can occur anywhere. Clinical presentations include:

- A greasy, brown/yellow, oval-shaped-plaque with a verruciform surface, appearing to be stuck onto the normal surrounding skin (**351**).
- A brown/black, dome-shaped tumour with a relatively smooth surface, punctuated with plugged follicular openings (**352**).
- A sandy brown, minimally scaly, irregular plaque (**353**).

INVESTIGATIONS

Atypical lesions, especially with deep pigmentation, should be removed or biopsied and sent for histological confirmation.

DIFFERENTIAL DIAGNOSIS

Pale, flat, pigmented facial lesions must be differentiated from lentigo maligna. Distinction from solar keratoses, atypical melanocytic naevi and, rarely, malignant melanoma may be difficult, particularly when the clinical appearances are altered by trauma or infection.

TREATMENT

Removal is usually undertaken on aesthetic grounds or due to pruritus. Superficial lesions may clear with liquid nitrogen cryotherapy. Larger lesions can be removed by curettage and cautery or electrodessication.

Dermatosis papulosa nigra

DEFINITION AND CLINICAL FEATURES

A pigmented papular eruption on the face and neck caused by a developmental defect in the pilo-sebaceous follicle, resembling seborrhoeic keratosis. The condition is extremely common in black races. Lesions consist of small, warty, dark macules and papules and are often numerous over the cheeks and forehead (**354**).

DIFFERENTIAL DIAGNOSIS

Lentigenes.

INVESTIGATION

None necessary.

TREATMENT

Most patients do not request treatment. Lesions can be removed by gentle electrocautery or diathermy.

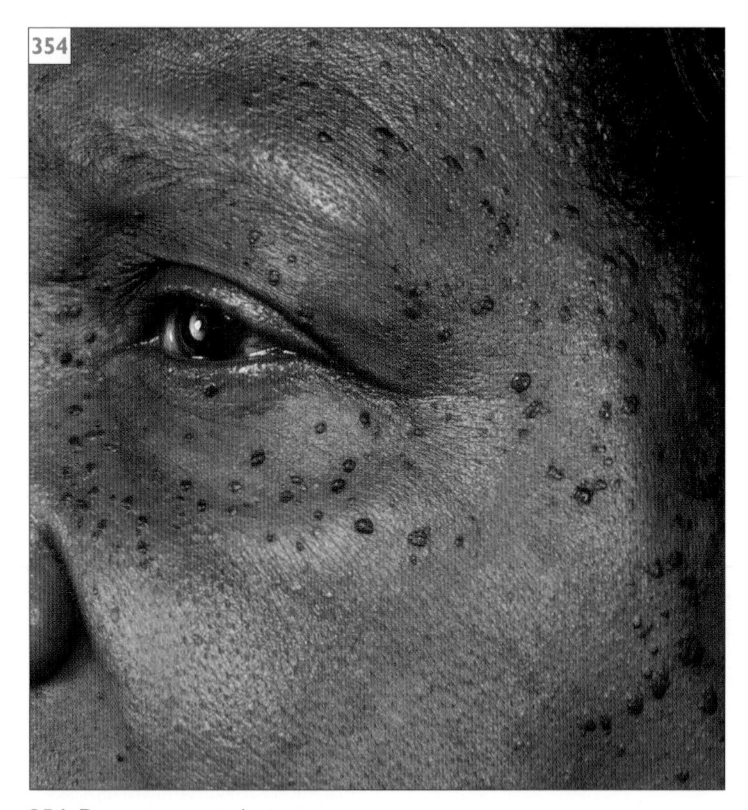

354 Dermatoses papulosis nigra.

Keratoacanthoma

DEFINITION AND CLINICAL FEATURES

A rapid proliferation of keratinocytes giving rise to a squamo-proliferative nodule which resolves spontaneously. Lesions occur on sun-exposed sites, particularly on the head and upper limbs. A solitary, firm, pink or skin-coloured papule rapidly enlarges over a period of days or weeks. At the end of this growth phase, the lesion forms a symmetrical, dome-shaped nodule with an overlying thinned, telangiectatic epidermis and a central keratin plug (**355, 356**). Spontaneous resolution occurs over a few months to leave a depressed scar.

EPIDEMIOLOGY

UV exposure is implicated in the development of keratoacanthoma though, in contrast to squamous cell carcinoma, keratoacanthomas occur predominantly in middle age, and the incidence does not increase in old age. Multiple lesions may occur in immunosuppressed individuals and those with underlying malignancy. Self-healing lesions occur in the Ferguson–Smith syndrome.

INVESTIGATION

Histology to exclude squamous cell carcinoma.

DIFFERENTIAL DIAGNOSIS

Distinction between invasive squamous cell carcinoma and keratoacanthoma may be clinically and histologically difficult; where doubt exists, the tumour should be treated as an invasive squamous cell carcinoma.

TREATMENT

Excision for histological confirmation.

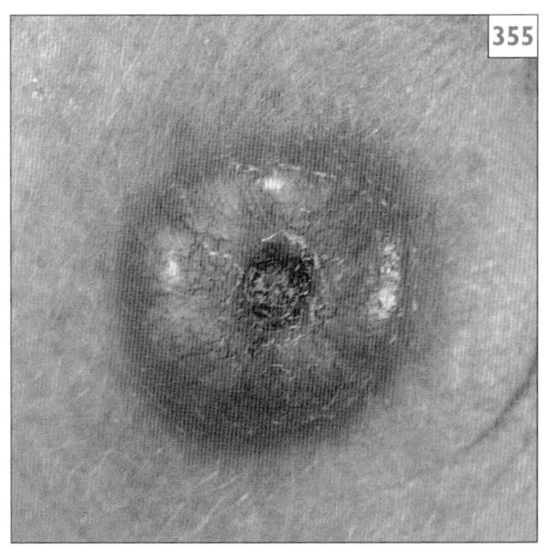

355 Keratoacanthoma with central keratin plug.

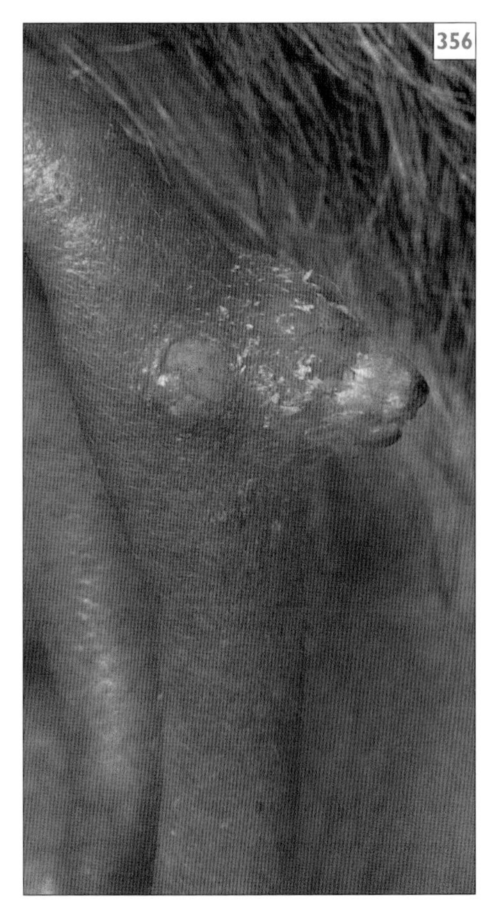

356 Keratoacanthoma.

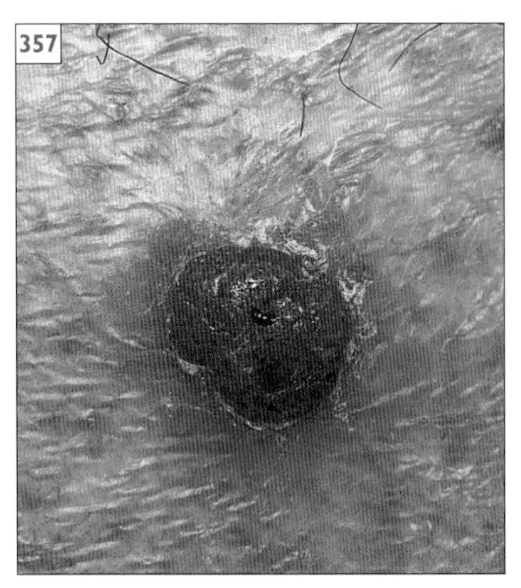

357 Clear cell acanthoma.

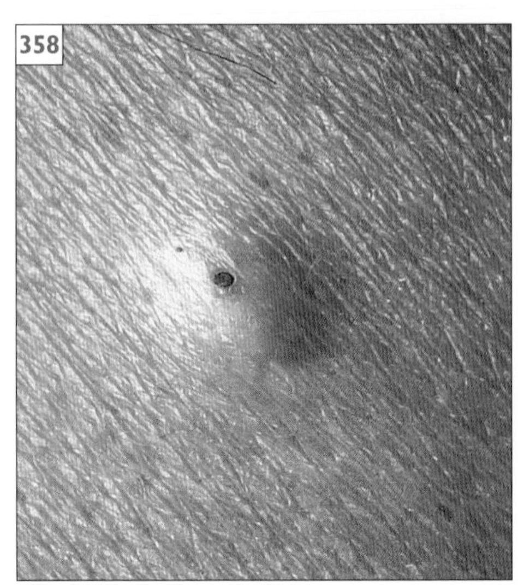

358 Epidermoid cyst.

Clear cell acanthoma

DEFINITION AND CLINICAL FEATURES

A scaly nodule on the lower leg derived from large, glycogen-containing keratinocytes. There is a solitary red (or less commonly brown), well-demarcated nodule, 0.5–2 cm in diameter, with very fine surface scale and occasional oozing (**357**). This benign tumour is relatively uncommon and occurs in middle-aged or elderly adults.

DIFFERENTIAL DIAGNOSIS

Dermatofibroma, pyogenic granuloma, seborrhoeic keratosis.

TREATMENT

Excision.

Epidermoid cyst

DEFINITION AND CLINICAL FEATURES

A cyst containing keratin, surrounded by a lining identical in its stratification to that of epidermis. These lesions are very common and present as a soft, mobile, dome-shaped protuberance, varying in size from a few millimetres to several centimetres, tethered to the overlying epidermis, often with a central punctum (**358**). They usually affect young or middle-aged adults, and are commonly distributed on the head, neck, shoulders, and chest. May become secondarily infected or spontaneously discharge white, cheesy, keratinous material. They may also arise following trauma, due to implantation of a small portion of the epidermis into the dermis. Multiple epidermoid cysts in childhood are a characteristic feature of Gardener's syndrome and the naevoid basal cell carcinoma syndrome (or Gorlin's syndrome).

TREATMENT

Symptomatic or unsightly lesions can be excised carefully when non-inflamed. Incomplete excision may lead to recurrence.

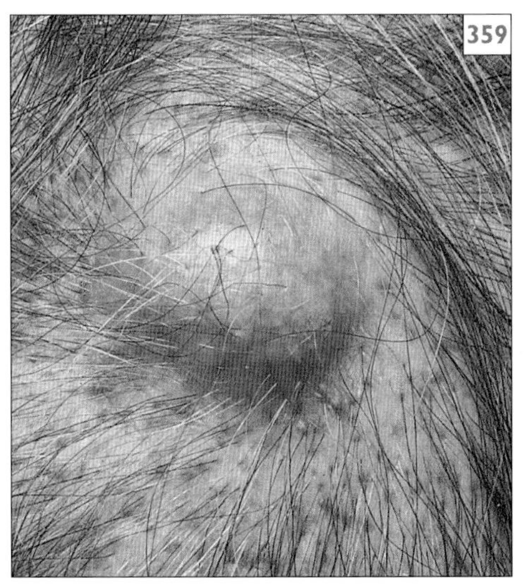

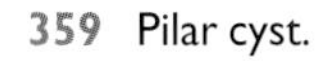

359 Pilar cyst.

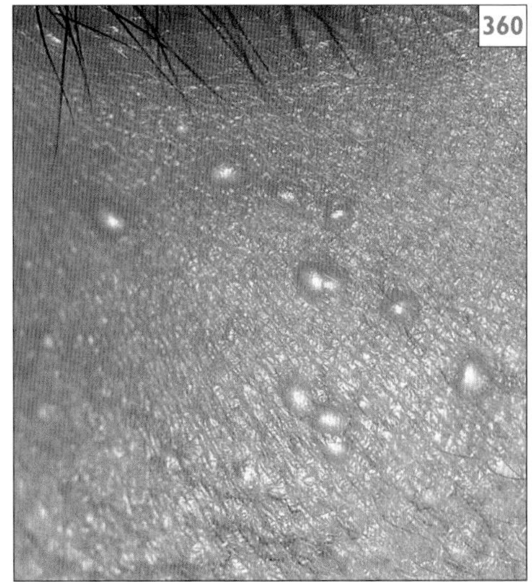

360 Milia.

Pilar cyst

DEFINITION AND CLINICAL FEATURES

A keratin-filled cyst on the scalp surrounded by a lining resembling the external hair root sheath. A firm, mobile nodule on the scalp (**359**), which may be tender if secondarily infected. These usually occur in young and middle-aged adults. Multiple cysts may be inherited as an autosomal dominant trait.

DIFFERENTIAL DIAGNOSIS

Dermal, appendageal tumours.

TREATMENT

Excision.

Milium

DEFINITION AND CLINICAL FEATURES

A small, subepidermal cyst. They are usually idiopathic and multiple (milia) and typically occur around the eyelids and cheeks of young women as small (1–2 mm in diameter), white papules (**360**). They may also occur in infancy. Milia arise either in underdeveloped sebaceous glands or within damaged ducts of eccrine sweat glands following subepidermal bulla formation (e.g. epidermolysis bullosa, porphyria cutanea tarda, bullous pemphigoid) or skin radiotherapy.

TREATMENT

Cosmetically troublesome facial lesions can often be removed carefully with a sterile needle without the need for local anaesthetic, or by fine point cautery.

BENIGN TUMOURS ARISING FROM THE DERMIS

Dermatofibroma

DEFINITION AND CLINICAL FEATURES

A dermal nodule comprised of an interwoven mesh of histocytes and collagen, with overlying epidermal hyperplasia. These common lesions usually affect the lower limbs of young adults (**361**) and are thought to represent an abnormal reaction to insect bites. They may be mildly pruritic. They present as a firm violaceous-pigmented papule or nodule with a characteristic peripheral ring of hyperpigmentation. Palpation reveals a larger dermal component than expected on initial inspection, with puckering overlying hyperkeratotic, pigmented epidermis.

DIFFERENTIAL DIAGNOSIS

Cellular naevus, malignant melanoma when lesion is deeply pigmented.

TREATMENT

Most patients are satisfied with reassurance that these lesions are benign and do not request their removal. Excision should be performed if there is diagnostic doubt.

Juvenile xanthogranuloma

DEFINITION AND CLINICAL FEATURES

A benign tumour of histiocytes that occurs mostly in early childhood and regresses spontaneously. Most patients develop solitary lesions although occasionally they are numerous. Lesions appear as red–yellow papules (**362**) and are commonest on the upper body and face. They resolve slowly to leave atrophic scars. Visceral involvement may occur and up to 10% of children have eye involvement with varied complications including glaucoma.

DIFFERENTIAL DIAGNOSIS

Papular urticaria, Langerhans cell histiocytoses.

INVESTIGATIONS

Histology and immunocytochemistry.

TREATMENT

No treatment is necessary. Ophthalmic examination should be performed.

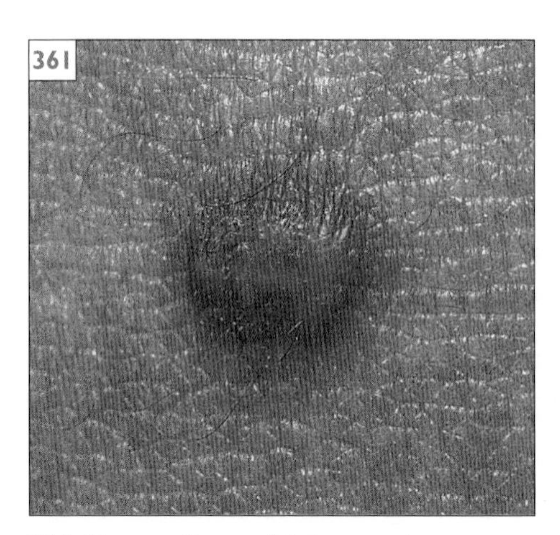

361 Dermatofibroma (histiocytoma).

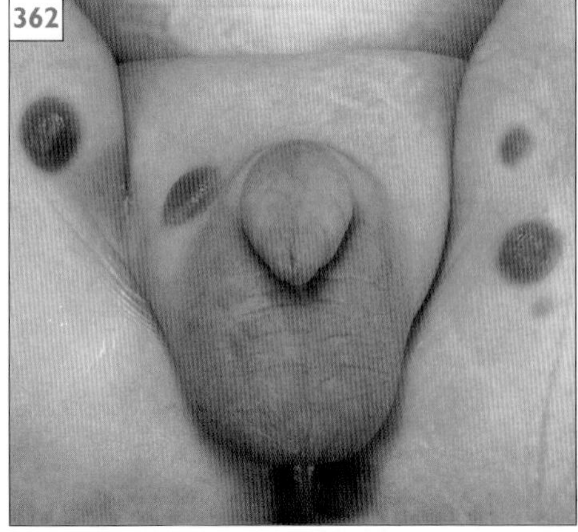

362 Juvenile xanthogranuloma.

Xanthelasma

DEFINITION AND CLINICAL FEATURES

Yellow papules and plaques caused by lipid deposits around the eyelids which may occur in association with hypercholesterolaemia (**363**).

DIFFERENTIAL DIAGNOSIS

The appearance is highly characteristic and unlikely to be confused with other dermatoses.

INVESTIGATIONS

Fasting lipid profile.

TREATMENT

Options include electrodessication and curettage under local anaesthetic, application of a saturated solution of trichloracetic acid, and ablative laser therapy.

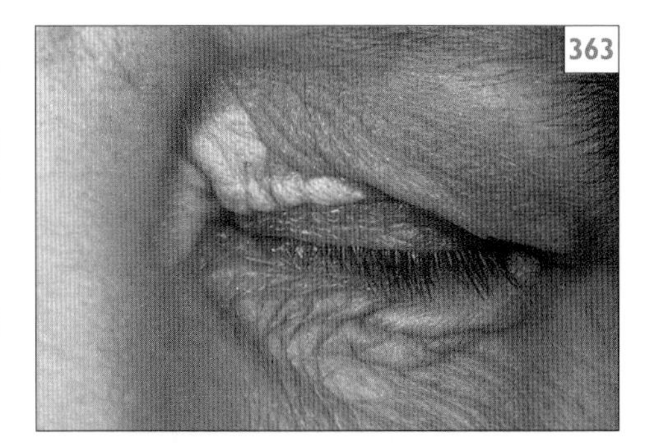

363 Xanthelasma.

Angiofibroma

DEFINITION AND CLINICAL FEATURES

A firm red papule comprised of fibrotic tissue centred around small blood vessels in the papillary dermis. Multiple smooth, red papules on the face, particularly around the nasolabial folds. Number and size increase during puberty (**364**). Multiple lesions are a pathognomonic feature of tuberous sclerosis, where misdesignated as sebaceous adenoma (adenoma sebaceum); angiofibromas are otherwise rare.

TREATMENT

The cosmetic appearance of angiofibromas may be improved by vascular lasers.

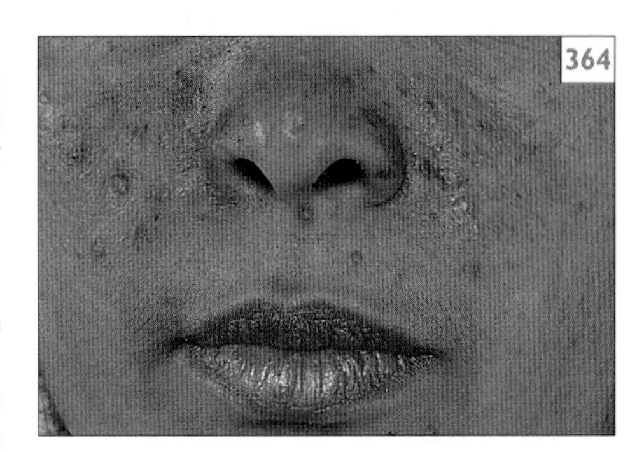

364 Angiofibromata.

Pyogenic granuloma

DEFINITION AND CLINICAL FEATURES

A rapidly expanding, painful vascular nodule that follows minor trauma, comprised of a capillary network within an oedematous stroma (**365**). These lesions are common in children and young adults and usually arise on the fingers. They may recur or develop satellite lesions following excision.

DIFFERENTIAL DIAGNOSIS

Atypical fibroxanthoma, amelanotic melanoma, squamous cell carcinoma.

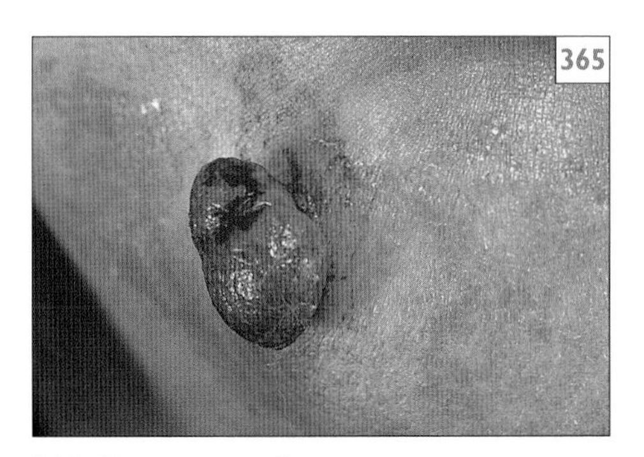

365 Pyogenic granuloma.

INVESTIGATIONS

Lesions should be sent for histological confirmation.

TREATMENT

Polypoid lesions may be removed by curettage and cautery, but recurrence is common. Excision with removal of the underlying deep dermis is usually more definitive.

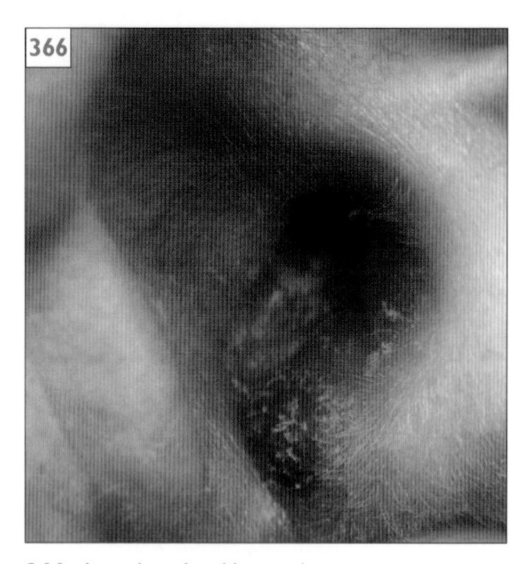

366 Angiolymphoid hyperplasia.

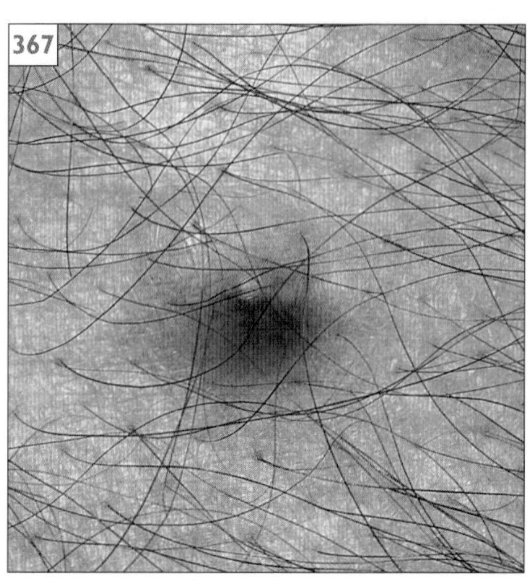

367 Glomus tumour.

Angiolymphoid hyperplasia with eosinophilia

DEFINITION AND CLINICAL FEATURES

A benign locally proliferating lesion composed of vascular channels lined with endothelial cells with abundant pink cytoplasm and vesicular nuclei and a perivascular eosinophil-rich infiltrate. These lesions are thought to arise as a reactive process and typically affect young adults. They appear as small erythematous translucent nodules on the head and neck, particularly around the ears (**366**).

DIFFERENTIAL DIAGNOSIS

Other haemangiomas, Kaposi's sarcoma.

INVESTIGATION

Biopsy for histological confirmation.

TREATMENT

Lesions often resolve spontaneously within 6 months. Surgery is effective, but recurrence is common.

Glomus tumour

DEFINITION AND CLINICAL FEATURES

A painful, vascular nodule comprised of cuboidal (glomus) cells arranged around endothelial-lined vascular channels. Glomus tumours are uncommon and may occur either as a solitary, vascular, subungual tumour or as multiple blue/black nodules on any body site (**367**). Multiple lesions are usually familial.

DIFFERENTIAL DIAGNOSIS

Malignant melanoma.

INVESTIGATIONS

Histology.

TREATMENT

Excision of solitary type is invariably required because of the associated pain.

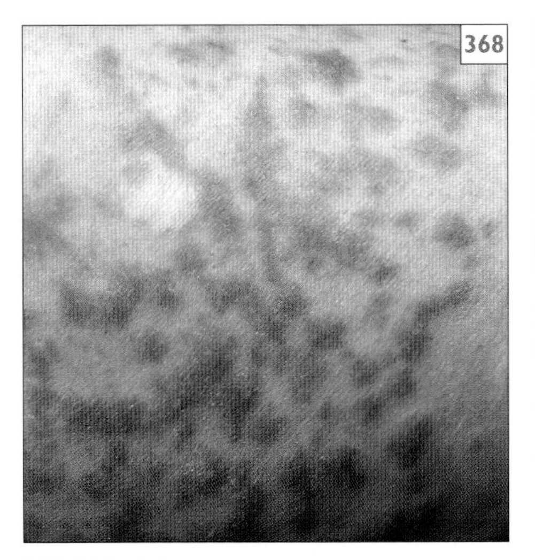

368 Multiple leiomyomas.

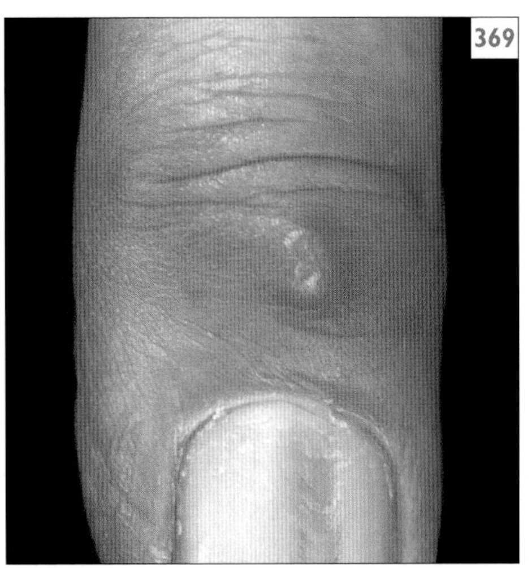

369 Myxoid cyst.

Leiomyoma

DEFINITION AND CLINICAL FEATURES

An uncommon benign tumour of smooth muscle. Lesions present as pink or dusky brown tender nodules (**368**) which become painful in the cold. Multiple lesions may be familial and associated with uterine leiomyomas and renal cancer. In these cases, an underlying defect in the gene for fumarate hydratase has been identified.

DIFFERENTIAL DIAGNOSIS

Other vascular tumours, dermatofibromas.

INVESTIGATIONS

Excision of lesion for histological confirmation; gynaecological evaluation for uterine fibroids in women with multiple cutaneous leiomyomas. Consider screening for renal malignancy.

TREATMENT

Solitary lesions can be excised. Treatment of symptomatic multiple cutaneous leiomyomas is difficult. Options include calcium antagonists, alpha blockers, and gabapentin.

Myxoid cyst

DEFINITION AND CLINICAL FEATURES

A benign pseudocystic cystic swelling with clear gelatinous contents probably arising from the localized mucoid degeneration of connective tissue or directly from the interphalangeal joint. They appear as solitary, circumscribed, soft, often transparent cystic structure, up to 5–10 mm in size, and are occasionally painful. They typically occur on the dorsa of the distal phalanges of the fingers or toes (**369**) in association with osteoarthritis, and are more common in women.

DIFFERENTIAL DIAGNOSIS

Ganglion, viral wart.

TREATMENT

Incision and drainage are often followed by recurrence. Definitive surgical therapy usually involves tracing the communication between the joint and cyst and tying it off.

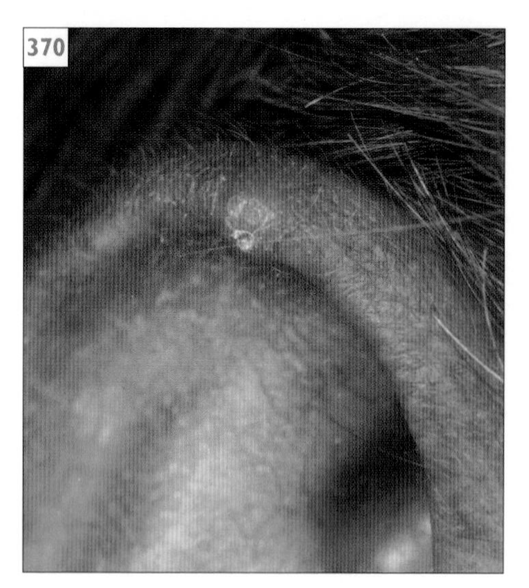

370 Chondrodermatitis nodularis.

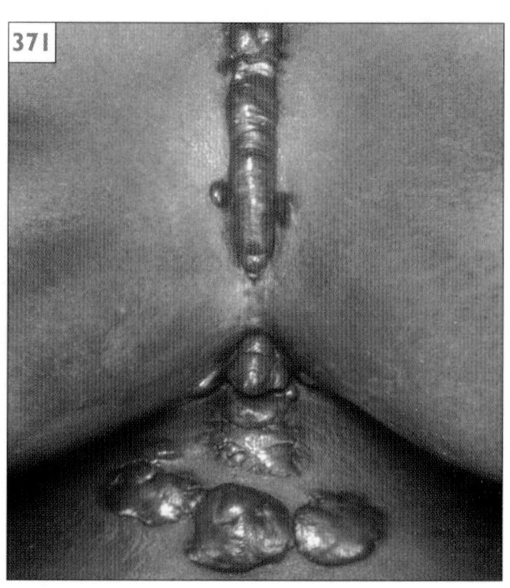

371 Keloids.

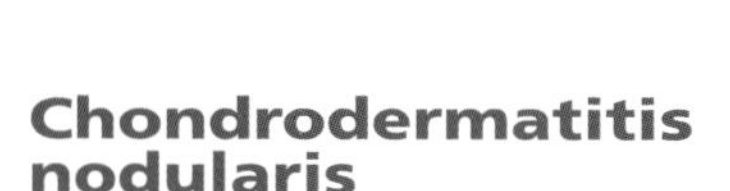

Chondrodermatitis nodularis

DEFINITION AND CLINICAL FEATURES

A painful or tender nodule on the ear associated with inflammation and degeneration of the underlying perichondrium and cartilage. The condition is commonest in elderly men and lesions usually present on the upper helix as an ulcerated or keratotic papule (**370**). They are tender on pressure and typically cause symptoms at night when resting on a pillow. The cause is unknown, but chronic sun damage and a compromised blood supply from cold, trauma, or pressure are thought to be factors.

DIFFERENTIAL DIAGNOSIS

Lesions are often misdiagnosed as basal cell carcinomas, squamous cell carcinomas, or solar keratosis, but their tenderness is characteristic.

INVESTIGATIONS

Histology.

TREATMENT

Excision of the affected underlying cartilage with or without an ellipse of overlying skin is the standard treatment. However, lesions may recur. Efforts should be made to reduce pressure on the affected ear and protect against cold and UV exposure.

Keloids and hypertrophic scars

DEFINITION AND CLINICAL FEATURES

These conditions represent an exaggerated connective tissue response to injury. Hypertrophic scars remain confined to the initial defect and tend to improve with time while keloids extend beyond the original site of damage. Keloids are commoner in Afro-Caribbeans and can reach a considerable size, with cosmetic disfigurement. Hypertrophic or keloidal scars are particularly common around the upper trunk, shoulders, neck, and ears (**371**) and non-essential surgery should be avoided at these sites in at-risk individuals. Scarring truncal acne may give rise to keloids.

DIFFERENTIAL DIAGNOSIS

Scar sarcoid, dermatofibrosarcoma.

INVESTIGATIONS

None.

TREATMENT

Silicone oil or gel sheeting is a simple and safe treatment for small lesions. Keloids usually recur following excision, but the chances of this may be reduced by postoperative radiotherapy, compression garments, or intralesional steroids.

BENIGN TUMOURS ARISING FROM SKIN APPENDAGES

Virtually every cellular component of hair follicles, apocrine and eccrine sweat glands and sebaceous glands may give rise to tumour formation. Most are rare and present as nondescript, dermal papules or nodules. These lesions are therefore rarely diagnosed clinically and invariably require histological evaluation. A few of the more commonly encountered lesions will be briefly described.

Hair follicle tumours

DEFINITION AND CLINICAL FEATURES

Tumours derived from a component of the hair follicle. Most are benign and occur on the face, and multiple lesions may be single or multiple. Trichodiscomas and tumours of the follicular infundibulum present as multiple, smooth, superficial, skin-coloured papules. Tufts of hair occasionally emerge from tricholemmomas and are invariably present in trichofolliculomas. Trichoepitheliomas predominantly affect the nasolabial folds, and have a pearly appearance. Multiple lesions may be inherited as an autosomal dominant trait (epithelioma adenoides cysticum) (**372**). Fibrofolliculomas are rare tumours of the perifollicular connective tissue. Multiple lesions are seen in the Birt–Hogg–Dubé syndrome which is associated with renal carcinoma. Pilomatricoma is the most commonly excised hair appendage tumour and typically presents in childhood. Lesions form hard, deep dermal nodules up to 3 cm in diameter.

DIFFERENTIAL DIAGNOSIS

Other appendageal tumours.

INVESTIGATIONS

Biopsy.

TREATMENT

Solitary lesions are usually excised for diagnostic confirmation. Treatment of multiple lesions is usually for cosmetic reasons. Destructive treatment with lasers or curettage may carry the risk of scarring and recurrence.

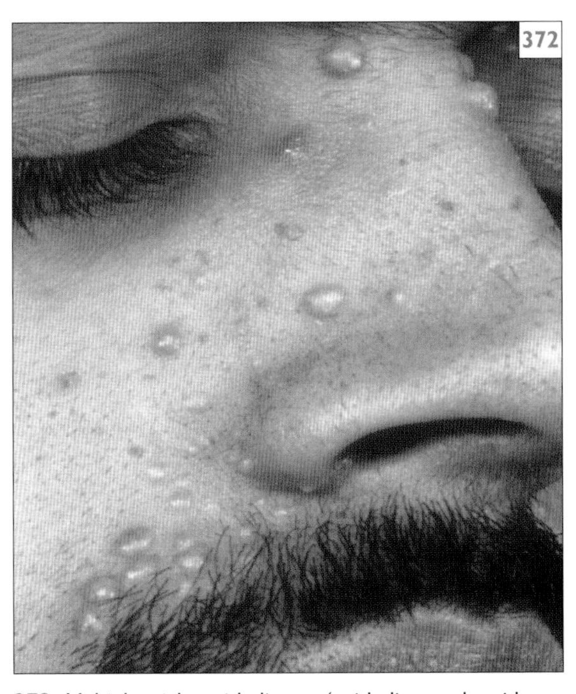

372 Multiple trichoepitheliomas (epithelioma adenoides cysticum).

Apocrine tumours

DEFINITION AND CLINICAL FEATURES

Tumours arising from the apocrine glands. Several benign variants exist including apocrine hidrocystoma, which presents as a grey blue cystic nodule, and syringocystadenoma papilliferum, which is composed of a cluster of proliferative papules. Cylindroma or turban tumour is a dome-shaped well-circumscribed nodule usually on the scalp. Multiple lesions may occur and involve large areas to produce a cerebriform appearance – hence 'turban tumour' (**373**). Apocrine carcinoma is very rare and may metastasize.

DIFFERENTIAL DIAGNOSIS

Other adnexal tumours. Basal cell carcinoma (early lesions particularly).

INVESTIGATIONS

Biopsy.

TREATMENT

Excision.

Eccrine gland tumours

DEFINITION AND CLINICAL FEATURES

Tumours arising from part of the eccrine sweat gland. Eccrine poroma presents as a moist, red, nodule on the palms and soles (**374**). Eccrine spiradenomas are painful and occur as isolated nodules on any body site. Eccrine hidrocystomas usually occur close to the eyelids and are cystic papules which may enlarge with sweating (**375**). Syringomata are invariably multiple and form small (1–2 mm diameter), soft, flat papules on and around the eyelids (**376**). They usually affect young women.

DIFFERENTIAL DIAGNOSIS

Syringomata may simulate plane warts, milia, or trichoepitheliomas.

INVESTIGATIONS

Biopsy for histological confirmation.

TREATMENT

Excision of solitary lesions. Syringomata may respond to careful elecrocautery or diathermy.

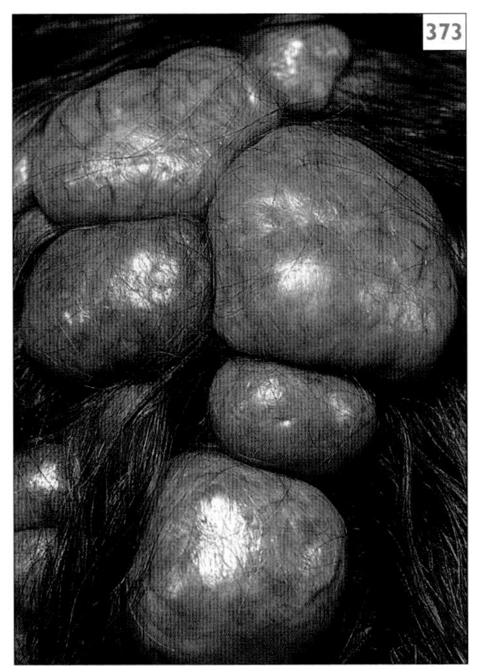

373 Cylindroma ('turban tumour').

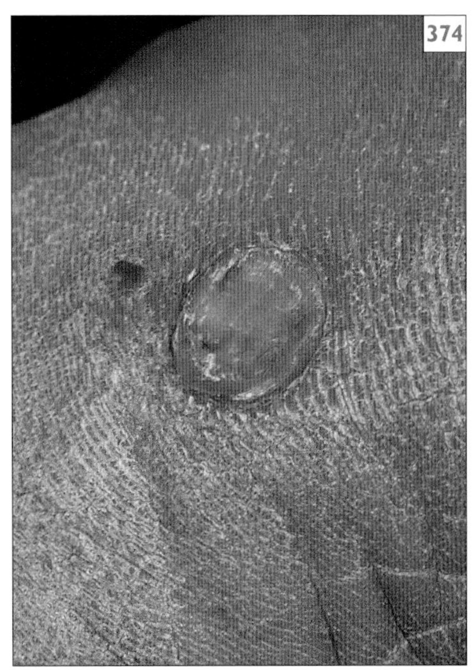

374 Eccrine poroma.

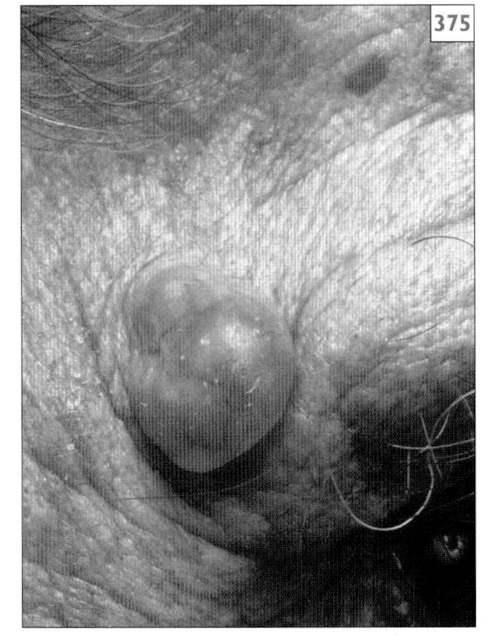

375 Eccrine hidrocystoma.

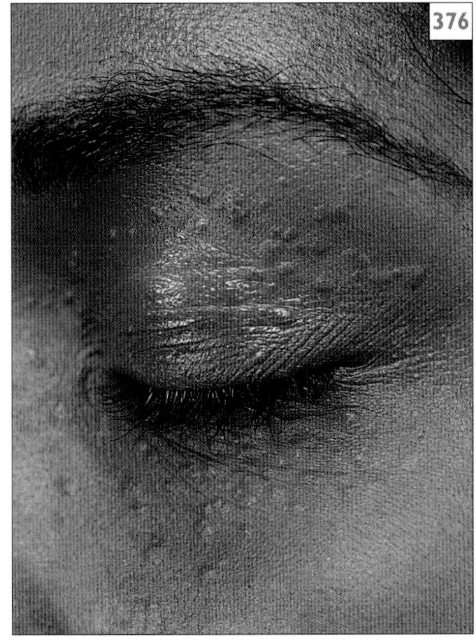

376 Syringomata.

BENIGN MELANOCYTIC LESIONS

Congenital melanocytic naevus

DEFINITION AND CLINICAL FEATURES

Pigmented naevus present at birth derived from melanocytes. Congenital naevi may be divided into small (less than 1.5 cm in diameter), medium (less than 20 cm in diameter), and giant (greater than 20 cm in diameter) (**377, 378**). The prevalence of small congenital naevi is estimated at approximately 1% of newborn infants; giant congenital naevi are rare (less than 0.002% of infants). During infancy, naevi may be pale brown; increasing pigmentation and excessive terminal hair growth characterize older lesions. Giant naevi may be associated with underlying spinal defects, pigmentation of leptomeninges, and numerous small congenital naevi elsewhere.

DIFFERENTIAL DIAGNOSIS

Vascular and epidermal naevi.

INVESTIGATIONS

Biopsy if malignant change is suspected.

TREATMENT

The risk of malignant transformation of small congenital melanocytic naevi is extremely small but they are sometimes excised in early childhood or adulthood for cosmetic reasons. Giant melanocytic naevi are associated with an estimated lifetime risk of malignant transformation of approximately 5%. Total excision may not be possible, but their appearance may be improved by shaving the lesion in the neonatal period.

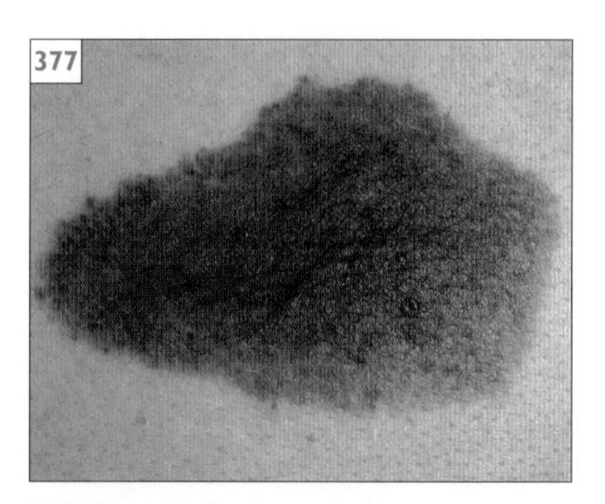

377 Congenital melanocytic naevus.

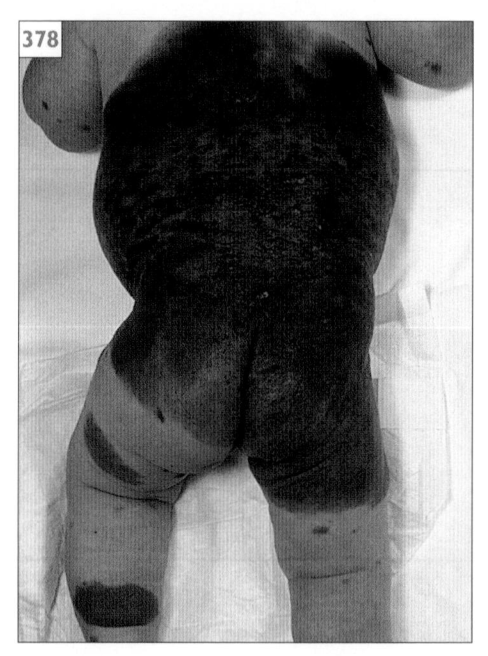

378 Giant congenital melanocytic naevus.

Blue naevus

DEFINITION AND CLINICAL FEATURES

A deep dermal aggregate of melanocytes. An evenly pigmented bluish macule or papule (**379**) on the face, less commonly on the limbs and buttocks. This condition occurs in older children and young adults. The dermal, spindle-shaped melanocytes are thought to represent melanocytes which have failed to migrate to the epidermis during foetal life. Malignant change is rare.

DIFFERENTIAL DIAGNOSIS

Density of pigment may cause confusion with malignant melanoma.

INVESTIGATIONS

Biopsy if diagnostic doubt or when growth occurs in a previously stable naevus.

TREATMENT

None is needed unless there is diagnostic doubt or requested on cosmetic grounds.

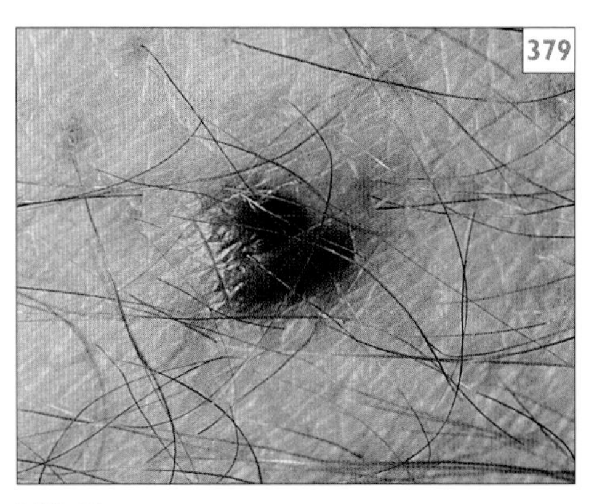

379 Blue naevus.

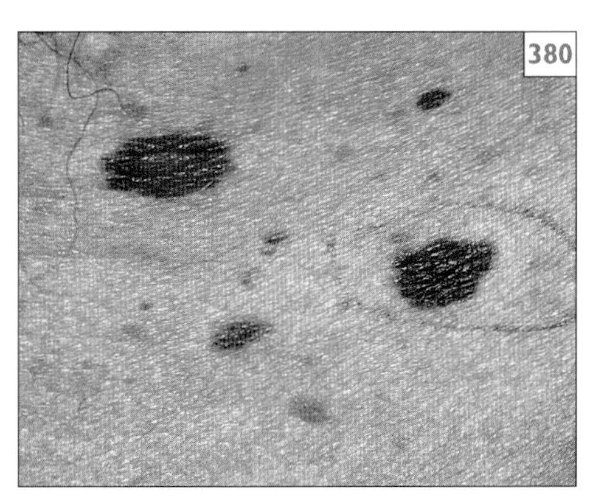

380 Atypical melanocytic (dysplastic) naevi.

Atypical melanocytic naevus

DEFINITION AND CLINICAL FEATURES

A compound (or less commonly junctional) melanocytic naevus with atypical clinical and/or histological features. These pigmented lesions show one or more of the following features (**380**):

- Size greater than 0.5 cm in diameter.
- Irregular, smudged border.
- Irregular pigmentation.
- Associated erythema.
- Both a papular and macular component.

The term 'dysplastic naevus' is reserved for naevi that fulfil histopathological criteria.

Individuals with the atypical mole syndrome (either familial or sporadic) have numerous atypical naevi distributed on non-sun-exposed sites (buttocks, genitalia, scalp, soles, dorsa of feet). The atypical mole phenotype may be inherited as an autosomal dominant trait or occur sporadically. Those with the very rare familial form, where first-degree relatives have atypical naevi and a history of multiple malignant melanoma, characteristically develop multiple primary malignant melanomas. Estimates of the prevalence of the sporadic form vary between 1 and 5% of the population. The risk of melanoma in these individuals may be increased by a factor of ten.

INVESTIGATIONS

Biopsy may demonstrate cytological melanocytic atypia, architectural atypia (bridging of rete ridges, lentiginous melanocytic hyperplasia), and host response (lymphocytic infiltrate, lamellar fibrosis).

TREATMENT

Atypical naevi that are difficult to distinguish from early malignant melanoma on clinical grounds should be excised. Photography or digital imaging may help in the follow-up of patients to identify any changing lesions.

Benign acquired melanocytic naevus

DEFINITION AND CLINICAL FEATURES

A benign proliferation of melanocytes. Clusters of melanocytes are initially confined to the basal layer of epidermis (junctional naevus) and then migrate into dermis (compound and intradermal naevi). Benign acquired melanocytic naevi are extremely common. The frequency of naevi increases slowly during childhood and sometimes sharply at puberty. Numbers reach a plateau in the third decade and slowly disappear thereafter to become rare in old age. Numbers may increase following sun exposure, pregnancy, or immunosuppression.

Junctional naevi present as small (0.1–1 cm in diameter), dark-brown, evenly pigmented, symmetrical macules or minimally elevated papules (**381**). The majority of naevi in children are junctional and occur on any body site – those found in adults are confined to the palms, soles, and genitalia. Compound naevi (where melanocytes are present in both the epidermis and the dermis) occur at any site and vary from light-brown, pigmented papules to dark-brown papillomatous and sometimes hyperkeratotic plaques (**382**). Intradermal naevi occur predominantly in the third decade, frequently on the face and may lack pigment. They are often dome-shaped or papillomatous nodules, or pedunculated skin tags (**383**). Malignant change in acquired benign melanocytic naevi is extremely rare.

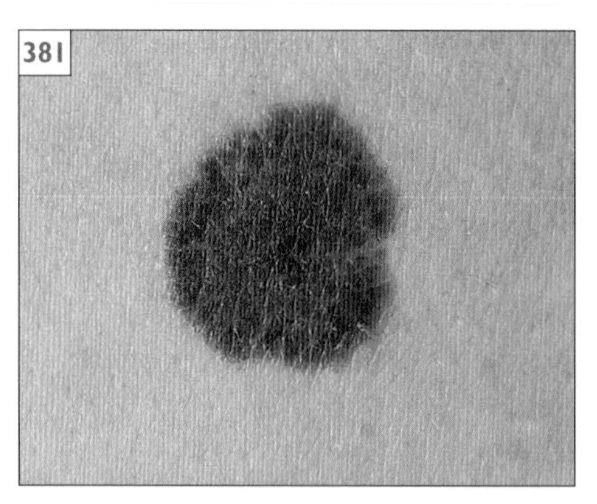

381 Junctional naevus.

DIFFERENTIAL DIAGNOSIS

Junctional and compound naevi may be confused with lentigines or seborrhoeic keratoses, respectively.

INVESTIGATIONS

Biopsy is required only where clinical differentiation from malignant melanoma is difficult.

TREATMENT

The great majority of lesions do not need to be excised on clinical grounds. Where removal is requested for cosmetic reasons the risk of scarring should be clearly discussed. Any melanocytic lesion which is removed must be sent for histological examination. Junctional and compound naevi should be excised with a narrow surgical excision. Protuberant skin coloured intradermal naevi may be removed by shave and cautery with good cosmetic results.

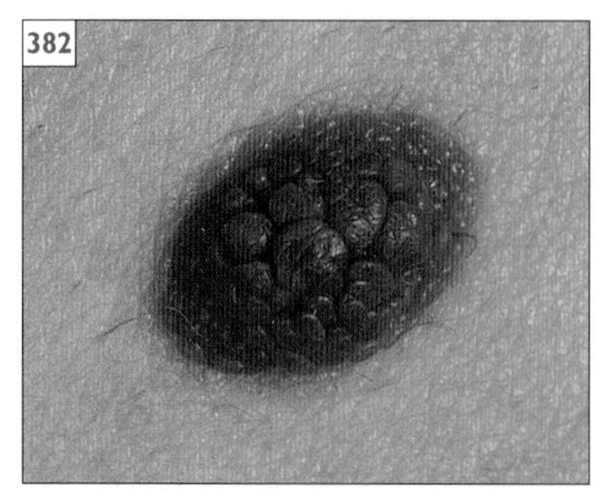

382 Compound naevus.

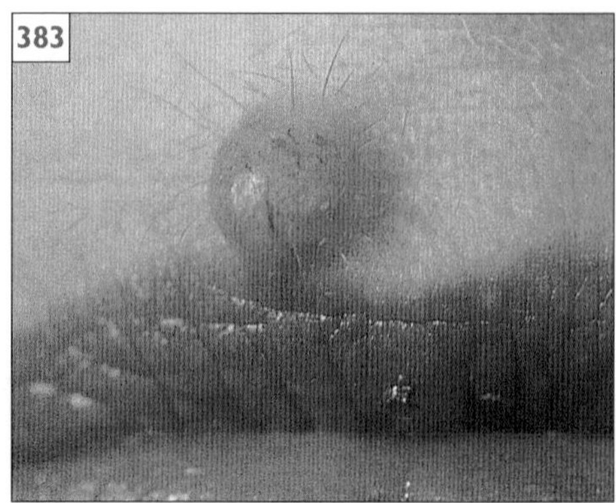

383 Intradermal naevus.

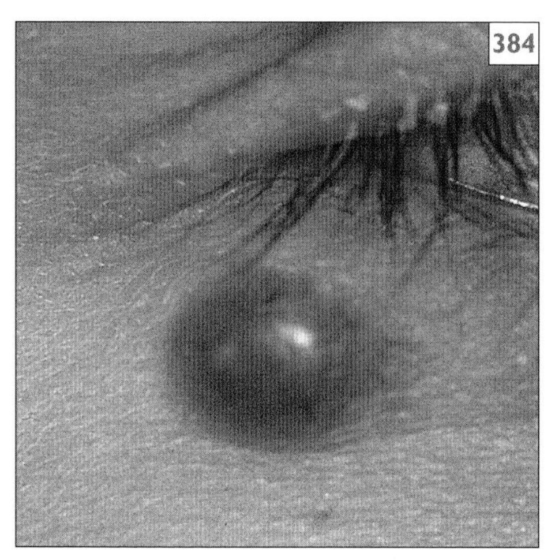

384 Spitz naevus.

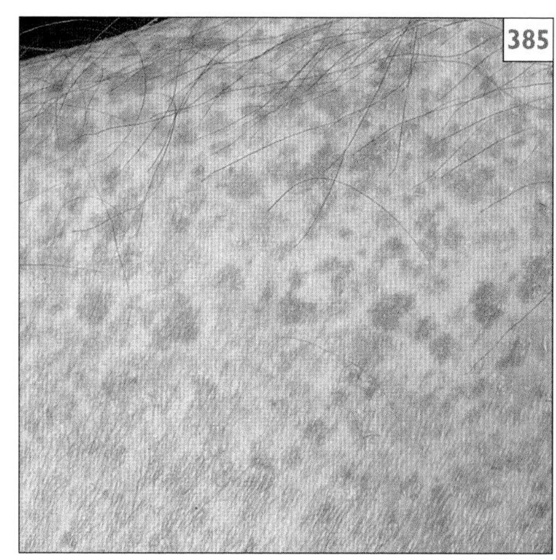

385 Freckles.

Spitz naevus

DEFINITION AND CLINICAL FEATURES

A benign compound naevus seen mostly in children clinically and histopathologically distinct from common acquired melanocytic naevi. These lesions are discrete, red-brown or pink papules and particularly affect the face (**384**) or limbs. The initial papule may increase rapidly to reach 1–2 cm in diameter but thereafter remains static.

DIFFERENTIAL DIAGNOSIS

Malignant melanoma, benign melanocytic naevus, juvenile xanthogranuloma, pyogenic granuloma.

INVESTIGATIONS

Histology shows a compound naevus variant with spindle or epithelioid naevus cells.

TREATMENT

Local excision with a narrow margin is usually required for diagnostic confirmation.

Freckles

DEFINITION AND CLINICAL FEATURES

Pale brown macules, less than 3 mm in diameter, due to the UV-induced production of melanin by a normal number of basal melanocytes. They are multiple and distributed on sun-exposed sites (**385**). Freckles are prominent during the summer, following UV exposure, and virtually disappear in the winter. They are very common, especially in children and individuals with Type I or II skin.

DIFFERENTIAL DIAGNOSIS

Lentigenes may be very similar in appearance but persist in the absence of UV stimulation.

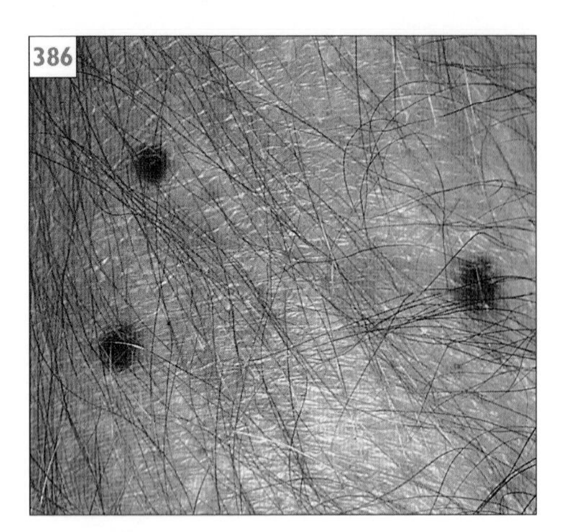

386 Lentigines.

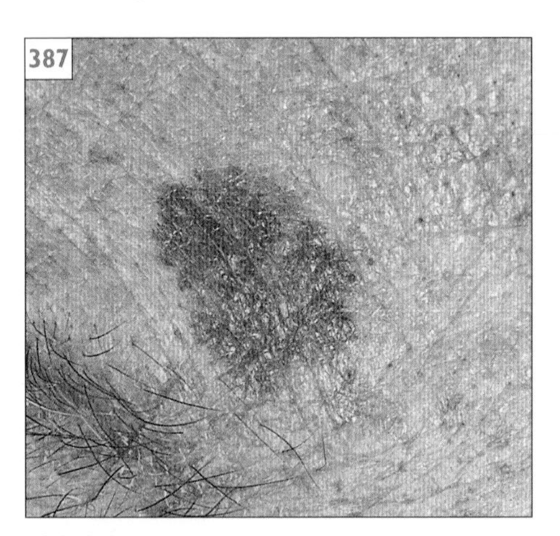

387 Solar lentigo.

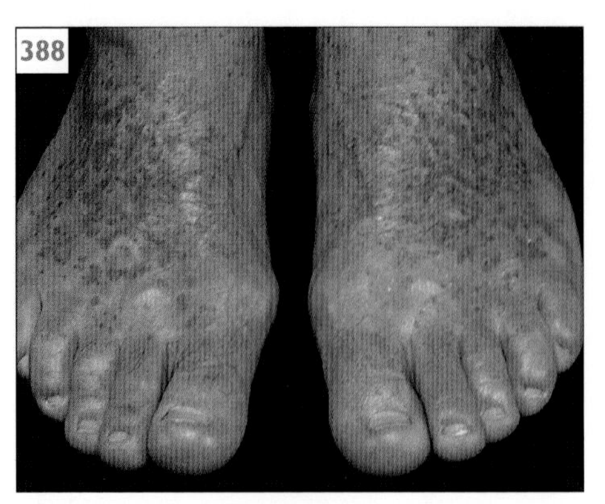

388 Multiple solar lentigines from PUVA therapy.

Lentigenes

DEFINITION AND CLINICAL FEATURES

These lesions are persistent brown macules due to a linear increase in the number of melanocytes within the basal layer of the epidermis (**386**). Lentigines may occur at any site on the skin, including the conjunctivae and mucocutaneous junctions. Multiple lentigenes are a common finding in people with fair skin, but may also rarely occur in rare hereditary multi-system disorders such as Peutz–Jeghers disease (particularly when distributed on the lips, buccal mucosae, and acral sites), centrofacial lentiginosis (associated with cardiac abnormalities), and the LEOPARD syndrome (i.e. lentigines, ECG abnormalities, ocular hypertelorism, pulmonary stenosis, abnormal genitalia, retarded growth, deafness). Lentigenes may also be caused by severe sunburn, especially on the upper back or from chronic sun exposure (solar or actinic lentigenes). They are common on the face and dorsal hands in middle-aged and elderly individuals (age spots or liver spots) (**387**). Multiple solar lentigines may result from PUVA therapy (**388**) or excessive sunbed use.

DIFFERENTIAL DIAGNOSIS

Freckle, junctional melanocytic naevus. Facial lesions may be difficult to differentiate from early lentigo maligna.

INVESTIGATIONS

None usually necessary. Atypical or rapidly enlarging solitary lesions should be biopsied.

TREATMENT

Prevention of further UV damage by sun avoidance and sunscreen use. Gentle cryotherapy may be used to fade benign facial lentigenes.

MALIGNANT NEOPLASMS AND THEIR PRECURSORS

Solar keratosis
(actinic keratosis)

DEFINITION AND CLINICAL FEATURES
A red, scaly plaque on light-exposed skin due to dysplastic epidermal keratinocytes. It may affect the face (including lower lip), bald pate (**389**), forearms, and dorsum of the hands, presenting as a red yellow or beige plaque, 0.5–1 cm in diameter, with surface scale or crust (**390**). It may ulcerate or develop a cutaneous horn. Frequently multiple. These lesions are common, especially in fair-skinned individuals over 40 years of age with a recreational or occupational history of chronic sun exposure. Enormous numbers may occur in those chronically immunosuppressed (e.g. renal transplant recipients). They carry a low risk of transformation to invasive squamous cell carcinoma.

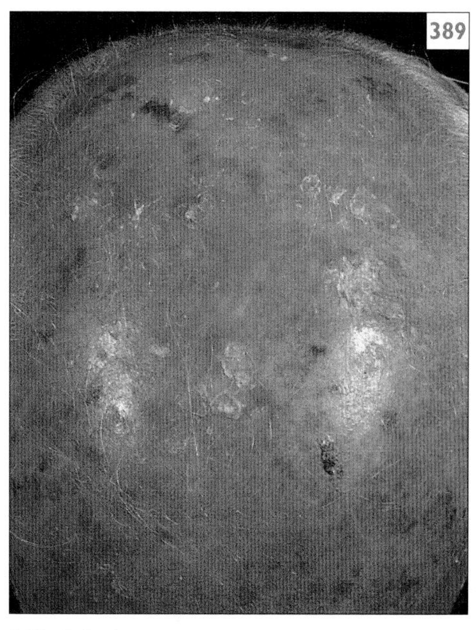

389 Solar keratoses.

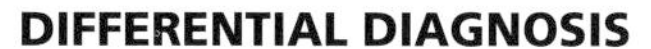

DIFFERENTIAL DIAGNOSIS
Seborrhoeic keratosis, viral warts, squamous cell carcinoma.

INVESTIGATIONS
Biopsy if diagnosis in doubt.

TREATMENT
Cryotherapy, curettage and cautery, topical 5-fluorouracil or diclofenac in imiquimod gel. Sun avoidance strategies including regular use of sunscreens reduce the rate of formation of new solar keratoses.

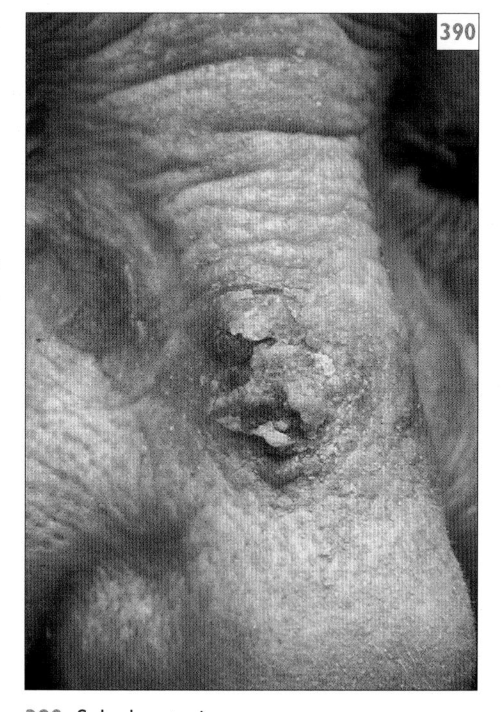

390 Solar keratosis.

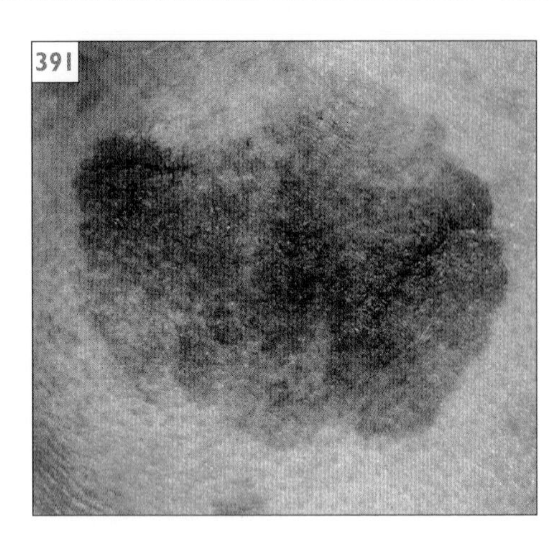

391 Lentigo maligna.

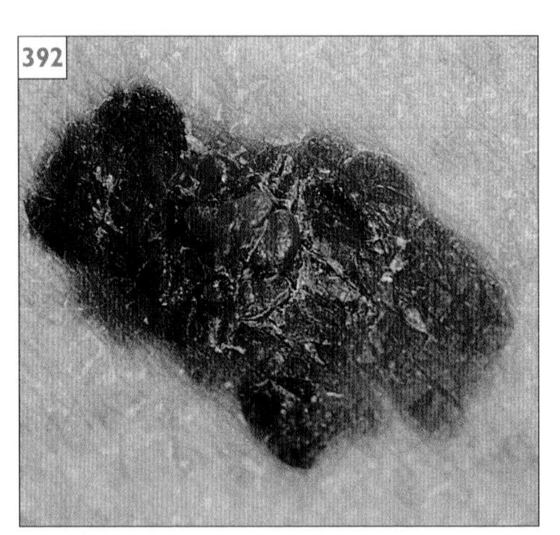

392 Superficial spreading melanoma.

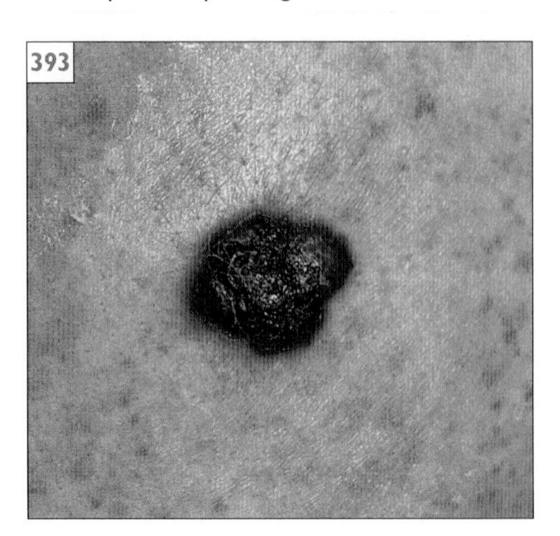

393 Nodular melanoma.

Malignant melanoma

DEFINITION AND CLINICAL FEATURES

A malignant proliferation of melanocytes. Features more commonly seen in malignant than in benign melanocytic lesions include a diameter greater than 1 cm, increasing size, variation in pigment, irregular edge, presence of inflammation, crusting or bleeding, altered sensation or itch. Any change in a pre-existing pigmented lesion should alert the clinician to the possibility of malignant melanoma.

The incidence of melanoma has increased dramatically in recent decades. The highest figures recorded are in white-skinned individuals in Australia and New Zealand. UV exposure is a major aetiological factor, particularly short, intense, exposure resulting in sunburn, and during childhood. Lentigo maligna contrasts with this pattern, where total cumulative exposure appears to be more relevant. Phenotypic risk factors include fair skin, red or blonde hair, blue eyes, inability to tan, freckles, lentigines, large numbers of benign melanocytic naevi, and the presence of atypical naevi. Melanoma most frequently involves the lower leg in women, and the back in men. It is very rare in childhood.

Four main clinical subtypes are recognized:

- Lentigo maligna – an irregularly pigmented macule, slowly enlarging over many years, commonly on the cheek or temple of an elderly person (**391**). Development of a more rapidly growing, deeply pigmented papule or nodule indicates dermal invasion by malignant melanocytes (lentigo maligna melanoma).
- Superficial spreading melanoma – a macule or papule, usually greater than 0.5 cm in diameter at presentation, with variable pigmentation from pale brown to blue-black, an irregular edge, and surface oozing or crusting (**392**).
- Nodular melanoma – a rapidly enlarging, frequently ulcerated, blue-black nodule (**393**).

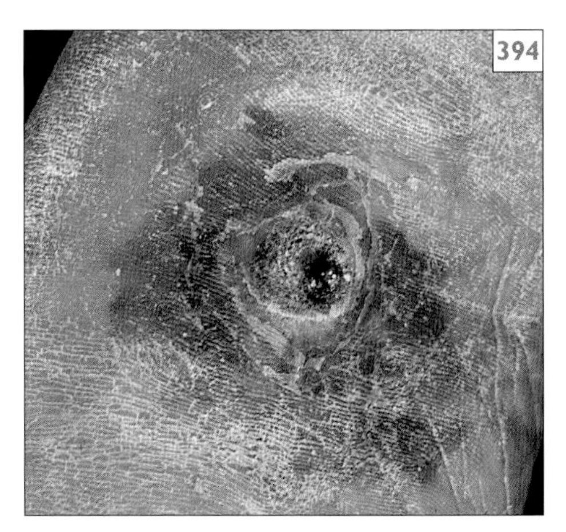

394 Acral lentiginous melanoma.

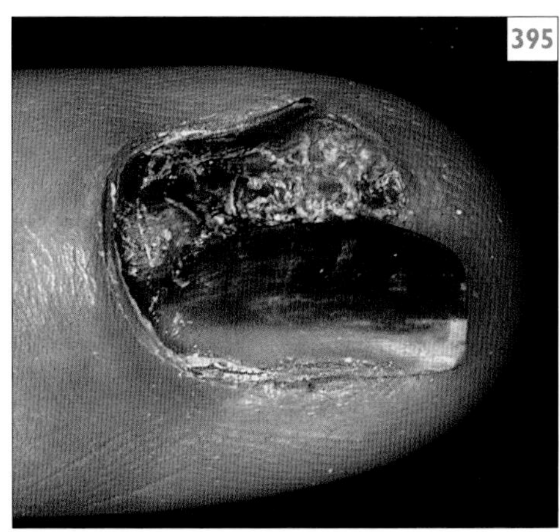

395 Subungual melanoma.

- Acral lentiginous melanoma – an irregularly pigmented macule on the sole of the foot or palm of the hand (**394**). Subungual or periungual melanoma (a variant of acral lentiginous melanoma) occurs either as a linear pigmented streak in the nail or an isolated nail dystrophy, accompanied by pigmentation of the proximal nail fold (Hutchinson's sign) (**395**).

DIFFERENTIAL DIAGNOSIS

Benign pigmented or vascular lesions. Particular difficulty may arise in differentiating lentigo maligna from simple lentigo, seborrhoeic keratosis, or pigmented solar keratosis; or differentiating nodular melanoma from a vascular tumour or pyogenic granuloma; or differentiating subungual melanoma from fungal infection or subungual haematoma.

INVESTIGATIONS

Histology of excised lesion. The prognosis of malignant melanoma is strongly correlated with the Breslow thickness (the depth of dermal invasion by malignant melanocytes from the granular cell layer) and therefore early diagnosis is crucial. An incisional biopsy may be taken from large lesions where the diagnosis is uncertain in order to avoid unnecessary excision of a benign lesion, such as a seborrhoeic keratosis.

Histology of sentinel (draining) lymph nodes may be performed to assess the need for further surgery to the lymph node basin. Computerized image analysis systems are being developed to aid the clinical diagnosis of melanoma but they are not yet used in routine practice.

TREATMENT

Surgical excision of the primary tumour with secondary excision of the scar depending on tumour depth (Breslow thickness). Recommendations are a 2–5 mm margin for *in situ* melanoma, 1 cm margin for invasive melanoma up to 1 mm depth, 2 cm margin for melanoma from 1–2 mm depth, and 3 cm for thicker tumours. Patients who have had surgery for primary melanoma with no evidence of secondary spread are usually followed up by dermatologists for 3–5 years. They should be informed about mole surveillance and self-examination for enlarged nodes. Patients who have palpable regional lymph nodes are likely to have metastatic spread and require combined care with surgical and oncology specialists.

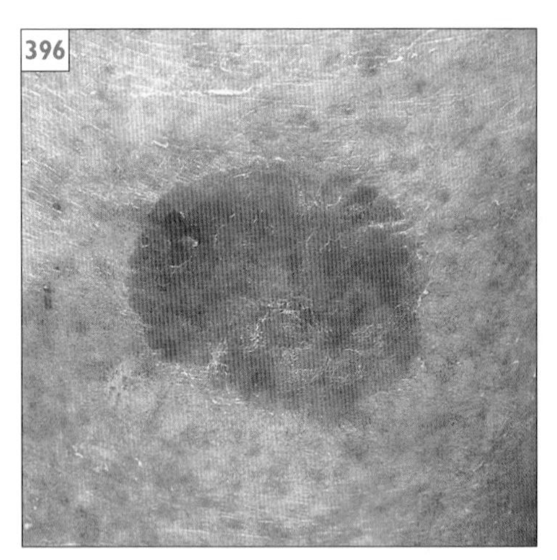

396 Bowen's disease.

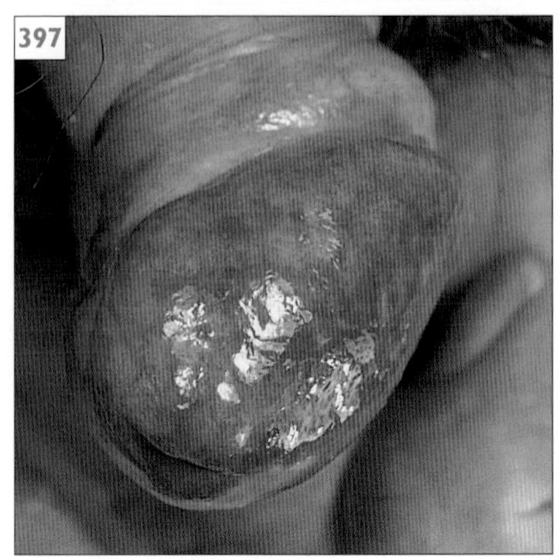

397 Erythroplasia of Queyrat.

Bowen's disease

DEFINITION AND CLINICAL FEATURES

An intraepidermal squamous cell cancer of the skin characterized by a persistent red scaly plaque. Lesions are usually found on the legs of elderly women and may be multiple. Their development is usually related to chronic UV exposure, but in some parts of the world chronic arsenic ingestion from contaminated water supplies is an important aetiological factor (**396**).

Erythroplasia of Queyrat (**397**) is a distinct clinical variant of intraepidermal squamous carcinoma, characterized by well-demarcated, red, shiny plaques on the genital mucosa (see also p.93).

DIFFERENTIAL DIAGNOSIS

Isolated plaque of psoriasis, discoid eczema multifocal basal cell carcinoma, actinic keratosis.

INVESTIGATIONS

Biopsy to confirm diagnosis.

TREATMENT

Destructive therapies like cryotherapy, curettage and cautery are usually effective, but slow healing may be a problem on the lower leg. Surgical excision is an alternative in this situation. Other treatments include topical 5-fluorouracil, imiquimod, and photodynamic therapy.

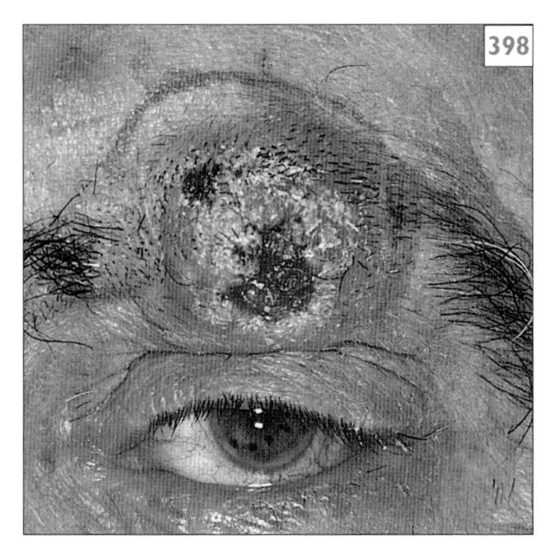

398 Squamous cell carcinoma.

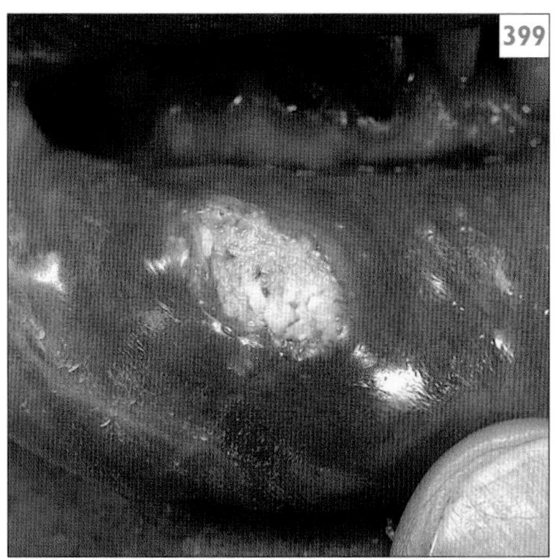

399 Squamous cell carcinoma on the lower lip.

Squamous cell carcinoma

DEFINITION AND CLINICAL FEATURES

A squamoproliferative lesion due to malignant, invasive, proliferation of epidermal keratinocytes. Tumours present as an expanding plaque or nodule with an ill-defined, indurated base, usually ulcerated, with surface scale and crust (**398**). Squamous cell carcinomas (SCC) occur predominantly on sun-exposed sites (dorsum of the hands, forearms, dorsal hands, neck and face – especially lower lips and pinna) in association with solar elastosis and multiple actinic keratoses. Local draining lymph nodes may be enlarged due to metastatic involvement.

Cutaneous SCC is predominantly a disease of white races and most prevalent in elderly males who have had chronic sun exposure. Other aetiological factors include topical (e.g. tar, cutting oils) and systemic (e.g. arsenic) carcinogens, photochemotherapy, human papilloma virus infection, and chronic immunosuppression. SCCs may arise at sites of long-standing radiation dermatitis, scarring (e.g. discoid lupus erythematosus), or ulceration (Marjolin's ulcer). Smoking is associated with lesions on the lip (**399**).

DIFFERENTIAL DIAGNOSIS

Keratoacanthoma, proliferative solar keratosis, Bowen's disease.

INVESTIGATIONS

Biopsy.

TREATMENT

The aims of treatment are to ensure complete removal of the tumour and prevent metastasis. Surgical excision with wide margins is the treatment of choice for most skin tumours but destructive therapies such as curettage and cautery may be appropriate for small slow-growing well-differentiated SCCs. Radiotherapy may be the preferred treatment for large or rapidly enlarging tumours in patients who are too frail to tolerate surgery.

Basal cell carcinoma

DEFINITION AND CLINICAL FEATURES

A slow growing, locally destructive, tumour due to proliferation of basal keratinocytes. Basal cell carcinoma (BCC) is the most common type of skin cancer – the ratio of basal to squamous cell carcinoma is approximately 4:1. Lesions predominantly affect fair-skinned individuals and are related to chronic sun exposure, but unlike SCCs they do not usually develop at sites of maximal UV exposure. BCCs may rarely arise in a pre-existing naevus sebaceus or in individuals with the basal cell naevus syndrome, or following arsenic ingestion (when lesions particularly arise on extrafacial sites).

Nodular or solid basal cell carcinoma arises on the forehead, nose, or adjacent to the inner canthus of the eye as a skin-coloured, pink or pigmented (**400**), translucent papule or nodule with surface telangiectasia. Gradual enlargement leads to central ulceration and a peripheral, 'rolled' pearly edge (**401**). Morphoeic basal cell carcinoma presents as a firm, indurated, skin-coloured, scar-like plaque (**402**) with ill-defined edges, commonly on the nasolabial fold or forehead. Superficial multifocal basal cell carcinoma tends to arise on extrafacial sites as red, scaly plaques (**403**).

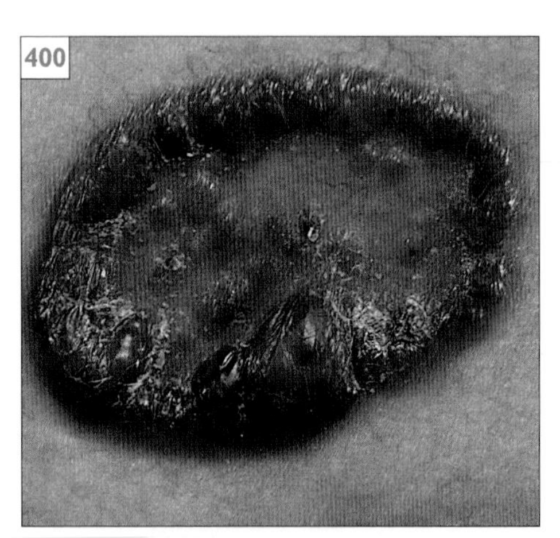

400 Pigmented basal cell carcinoma.

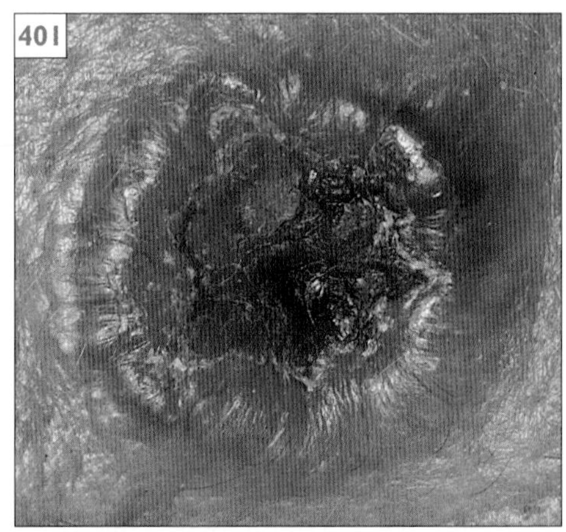

401 Basal cell carcinoma showing the 'rolled' pearly edge.

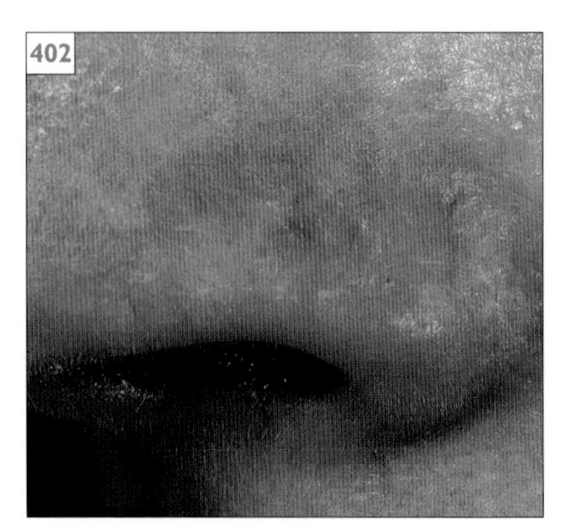

402 Morphoeic basal cell carcinoma.

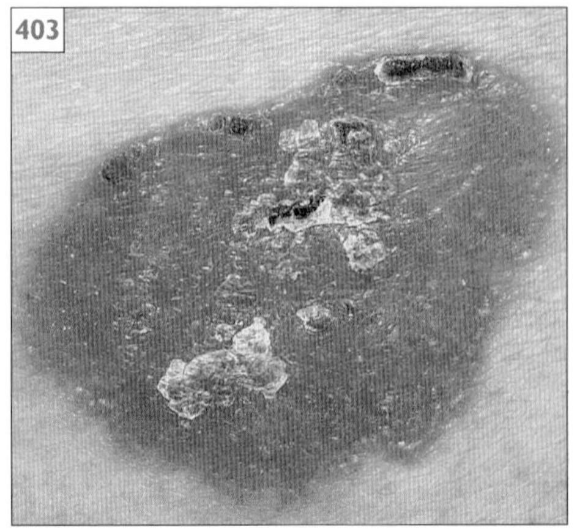

403 Superficial basal cell carcinoma.

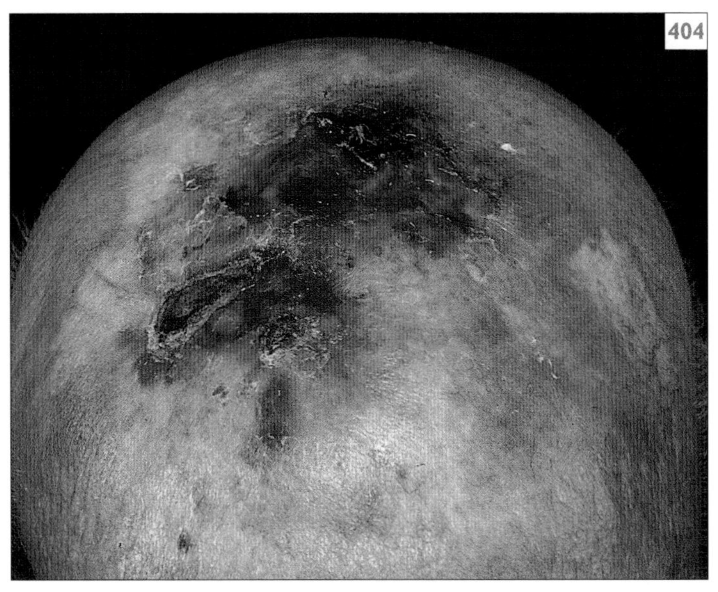

404 Angiosarcoma.

DIFFERENTIAL DIAGNOSIS

Superficial basal cell carcinoma may mimic Bowen's disease, and morphoeic-type basal cell carcinomas may be dismissed as scar tissue. Deeply pigmented lesions should be differentiated from malignant melanoma.

INVESTIGATIONS

Biopsy.

TREATMENT

The choice of treatment depends on the tumour size, location, clinical subtype, and previous treatment. For most nodular BCCs primary excision with a wide margin is the treatment of choice and provides a specimen for histology and evaluation of lateral and deep margins. Moh's micrographic surgery is indicated for recurrent BCCs and morphoeic (infiltrative) subtypes. Destructive modalities such as curettage and cautery, cryotherapy, and topical imiquimod are alternatives for superficial tumours in non-critical sites.

Angiosarcoma

DEFINITION AND CLINICAL FEATURES

A rare, aggressive, malignant tumour of blood vessels. Most cases occur on the face and scalp in the elderly. They may also be associated with chronic lymphoedema (Stewart–Treves' syndrome) and previous radiotherapy. The initial change is a bruise-like discolouration, followed by the appearance of dusky red nodules, ulceration, and oedema (**404**). Metastases and death are usual.

DIFFERENTIAL DIAGNOSIS

Early signs are subtle and may be mistaken for bruising or erysipelas.

INVESTIGATIONS

Histology shows disorganized vessels with plump endothelial cells.

TREATMENT

Treatment includes wide excision and radiotherapy but the prognosis is poor.

CUTANEOUS LYMPHOPROLIFERATIVE DISORDERS

Benign lymphocytic infiltrate of Jessner

DEFINITION AND CLINICAL FEATURES

A chronic, benign disorder of unknown cause, characterized by multiple, smooth, cherry-pink papules on the head and neck (**405**). Lesions may coalesce and are non-scarring. Histology shows a perivascular infiltrate of T-lymphocytes in the superficial and mid-dermis, with a normal overlying epidermis. Females are affected more often than males and childhood and familial cases have been reported.

INVESTIGATIONS

Histology usually helps support the diagnosis, although there is much overlap with other diseases characterized by dermal lymphocytic infiltrates. Direct immunofluorescence and serum autoimmune profile are negative and can help exclude lupus erythematosus (see p. 163).

DIFFERENTIAL DIAGNOSIS

Lupus erythematosus, pseudolymphoma, and malignant lymphocytic infiltrates such as chronic lymphocytic leukaemia and lymphoma.

TREATMENT

The condition often proves unresponsive to therapy, but potent topical corticosteroids, dapsone, and antimalarial drugs may help.

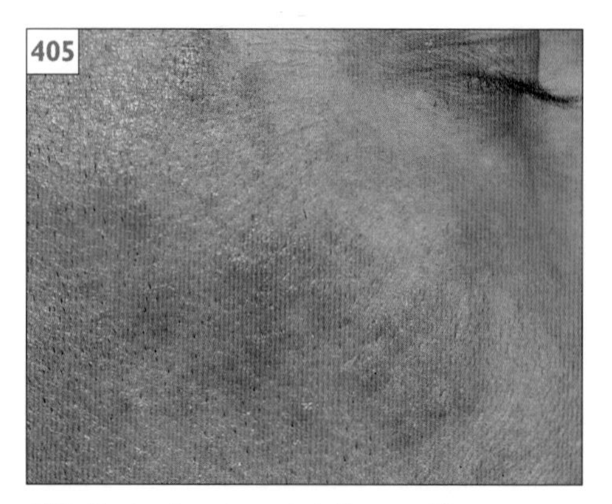

405 Benign lymphocytic infiltrate of Jessner.

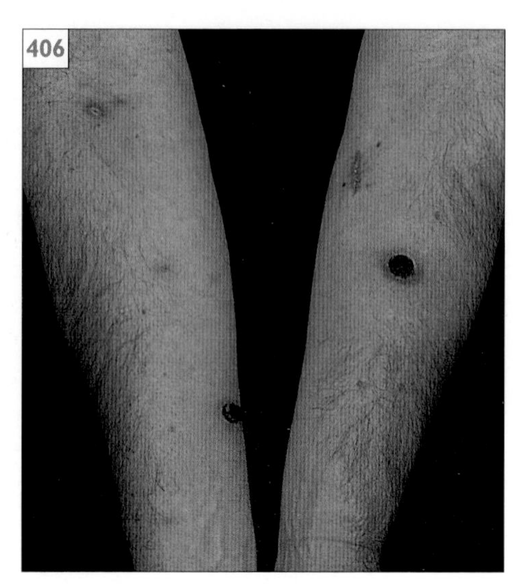

406 Lymphomatoid papulosis.

Lymphomatoid papulosis

DEFINITION AND CLINICAL FEATURES

A rare benign lymphoproliferative disorder characterized by recurrent, scaly papules which heal with scars. There are recurrent, well-circumscribed, red-brown indurated papules with a collarette of scale, of variable size, up to 2 cm in diameter, which may heal slowly to leave depigmented, atrophic scars (**406**). Lesions are distributed predominantly on the trunk and inner flexural aspects of the limbs. Long-term follow up is necessary because approximately 5% of patients progress to a more aggressive lymphoma.

DIFFERENTIAL DIAGNOSIS

Pityriasis lichenoides chronica, cutaneous B cell lymphoma.

INVESTIGATIONS

Histology. Lymphomatoid papulosis can be classified into histological subtypes. Atypical CD30 + lymphocytes may be prominent in the dermal infiltrate and T-cell receptor gene rearrangement studies often show clonality.

TREATMENT

There is no treatment that alters the disease course, but healing may be accelerated by phototherapy, low dose methotrexate, or dapsone.

Mycosis fungoides

DEFINITION AND CLINICAL FEATURES

Mycosis fungoides is the commonest form of cutaneous T-cell lymphoma. It is a rare disease which mainly affects older adults and usually runs a chronic indolent course. The initial presentation is usually with asymptomatic or slightly scaly erythematous patches of variable size. These may be distributed anywhere but occur especially on the trunk and buttocks (**407**). In dark-skinned individuals, hypopigmentation may be prominent (**408**). The majority of patients do not progress beyond this stage. Patches may develop into infiltrated, purplish-red plaques and, rarely, ulcerating plaques or nodules (tumour stage) (**409**). All three stages may occur concurrently.

Involvement of the scalp may lead to alopecia. Peripheral lymphadenopathy and, rarely, hepatosplenomegaly and systemic lymphomatous infiltration may develop.

Pagetoid reticulosis (Woringer–Kolopp disease) is a localized solitary plaque of cutaneous T-cell lymphoma which tends to occur on acral sites in younger adults. The lesion presents as a slowly expanding scaly plaque.

DIFFERENTIAL DIAGNOSIS

Eczema, psoriasis, and chronic superficial scaly dermatitis.

INVESTIGATIONS

Biopsy of lesional skin for routine histology. T-cell receptor gene rearrangement studies may confirm early skin or lymph node involvement. Radiological and haematological investigation to exclude systemic involvement where extensive plaque or tumour stage disease is present.

TREATMENT

The choice of treatment depends on the disease stage and patient fitness, as patients are often elderly and frail. Potent topical corticosteroids and phototherapy are commonly used for early disease. Other options include topical chemotherapy (nitrogen mustard or carmustine), retinoids, radiotherapy, and electron beam therapy.

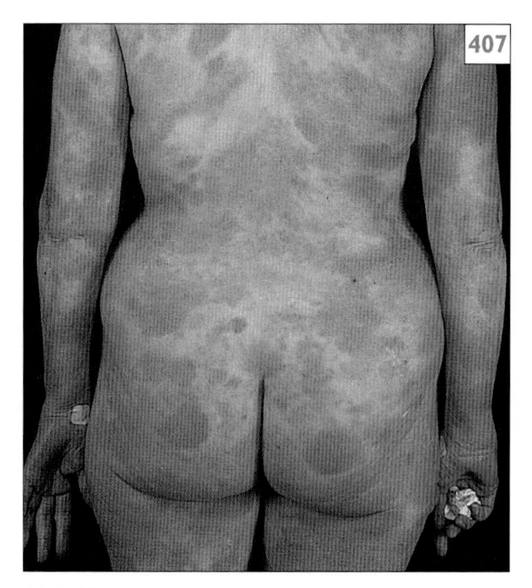

407 Plaque stage mycosis fungoides.

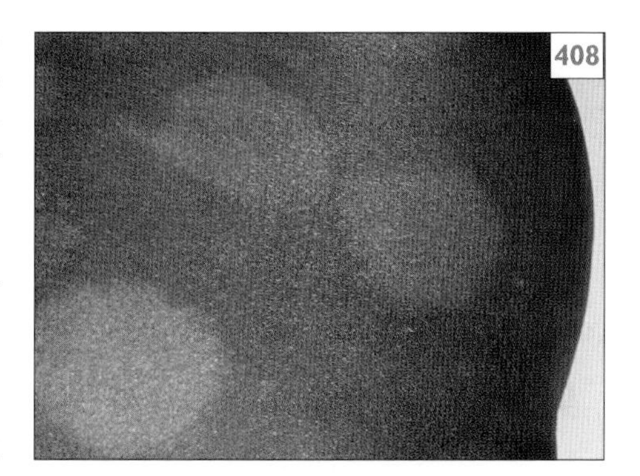

408 Hypopigmented mycosis fungoides.

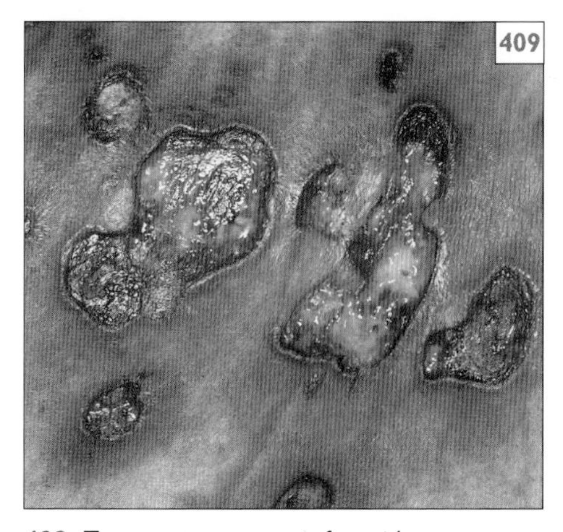

409 Tumour stage mycosis fungoides.

Sézary syndrome

DEFINITION AND CLINICAL FEATURES

A rare T-cell lymphoma/leukaemia characterized by erythroderma (**410**), lymphadenopathy, and atypical circulating lymphocytes (Sézary cells) comprising 5% of more of the peripheral lymphocyte count. This disease predominantly affects elderly men and may occur de novo or evolve from mycosis fungoides. Hepatomegaly, alopecia, nail dystrophy, and keratoderma may occur.

DIFFERENTIAL DIAGNOSIS

Other causes of erythroderma.

INVESTIGATIONS

Biopsy of skin and lymph node. Blood film for Sézary cells.

TREATMENT

The oral retinoid bexarotene may be used as monotherapy or in combination with interferons and phototherapy. Extracorporeal photopheresis involves administration of oral psorialen followed by UVA irradiation of the patient's lymphocytes *ex vivo*.

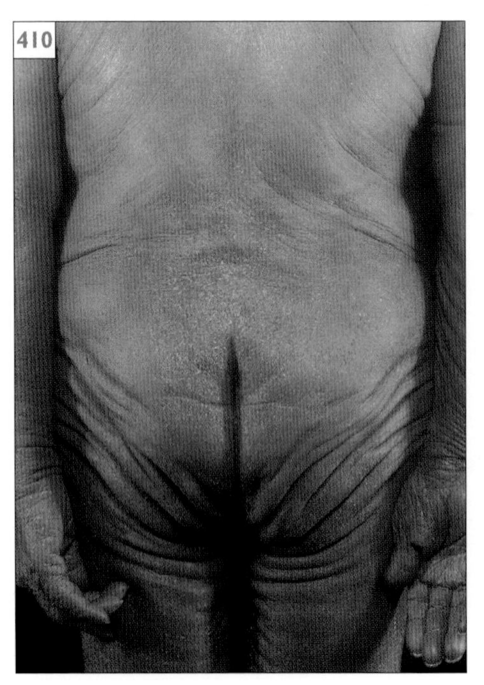

410 Erythroderma in Sézary syndrome.

Lymphocytoma cutis

DEFINITION AND CLINICAL FEATURES

A chronic benign cutaneous B-lymphoproliferative disorder which presents with erythematous or violaceous nodules or plaques on the head and neck (**411**). Lesions are asymptomatic and often expand slowly. The cause is unknown and it appears commoner in females. A small proportion of patients may progress to cutaneous B-cell lymphoma.

DIFFERENTIAL DIAGNOSIS

Jessner's lymphocytic infiltrate, polymorphic light eruption, cutaneous B-cell lymphoma, granulomatous disorders, and insect bites.

INVESTIGATIONS

Histology.

TREATMENT

There is no established treatment, but topical or intralesional corticosteroids and antimalarials may be used.

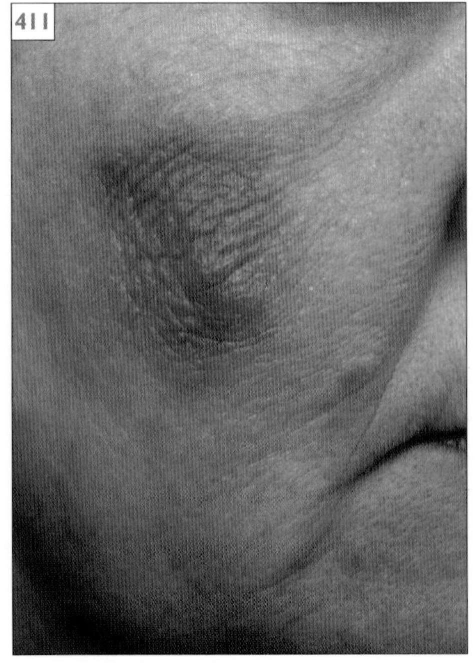

411 Lymphocytoma cutis.

Primary cutaneous B-cell lymphoma

DEFINITION AND CLINICAL FEATURES

A malignant proliferation of B lymphocytes within the skin that presents as multiple, smooth, red-purple, indurated plaques and grouped nodules of variable size. Cutaneous B-cell lymphomas comprise approximately a quarter of all cutaneous lymphomas and are rare. Different subtypes include follicle centre cell lymphoma which is commonest on the head and neck (**412**), marginal zone lymphoma which often affects the trunk, and large B-cell lymphoma which typically affect the legs of elderly women (**413**). Lesions may heal spontaneously, and the prognosis is usually excellent, which is in contrast to systemic B-cell lymphomas occurring at extracutaneous sites.

DIFFERENTIAL DIAGNOSIS

Benign lymphocytic infiltrates.

INVESTIGATIONS

Histology and immunophenotyping of lymphocytes. Full staging investigations are required to exclude systemic B-cell lymphomas.

TREATMENT

Solitary lesions may be excised. Superficial radiotherapy is often effective, but multi-agent chemotherapy is often required for large B-cell lymphoma of the leg.

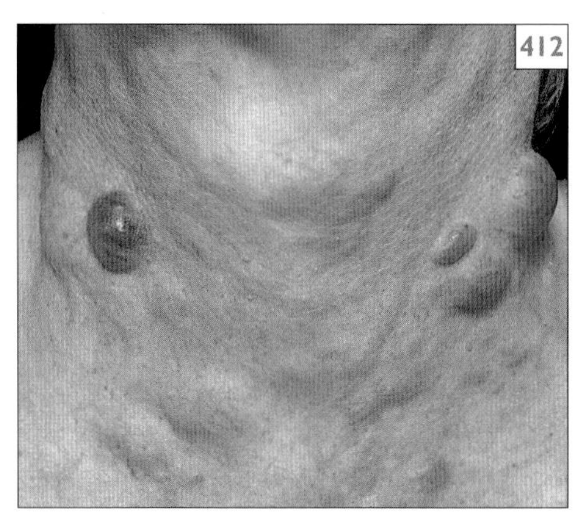

412 Cutaneous B-cell lymphoma.

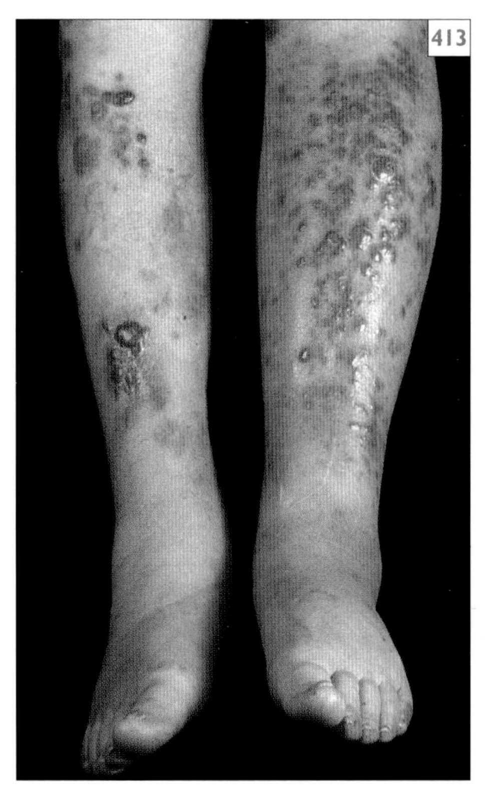

413 Large B-cell lymphoma.

PART 3

Infections and infestations

- **Bacterial infections**
- **Fungal diseases**
- **Viral infections**
- **Human immunodeficiency virus (HIV) infection**
- **Infestations**
- **Tropical infections**

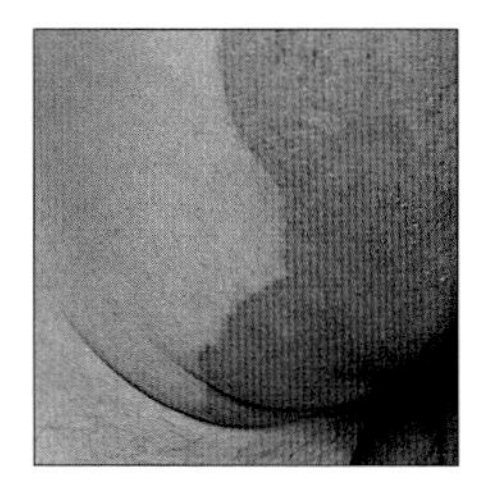

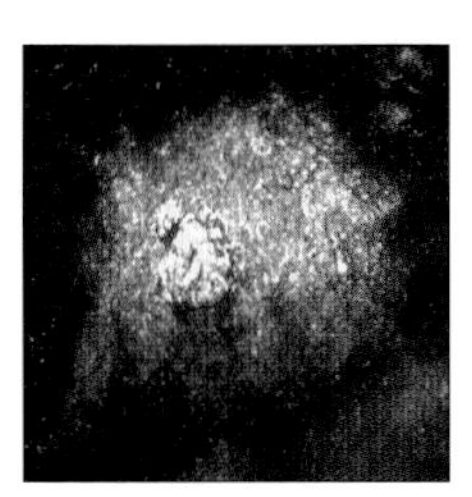

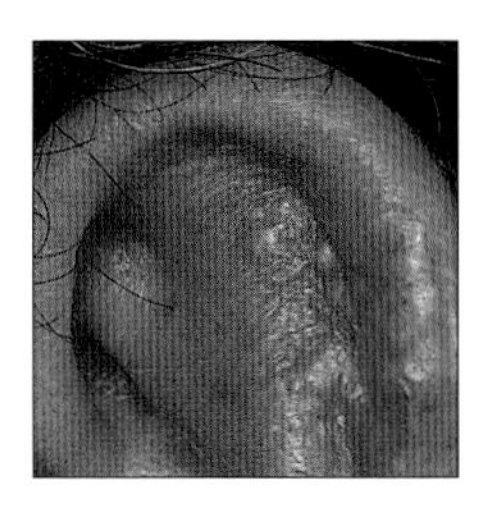

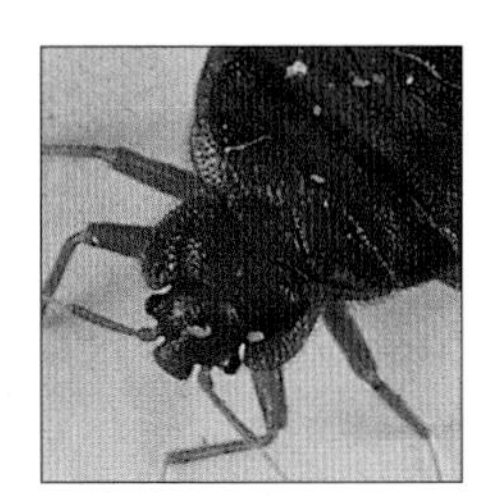

BACTERIAL INFECTIONS

Impetigo

DEFINITION AND CLINICAL FEATURES

Impetigo is a contagious acute superficial infection of the skin caused by *Staphylococcus aureus* or, less commonly, streptococci, particularly Lancefield group A. Young children are most commonly affected but no age group is exempt. Overcrowding, poor hygiene, hot humid climates, and pre-existing skin disease including eczema and scabies predispoe to impetigo.

It presents as golden-yellow crusts, formed from exuding serum, usually affecting the face (**414**). The lesions spread locally and may coalesce; multiple lesions are common. Infection with epidermolytic toxin-producing strains of staphylococci can result in blister formation (**415**) (bullous impetigo). After rupture these leave brown crusts which tend to heal centrally, forming annular lesions. Systemic upset is not usual but glomerulonephritis has been reported following streptococcal impetigo.

DIFFERENTIAL DIAGNOSIS

Fungal infections, herpes simplex, eczema.

INVESTIGATIONS

Bacterial swab should be taken from lesions to determine antibiotic sensitivities.

TREATMENT

Treatment with a topical antibiotic such as mupirocin or fusidic acid is effective for localized impetigo, but fucidin-resistant staphylococci have become more frequent due to widespread use of this antibiotic. For more extensive lesions or if there is lymphadenopathy or reason to suspect nephritogenic streptococci, an oral antibiotic such as erythromycin or flucloxacillin should be prescribed. Topical antiseptics such as chlorhexidine or povidone iodine may be useful adjuncts.

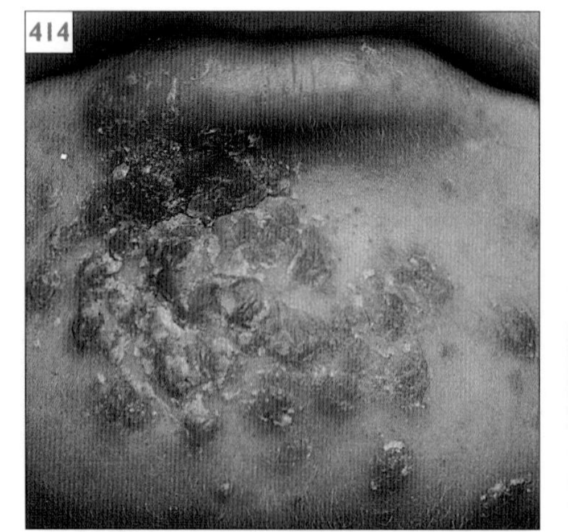

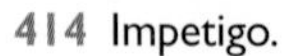

414 Impetigo.

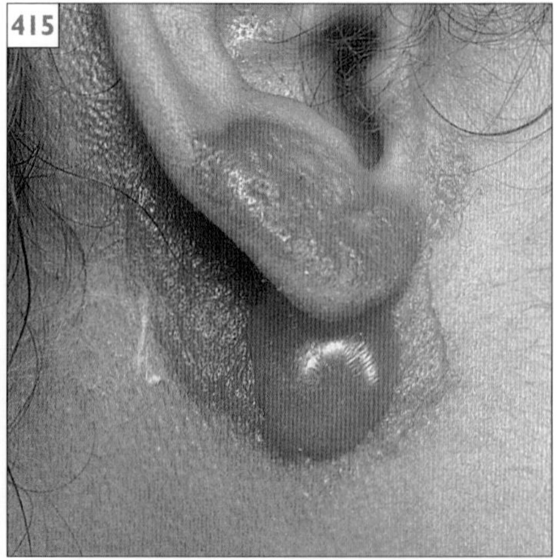

415 Bullous impetigo.

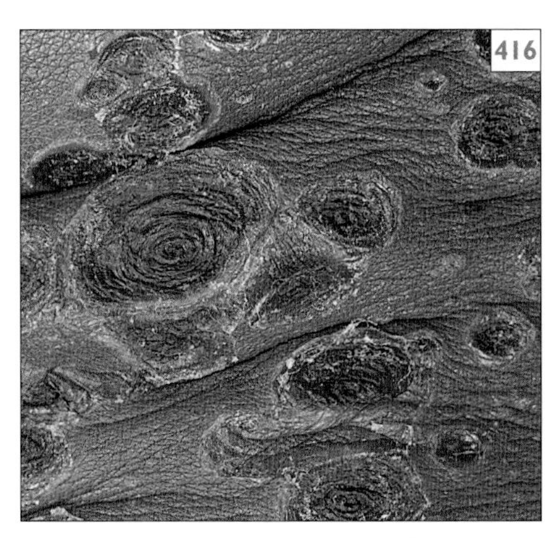

416 Ecthyma.

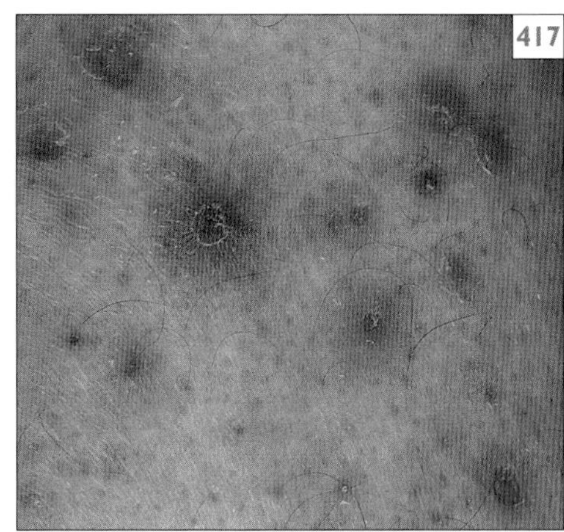

417 Folliculitis.

Echthyma

DEFINITION AND CLINICAL FEATURES

Ecthyma is a deeper infection than impetigo and is also caused by *Staphylococcus aureus* and *Streptococcus* species. It is uncommon in temperate climates where it occurs mostly in children, but in the tropics it may affect any age. Poor hygiene and malnutrition are predisposing factors. The condition presents as hard dark crusts and eschars overlying localized areas of necrotic skin, with a surrounding halo of inflammation (**416**). Lesions usually occur on the limbs and bullae are sometimes seen. Healing takes 2–3 weeks and leaves scars.

DIFFERENTIAL DIAGNOSIS

Vasculitis, pityriasis lichenoides.

INVESTIGATIONS

Bacterial swabs for antibiotic sensitivities.

TREATMENT

Oral antibiotics are indicated and any underlying disease or associated skin disease such as scabies should be treated.

Folliculitis

DEFINITION AND CLINICAL FEATURES

Folliculitis is a superficial inflammation within hair follicles. It may be caused by a range of pathogens including *Staphylococcus aureus*, coagulase-negative *Staphylococcus*, *Pseudomonas aeruginosa*, Gram-negative bacteria, and *Pityrosporum* yeasts. Non-microbial causes of folliculitis include a variety of chemicals and traumatic factors. This common problem is seen most often in young adults, but all ages are susceptible depending on the aetiology. It is characterized by small pustules which, on close inspection, can be seen to be centred on hair follicles (**417**). There are variable degrees of inflammation in surrounding skin.

DIFFERENTIAL DIAGNOSIS

Other follicular disorders, such as lichen planopilaris, and non-follicular pustules, as in psoriasis.

INVESTIGATIONS

Skin swabs for microbiology. A nasal swab may be taken in recurrent cases to identify staphylococcal carriage.

TREATMENT

Mild staphylococcal follicultis is often self-limiting, and may be treated with topical antiseptics. In more severe cases, topical or oral antibiotics are indicated. Chemical or traumatic folliculitis responds to removal of the external irritant.

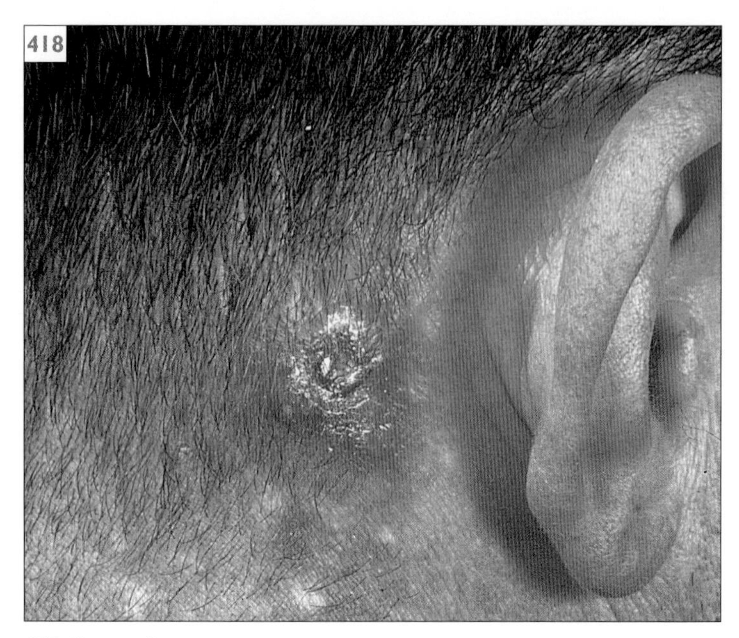

418 Furunculosis.

Furuncles and carbuncles

DEFINITION AND CLINICAL FEATURES

A furuncle (or boil) is an abscess caused by *Staphylococcus aureus* within a hair follicle. Carbuncles are more extensive lesions with infection and necrosis spreading to several follicles and to surrounding soft tissues. An inflammatory nodule develops into a follicular pustule which will point and discharge (**418**). Furuncles are often multiple; carbuncles are similar but more extensive with multiple openings – they may reach more than 1 cm in diameter. Discharge leaves a deep ulcer. Fever and malaise can occur with both furuncles and carbuncles but are usually more severe with the latter. Furuncles typically affect healthy, young adults although recurrent boils can be a sign of poorly controlled diabetes. Carbuncles usually affect older patients with concurrent illness.

DIFFERENTIAL DIAGNOSIS

Severe acne may also show inflammatory cysts and papules, but close inspection shows comedones. Hidradenitis suppurativa is typically localized to the inguinal folds, axillae, and breast areas.

INVESTIGATIONS

Microbial swabs of the skin and carrier sites to determine antibiotic sensitivities. In recurrent cases further investigations such as fasting blood glucose should be performed to exclude underlying illness.

TREATMENT

A course of oral flucloxacillin or a penicillinase-resistant antibiotic should be given. Topical antiseptics may also be helpful. In recurrent cases eradication of *Staphylococcus* from carriage sites such as the nose and perineum should be attempted. Any underlying systemic disease or debility should be treated.

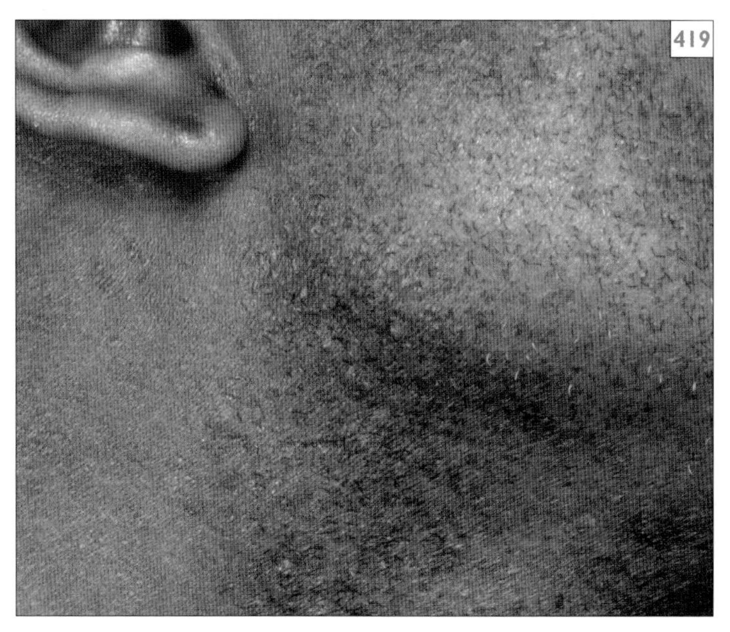

419 Pseudofolliculitis.

Pseudofolliculitis

DEFINITION AND CLINICAL FEATURES

Pseudofolliculitis is an inflammatory perifollicular disorder caused by an ingrowth of hair into the skin. It is most liable to occur with coarse curly hair, and is a common problem in Afro-Caribbean men. Close shaving and plucking aggravate the problem. The beard area and nape of the neck are typically affected with multiple firm papules and pustules (**419**). These may develop into hypertrophic scars and keloids – acne keloidalis nuchae (**420**).

INVESTIGATIONS

None are routinely necessary. Microbial swabs may be taken from pustular lesions.

TREATMENT

The most important aspect of management is to stop any methods of hair removal until the complaint settles. This is seldom popular with men. Simply changing shaving technique may help, e.g. using an electric razor rather than wet shaving, or using a depilatory cream. Antiseptics may help reduce secondary infection, and potent topical corticosteroids can be of benefit in flattening keloidal lesions.

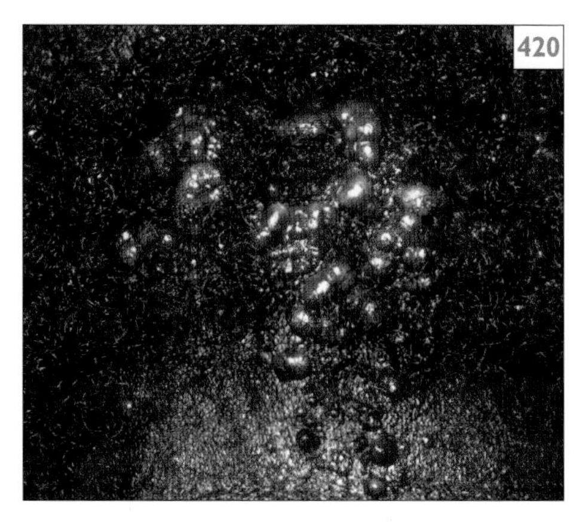

420 Acne keloidalis nuchae.

Erysipelas, cellulitis, and necrotizing fasciitis

DEFINITION AND CLINICAL FEATURES

Erysipelas and cellulitis are infections of the dermis and subcutaneous tissue and are usually caused by streptococci, although a variety of other bacteria may be implicated especially in the immunocompromised. There is no clear distinction between cellulitis and erysipelas: in the latter the infection is more superficial. In necrotizing fasciitis the infection is deeper still, reaching the fascia. In all three conditions predisposing factors such as trauma and diabetes are important, with both systemic and local disease allowing infection to become established. Oedema, particularly lymphoedema, is an important predisposing factor and can lead to recurrent attacks.

Infection is heralded by malaise and fever, and after a few hours to days the affected area becomes red, tender, and swollen (**421**). Bullae, sometimes haemorrhagic, can appear in acute cases. Red streaks of lymphangitis and tender lymphadenopathy are common. In erysipelas the margins of erythema are usually more clearly demarcated than in cellulitis (**422**). In necrotizing fasciitis the erythema is often dusky, and deep haemorrhagic bullae develop with necrosis of the skin and soft tissues (**423**).

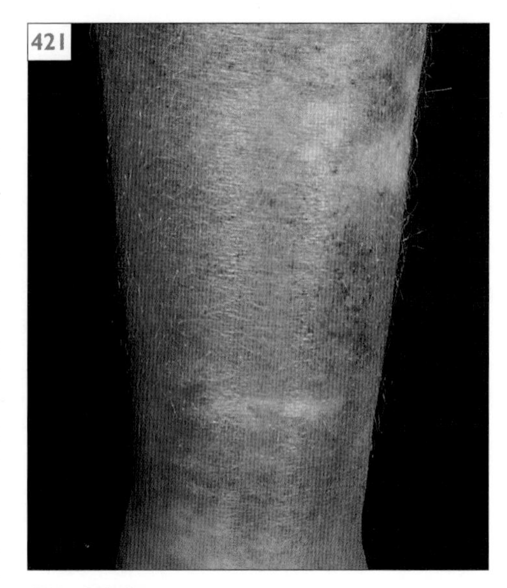

421 Cellulitis.

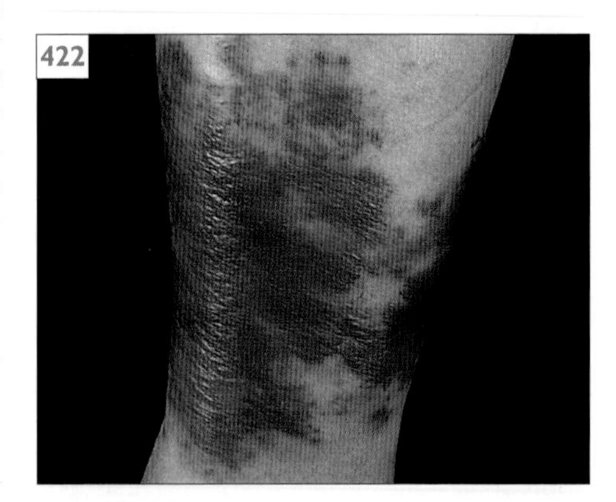

422 Erysipelas.

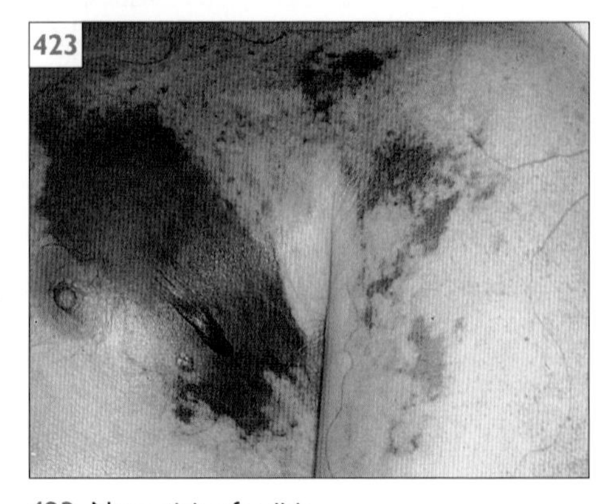

423 Necrotizing fasciitis.

DIFFERENTIAL DIAGNOSIS

Deep venous throumbosis of the lower legs, eosinophilic cellulitis (Wells' syndrome).

INVESTIGATIONS

Skin swabs should be taken from nany eroded or ulcerated areas in addition to blood cultures, but these are often negative. Serological studies may provide evidence of streptococcal infection (ASOT; anti-DNAase B).

TREATMENT

Treatment of all three conditions is with systemic antibiotics; these often need to be given parenterally. Necrotizing fasciitis may progress rapidly and carries a high mortality. Urgent surgery is essential to debride necrotic tissue. Management of recurrent cellulitis may require long-term antibiotics, and skin care to avoid entry portals such as toe-web tinea infection.

Scarlet fever

DEFINITION AND CLINICAL FEATURES

Scarlet fever (scarlatina) is an acute infection with a toxin-producing strain of *Streptococcus pyogenes*. The usual portal of entry of the streptococcus is the upper respiratory tract, hence the disease presents with sore throat and lymphadenopathy. An erythematous rash appears on the trunk and becomes generalized. The face is flushed but the perioral area shows relative pallor. The tongue becomes red with swollen papillae, the strawberry tongue. Scarlet fever is usually seen in children, and it has become less common and milder than in previous decades. Complications caused by the toxin or bacterial invasion include meningitis, osteomyelitis, rheumatic fever, and glomerulonephritis.

DIFFERENTIAL DIAGNOSIS

Staphylococcal toxic shock syndrome, Kawasaki disease, viral exanthems, and drug eruptions.

INVESTIGATIONS

Throat swab for bacteriology.

TREATMENT

A full-dosage course of penicillin should be started as soon as the diagnosis is suspected.

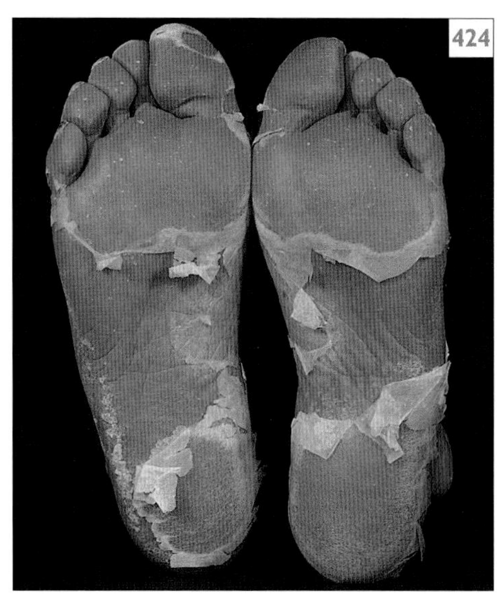

424 Skin peeling following toxic shock syndrome.

Toxic shock syndrome

DEFINITION AND CLINICAL FEATURES

This occurs as a consequence of infection with an exotoxin-producing strain of group A streptococcus or *Staphylococcus aureus*. The clinical features are fever, malaise, and a widespread sunburn-like rash followed by circulatory collapse and multisystem failure. Streptococcal toxic shock syndrome carries a higher mortality and usually follows severe invasive infection sugh as surgical wounds or post-partum infection. Staphylococcal toxic shock syndrome may occur following trivial, or asymptomatic infections and has been linked with the use of superabsorbent vaginal tampons. The rash fades within a few days and peeling of the hands and feet may occur after a week (**424**).

DIFFERENTIAL DIAGNOSIS

Other toxin-mediated erythemas. Kawasaki disease can usually be differentiated by its prolonged fever, cardiac involvement, generalized lymphadenopathy, and lack of circulatory shock.

INVESTIGATIONS

Microbiological examination of swabs from appropriate sites including blood cultures.

TREATMENT

High-dose parenteral antibiotics and intensive general support measures are essential.

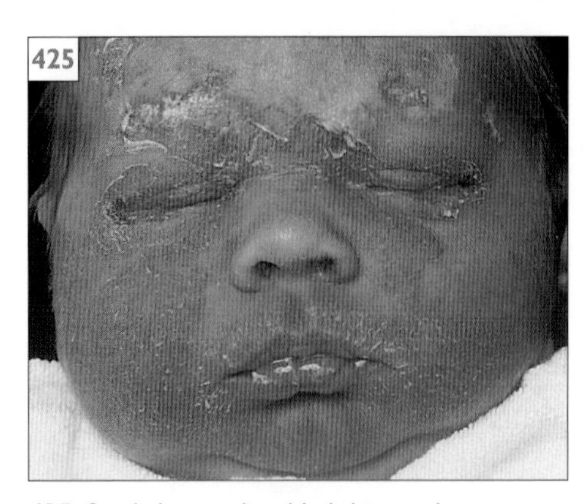

425 Staphylococcal scalded skin syndrome.

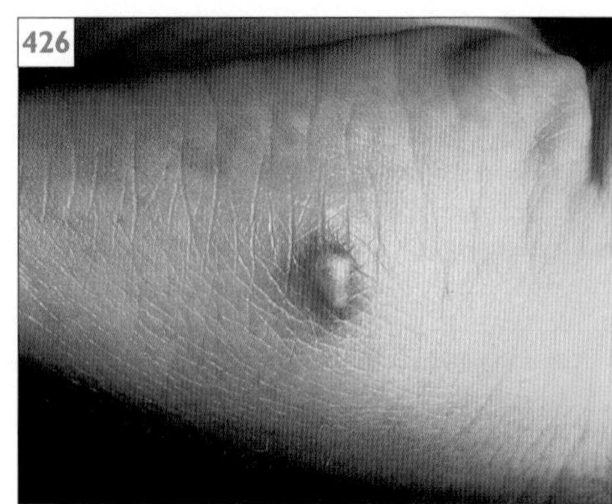

426 Haemorrhagic pustule in gonococcal septicaemia.

Staphylococcal scalded skin syndrome

DEFINITION AND CLINICAL FEATURES

Staphylococcal scalded skin syndrome (SSSS) is a widespread exfoliative dermatosis following infection with epidermolytic toxin-producing strains of *Staphylococcus aureus*. The same toxins are involved as in bullous impetigo. The causative *Staphylococcus* can be on the skin (or an occult infection) which becomes red and tender and peels away to form raw areas on the trunk, flexures, and face (**425**). Healing takes place in about a week. SSSS usually affects children, but adults may develop localized areas, usually in the context of renal failure or alcoholism.

DIFFERENTIAL DIAGNOSIS

In toxic epidermal necrolysis splitting of the skin occurs more deeply at the dermo-epidermal junction and this results in a higher morbidity and mortality.

INVESTIGATIONS

Histopathology of lesional skin shows splitting of the epidermis between the granular and prickle layers in SSSS which differentiates SSSS from toxic epidermal necrolysis. A frozen skin section may be taken for emergency diagnosis. Skin swabs and blister fluid do not usualy grow the causative bacterium as lesions are toxin mediated.

TREATMENT

The prognosis is good if treated promptly with parenteral antibiotics.

Gonococcal septicaemia

DEFINITION AND CLINICAL FEATURES

Chronic occult infection with *Neisseria gonorrhoeae* can result in bacteraemia and give rise to a multisystem illness. Skin lesions, fever, and arthralgia are presenting features. Haemorrhagic pustules and vesicles appear in crops, typically on the fingers (**426**).

DIFFERENTIAL DIAGNOSIS

Meningococcal septicaemia, vasculitis, and subacute bacterial endocarditis.

INVESTIGATIONS

Microbiological swabs should be taken from the genitalia, pharynx, and rectum as asymptomatic infection is common. Blood cultures may be positive, but gonococci are rarely cultured from skin lesions.

SPECIAL POINTS

Sexual contacts need to be traced and screened for infection.

TREATMENT

Parenteral antibiotics.

Meningococcal infection

DEFINITION AND CLINICAL FEATURES

Infection with the Gram-negative coccus *Neisseria meningitidis*. This bacterium may colonize the upper respiratory tract of healthy carriers. Mild localized forms of infection include conjunctivitis or otitis media or, following bacteraemia, severe disease may occur in the form of meningitis or septicaemia. The latter present acutely and may run a fulminant course. Early skin lesions are discrete small pink macules and papules and are *not* necessarily haemorrhagic. Transient urticarial or morbilliform rashes may also occur. Widespread purpura is characteristic, expecially on the limbs and trunk (**427**). Large purpuric, necrotic lesions with ragged edges and ecchymoses may occur. Vasculitic lesions may develop several days later, presenting with nodules or bullae on the limbs. Children and young adults are most commonly affected. Cases are usually sporadic but small epidemics may occur.

DIFFERENTIAL DIAGNOSIS

Viral meningitis and other causes of acute vasculitis.

INVESTIGATIONS

The diagnosis is confirmed by identifiying meningococci in blood, CSF, and skin lesions.

TREATMENT

Infection is rapidly progressive (**428**) and death can occur in the early stages. Parenteral antibiotic treatment should be given as soon as the diagnosis is suspected and the patient admitted to hospital.

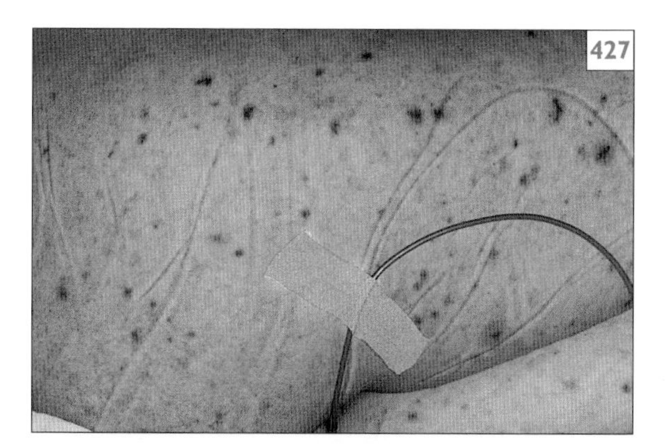

427 Purpuric lesions in meningococcal septicaemia.

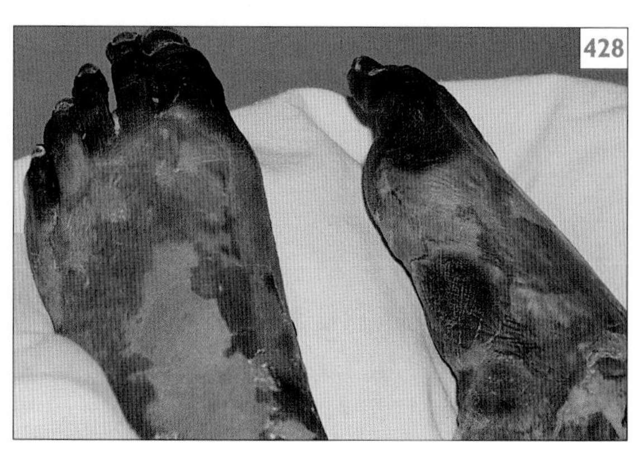

428 Gangrenous lesions in meningococcal septicaemia.

Erythrasma

DEFINITION AND CLINICAL FEATURES

Erythrasma is a mild, chronic superficial infection with the bacterium *Corynebacterium minutissimum*. These Gram-positive rods are part of the normal flora in the toe clefts, and their overgrowth in flexures can be triggered by warm humid climates. The rash consists of red or brown, well-marginated, slightly scaly or glazed patches (**429**). Sites most commonly affected are the axillae and groins. Lesions are asymptomatic or mildly pruritic. Adults are affected more often than children, and it is more common in tropical climates and in diabetics. Asymptomatic carriage of *C. minutissimum* is common.

DIFFERENTIAL DIAGNOSIS

Pityriasis versicolor does not usually affect flexures; tinea cruris and candidiasis are more inflammatory. In flexural psoriasis the lesions are usually deeper red and there are usually additional plaques on non-flexural sites. Seborrhoeic dermatitis.

INVESTIGATIONS

Coral red fluorescence under Wood's light is diagnostic.

TREATMENT

Topical azoles or fucidic acid are usually effective unless infection is extensive.

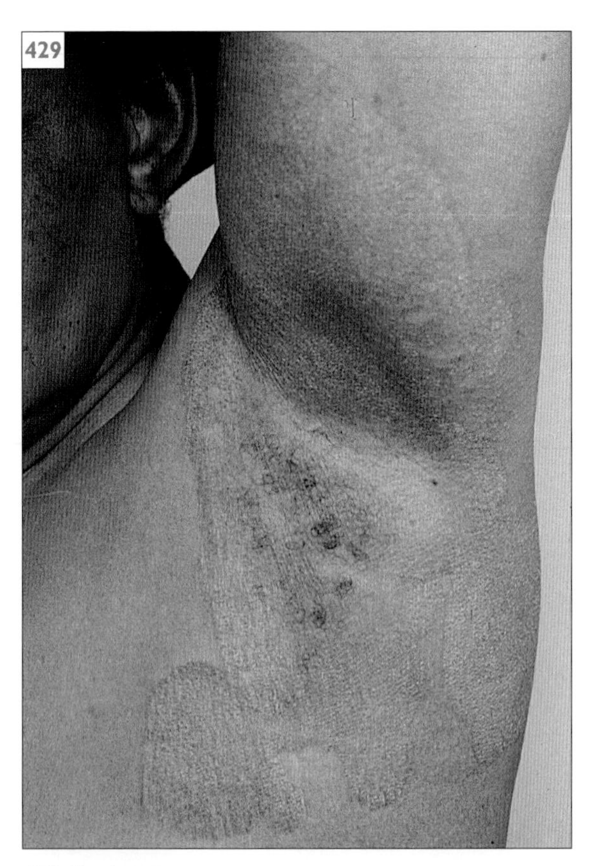

429 Erythrasma.

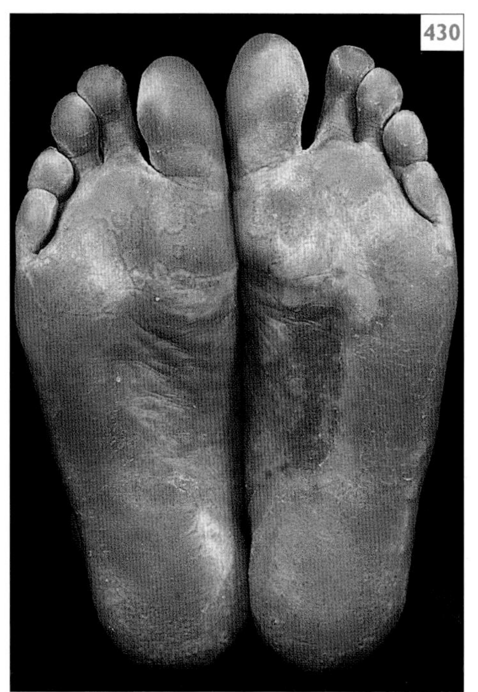

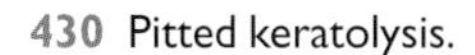

430 Pitted keratolysis.

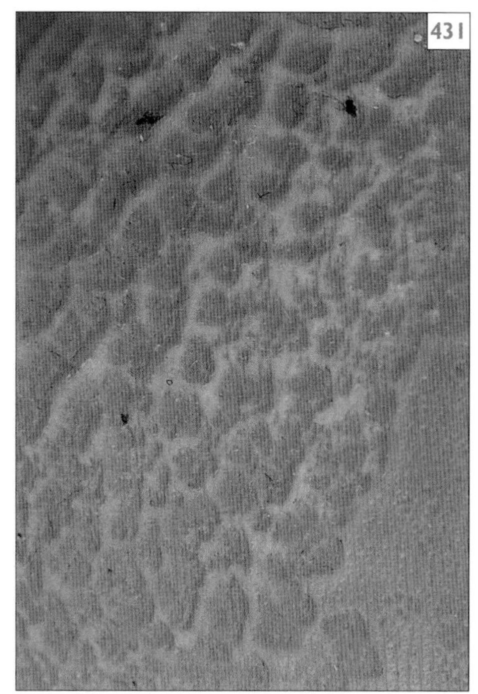

431 Pitted keratolysis.

Pitted keratolysis

DEFINITION AND CLINICAL FEATURES

This chronic superficial infection of the soles of the feet is due to infection with a *Corynebacterium* and possibly other organisms. The appearance is characteristic with small, round pitted/punched-out erosions in the skin surface (**430**, **431**). Occlusive footwear and hyperhidrosis of the feet usually precipitate the problem, which is most common in young men. It is usually asymptomatic.

INVESTIGATIONS

None are usually necessary.

TREATMENT

Reducing sweating of the feet helps to control the condition and can be combined with topical antibacerials.

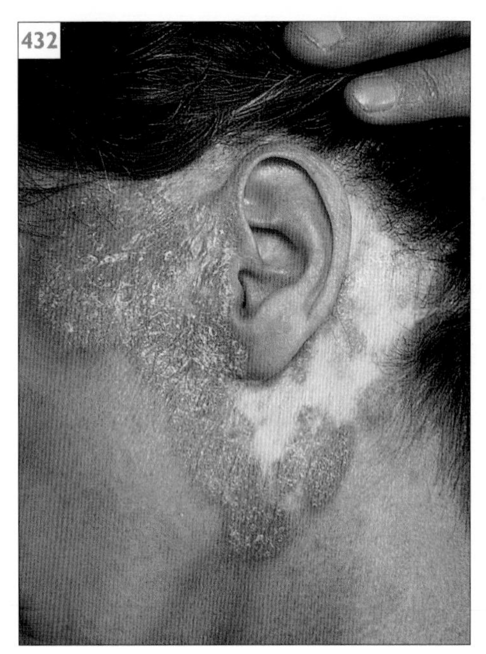

432 Lupus vulgaris.

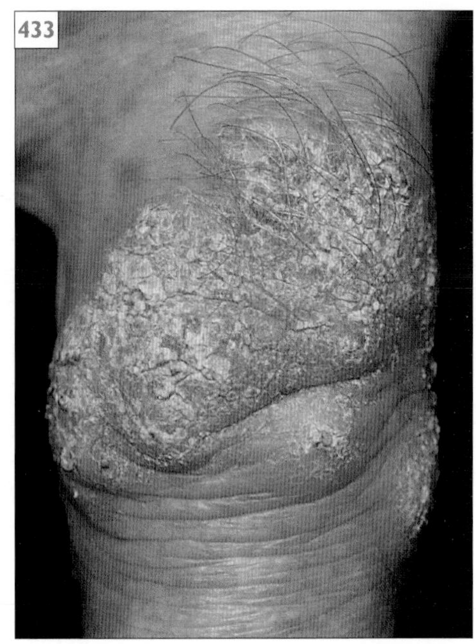

433 Warty TB.

Cutaneous tuberculosis (TB)

DEFINITION AND CLINICAL FEATURES

Infection with *Mycobacterium tuberculae* can produce a range of cutaneous lesions depending on host immunity and the mode of infection, which may be direct, metastatic, or from draining lymph nodes. Lupus vulgaris is the most frequent clinical variant and typically affects the head and neck. It may also arise at the site of BCG vaccination. It presents as progressive red–brown, soft papules and plaques, described as 'apple jelly' nodules (**432**). Disease spreads slowly over many years with resultant scarring. Tuberculous chancre, warty TB (**433**) (both from direct contact), and cutaneous spread from infected lymph nodes and bones are rarely seen. Cutaneous TB was rare in the UK, but the number of notified cases has increased in recent decades, mostly in people from the Indian subcontinent and those with HIV infection.

DIFFERENTIAL DIAGNOSIS

Lupus erythrmatosus, leprosy, sarcoid, and deep fungal infections.

INVESTIGATIONS

Culture of *Mycobacterium* from lesional skin is not usually successful. Histology shows granuloma but caseation is unusual in lupus vulgaris and tubercle bacilli may be hard to identify.

TREATMENT

Treatment is with standard antituberculous therapy.

SPECIAL POINTS

Squamous cell carcinoma can occur in long-standing lupus vulgaris.

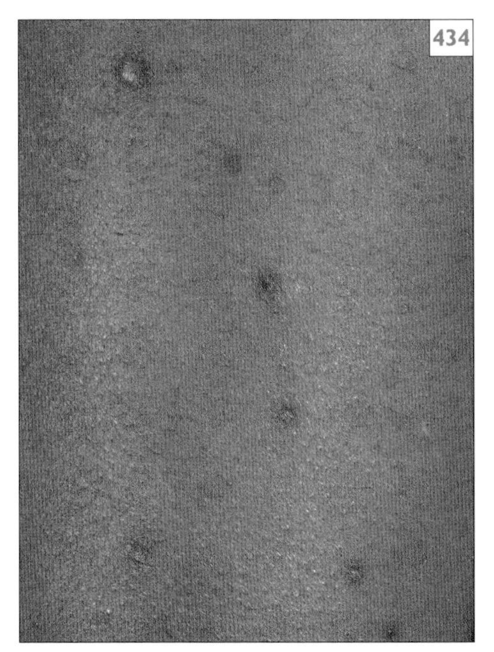

434 Papulonecrotic tuberculide.

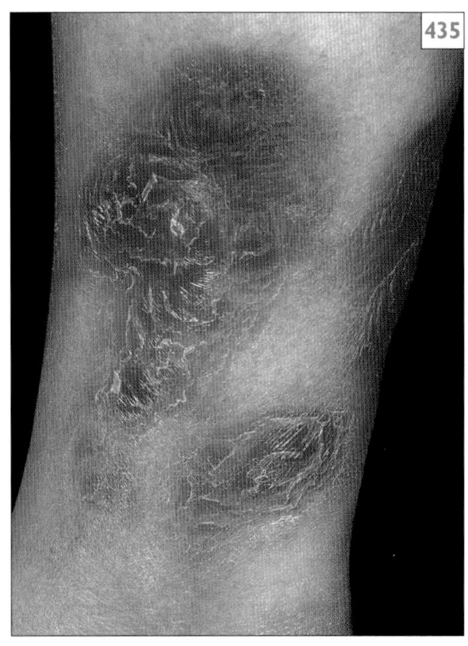

435 Erythema induratum (of Bazin).

Tuberculides

DEFINITION AND CLINICAL FEATURES

The tuberculides are a group of diseases which arise as a hypersensitivity reaction to haematogenous spread of *Mycobacterium tuberculosis* or its antigens in a host with high immunity. They comprise lichen scrofulosorum, papulonecrotic tuberculide, and erythema induratum. Bacteria are not identifiable in histology or culture of lesional skin, although polymerase chain reaction has detected mycobacterial DNA in some cases. Lichen scrofulosorum is rarely seen in Europe, and most cases occur in children in association with TB of the lymph nodes or bones. The eruption consists of small grouped lichenoid papules which are skin coloured or light brown, and is caused by superficial granulomatous inflammation around the sweat ducts, hair follicles, and dermal papillae. Papulonecrotic tuberculide is an eruption of necrotic papules usually on the extensor surfaces of the distal limbs. It mainly affects children and young adults. Lesions occur in crops and ulcerate leaving pigmented scars (**434**). In this tuberculide, granulomatous inflammation involves the thickness of the dermis to the subcutis. Erythema induratum (of Bazin) is characterized by ulcerative nodules on the lower legs and typicall affects overweight women (**435**). There is an underlying granulomatous panniculitis and associated neutrophilic vasculitis.

DIFFERENTIAL DIAGNOSIS

Sarcoid and other granulomatous disorders.

INVESTIGATIONS

Histology of lesional skin supports the diagnosis, but other causes of granulomatous inflammation may share overlapping features. A search should be made for active TB elsewhere in the body. Consider screening for HIV infection in at-risk groups as this predisposes to TB and increases its mortality.

TREATMENT

Standard antituberculous drug therapy should be given.

SPECIAL POINTS

TB may also invoke erythema nodosum, panniculitis, and nodular vasculitis, although other causes are more common.

Leprosy

DEFINITION AND CLINICAL FEATURES

A chronic granulomatous disease caused by *Mycobacterium leprae* primarily affecting the peripheral nerves and skin. The clinical features depend on the underlying immunity of the affected person.

Tuberculoid leprosy is seen in those with high immunity. Lesions are few, and consist of a well-defined plaque with an erythematous raised border and a hypopigmented, dry, anaesthetic centre (**436**). Thickened peripheral nerves may be palpated. Lepromatous leprosy occurs in individuals with poor cell-mediated immunity. Lesions are multiple, infiltrating dermal papules, nodules, and plaques favouring cooler body sites (**437**). Various degrees of intermediate forms exist (**438**) which are at risk of tissue damaging immunological complications.

Leprosy is one of the commonest skin diseases world-wide, with 70% of cases occurring in India. The young are most susceptible to acquiring infection, and spread occurs mainly via the oro-nasal route. The incubation period may last for several years.

DIFFERENTIAL DIAGNOSIS

Post-inflammatory hypopigmentation may be mistaken for tuberculoid leprosy, but such changes resolve after a few months. Vitiligo is depigmented rather than hypopigmented. Other granulomatous diseases, such as TB, leishmaniasis, syphilis, yaws, and sarcoidosis, should be ruled out by histology, microbiology, and skin testing.

INVESTIGATIONS

Skin smear, skin biopsy, nasal scrape, nerve biopsy, and lepromin test.

TREATMENT

All patients with leprosy should receive appropriate multidrug therapy as recommended by the World Health Organization. The first-line drugs are rifampicin, dapsone, and clofazimine. Paucibacillary disease is treated for 6 months, and multibacillary disease for 24 months with follow up of 2 and 5 years respectively. Neuritis or inflammation of skin lesions should be treated with additional oral corticosteroids.

Rapidly growing mycobacteria

DEFINITION AND CLINICAL FEATURES

These are a group of mycobacteria that can produce skin, soft tissue, and bone infections. They include *Mycobacterium fortuitum*, *M. chelonae/abscessus*, and *M. smegmatis*. They are widely found in the environment and may contaminate hospital equipment via water supplies. Skin infection in the immunocompetent individual usually occurs after a penetrating injury and leads to localized abscess formation, while in immunocompromised individuals disseminated skin lesions may occur in association with systemic infection.

DIFFERENTIAL DIAGNOSIS

Deep fungal infection.

INVESTIGATIONS

Culture of skin biopsy material such as an abscess wall is more reliable in identifying the organism than aspirated pus.

TREATMENT

Systemic antimicrobial therapy is needed. Localized skin disease usually responds to monotherapy but systemic disease requires multiple drugs.

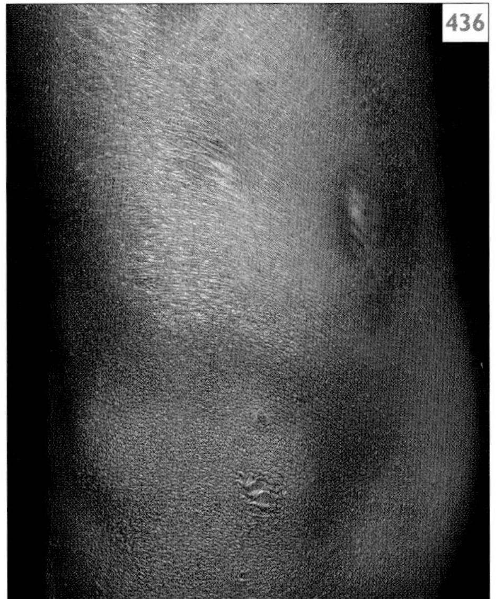

436 Tuberculoid leprosy.

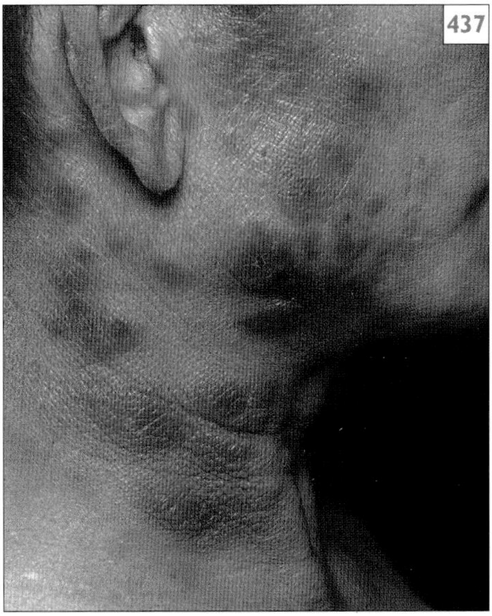

437 Lepromatous leprosy.

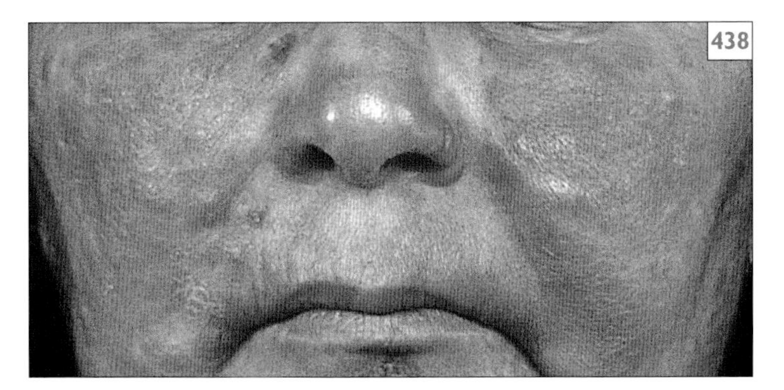

438 Intermediate form of leprosy.

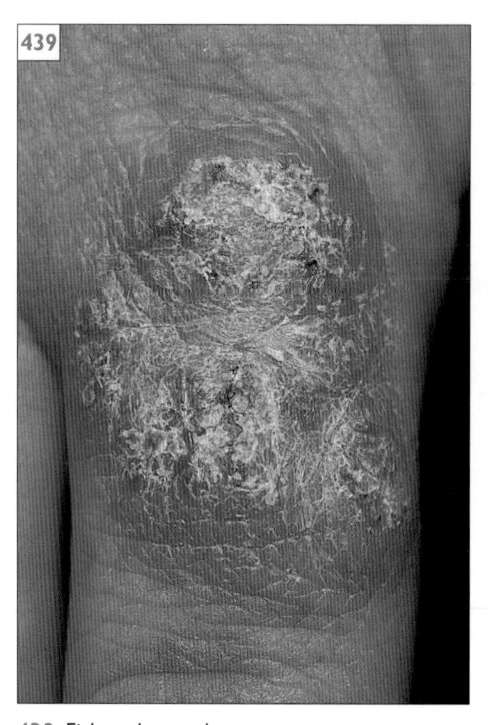

439 Fish-tank granuloma.

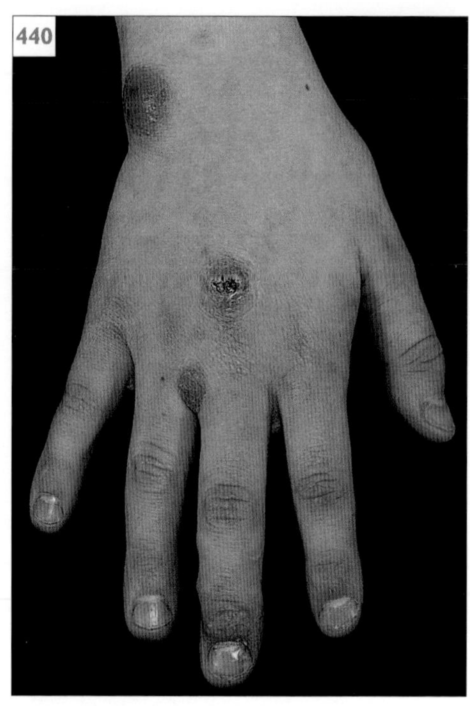

440 Sporotrichoid spread.

Mycobacterium marinum
(fish tank granuloma)

DEFINITION AND CLINICAL FEATURES

This chronic cutaneous infection is caused by the non-tuberculous (atypical) mycobacteria, *Mycobacterium marinum*, an organism that occurs in warm water, especially tropical aquaria. The organism is endemic in most tropical fish and this uncommon condition is usually seen in fish fanciers. Lesions arise in broken skin on exposed areas such as the hands. Pustules or nodules become crusted and warty (**439**). Spread along lymphatics may cause lines of nodules and lymphadenopathy (**440**) as in sporotrichosis (see p. 225). The lesions may heal over a period of months. Growth of the bacterium is inhibited at 37 °C, which is why infections rarely spread systemically.

DIFFERENTIAL DIAGNOSIS

Sporotrichosis, leishmaniasis.

INVESTIGATIONS

Culture of lesional skin is often positive and can help define antibiotic sensitivities. Histology is helpful but does not always distinguish from sporotrichosis.

SPECIAL POINTS

It is important to alert the microbiologist to the possibility of *Mycobacteria marinum* infection so samples can be cultured in the optimum conditions.

TREATMENT

The optimum oral antibiotic is not clear. Treatment options include minocycline, trimethoprim, clarithromycin, and rifampicin for 3–4 months.

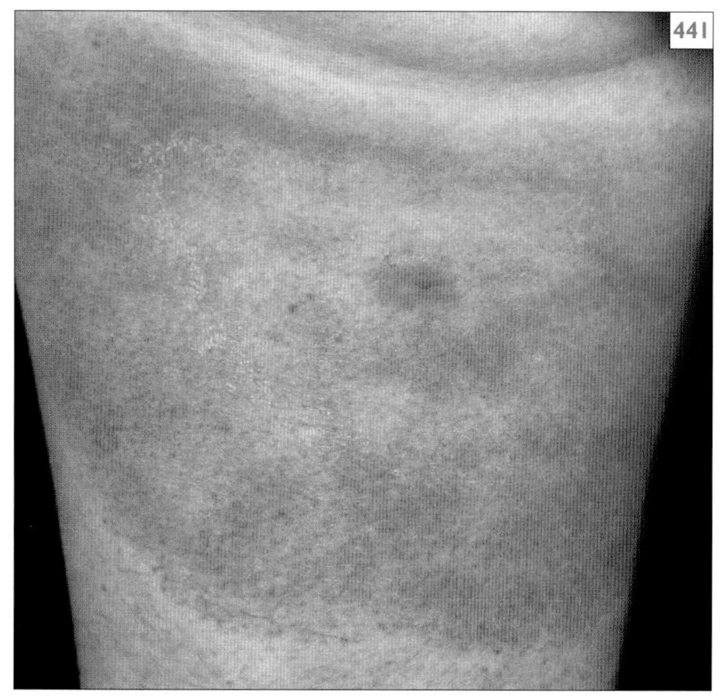

441 Erythema chronicum migrans.

Lyme disease

DEFINITION AND CLINICAL FEATURES

Lyme disease (lyme borreliosis) is caused by *Borrelia burgdorferi*, a tick-borne spirochete. It is named after the town of Lyme in Connecticut, USA, where it was first recognized. It occurs in many other parts of the world, especially central Europe and Scandinavia. Lyme disease is a chronic multisystem infection that often presents with dermatological changes and progresses to involve the joints and nervous system. The early signs of infection are seen in the skin around the site of the bite, as a spreading annular erythema known as erythema chronicum migrans (**441**). The degree of erythema is highly variable, and may be faint. The lesion expands slowly over at a rate of several centimetres a week, and if untreated will fade. There may be associated lymphadenopathy and constitutional symptoms. Dissemination of infection may occur within days or weeks of inoculation and can lead to neurological disease, including meningitis and nerve palsies, carditis, and arthritis. Another cutaneous manifestation, acrodermatitis chronica atrophicans, may occur in the later stages. This is seen as nodules and plaques, usually on the feet or hands, that spread leaving central atrophy.

DIFFERENTIAL DIAGNOSIS

Other causes of annular erythema. The lesions of tinea corporis are usually more scaly than erythema chronicum migrans.

INVESTIGATIONS

B.burgdorferi serology usually confirms the diagnosis but may be negative in the early stages of disease. A Warthin–Starry stain may identify spirochaetes in lesional skin.

SPECIAL POINTS

Adequate treatment with antibiotics is important to prevent later multisystem illness.

FUNGAL DISEASES

Dermatophyte infection and tinea

DEFINITION AND CLINICAL FEATURES

Dermatophytes are fungi that infect the stratum corneum of the skin producing ringworm. There are three genera – *Microsporum*, *Trichophyton*, and *Epidermophyton*.

Skin signs vary with the site of infection and species of infecting fungus, but fungi transmitted from animals usually produce more inflammation than those that are exclusively human pathogens. The endemic species of fungi varies from country to country.

Tinea corporis refers to infection of the body and limbs excluding the palmo-plantar skin and scalp, which may be the original source of infection. It can be caused by any of the dermatophytes. *Trichophyton rubrum* and *Microsporum canis* are frequent offenders. Lesions are pruritic and circular, becoming annular, clearly defined and with a raised, scaly edge (**442**). Inappropriate treatment with topical or systemic corticosteroids can modify the appearance reducing inflammation and temporarily relieving pruritus. Lesions are ill defined, less scaly and slowly spread peripherally. This leads to tinea incognito (**443**).

Tinea cruris, affecting the groins and natal cleft (**444**), is often more itchy than tinea corporis but is otherwise similar. Tinea pedis (athlete's foot) is extremely common. The moist skin of the web spaces provides ideal conditions for *Trichophyton interdigitale*, *T. rubrum*, and *Epidermophyton floccosum*, often coexisting with bacteria (**445**). Moist scaling and fissuring spreads from the toe webs to the soles and dorsae of the feet. Shared showering or bathing facilities encourage the spread of this infection.

Tinea capitis is mainly a disease of children and results from fungal invasion of the hair shafts with *Microsporum canis*, *M. audounii*, and some species of *Trichophyton*. The inflammatory reaction depends on the type of infecting fungus. *M. canis* produces patches of alopecia with broken hairs, scaling, and inflammation (**446**). Animal dermatophytes such as *T. verrucosum* cause the most inflammation, producing a painful, swollen, boggy, purulent plaque known as a kerion (**447**). Malaise, lymphadenopathy, and scarring alopecia are common.

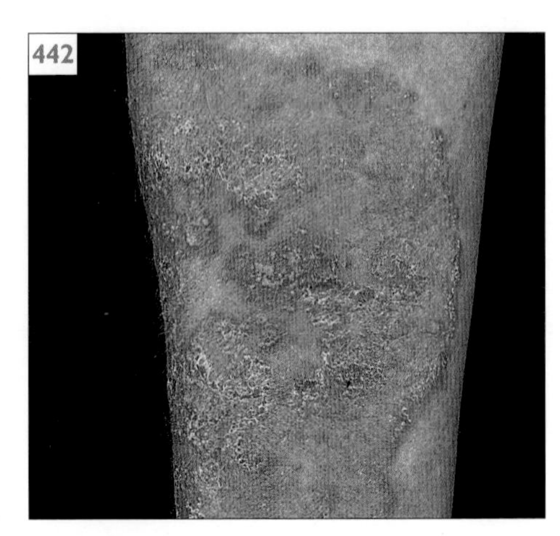

442 Tinea corporis.

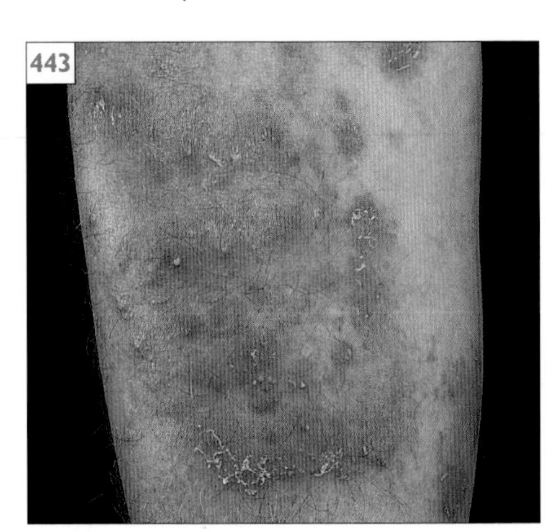

443 Tinea incognito.

Infection of the beard, tinea barbae, causes similar problems to tinea capitis, but, as the infecting agent is often an animal dermatophyte, inflammatory reactions can be marked (**448**).

Tinea manuum, affecting the hands, is usually caused by *T. rubrum* and causes particular diagnostic difficulties. Inflammation is often minimal. The palm becomes dry with mild scaling which is most obvious in the palmar creases (**449**). Infection is often unilateral.

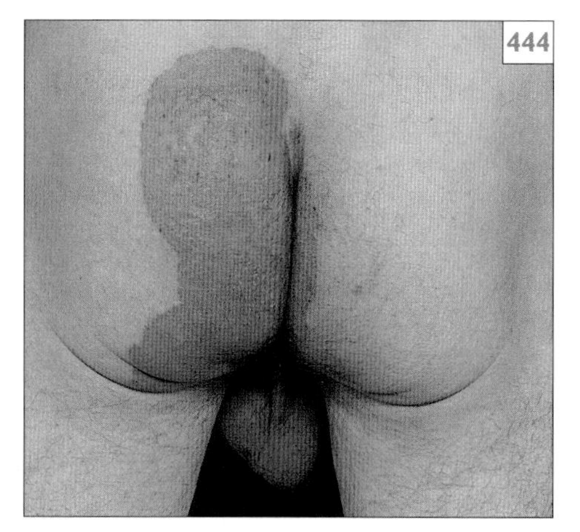

444 Tinea cruris.

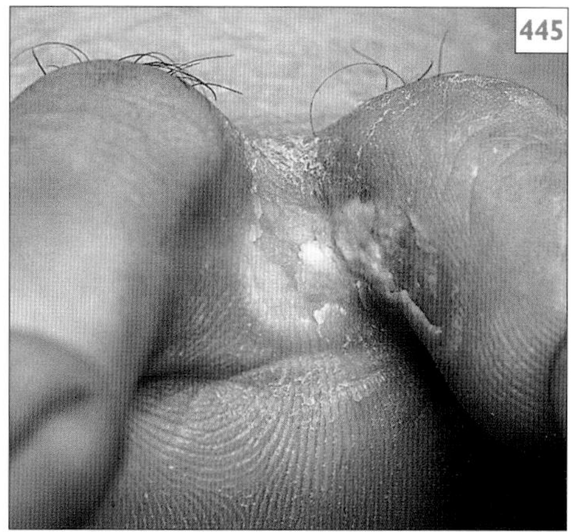

445 Tinea pedis ('athlete's foot').

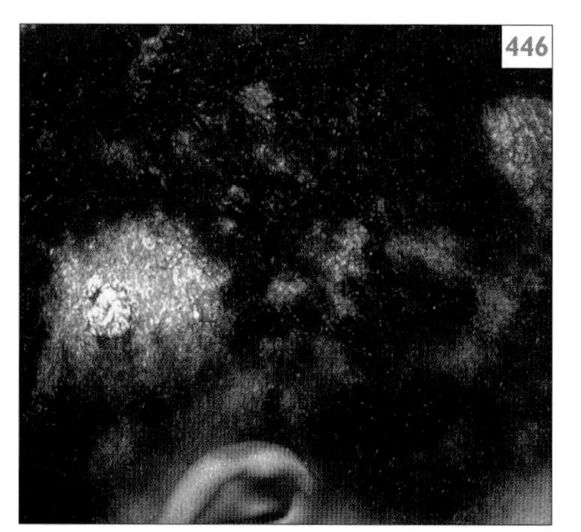

446 Tinea capitis.

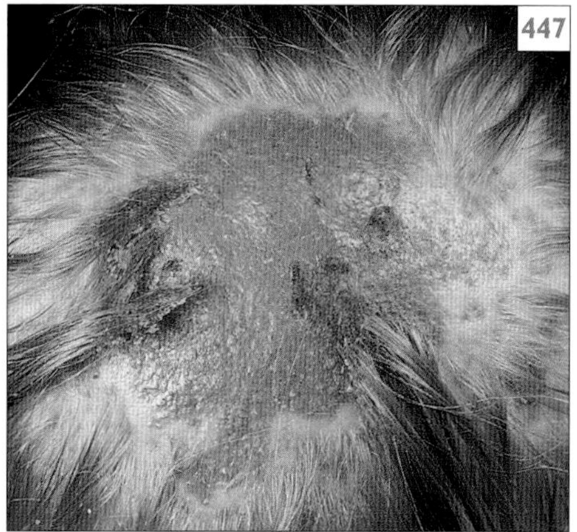

447 A kerion.

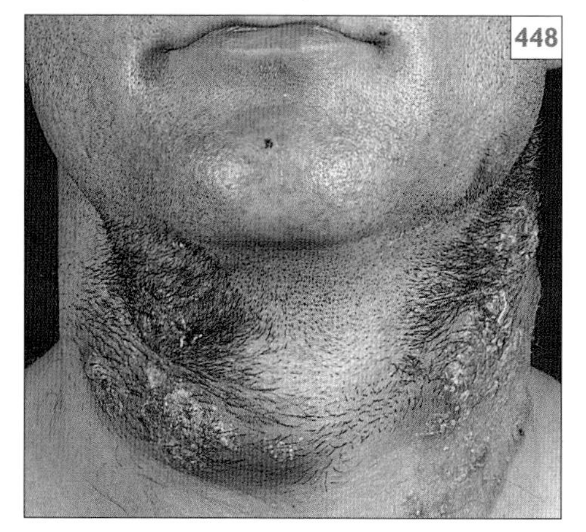

448 Tinea barbae.

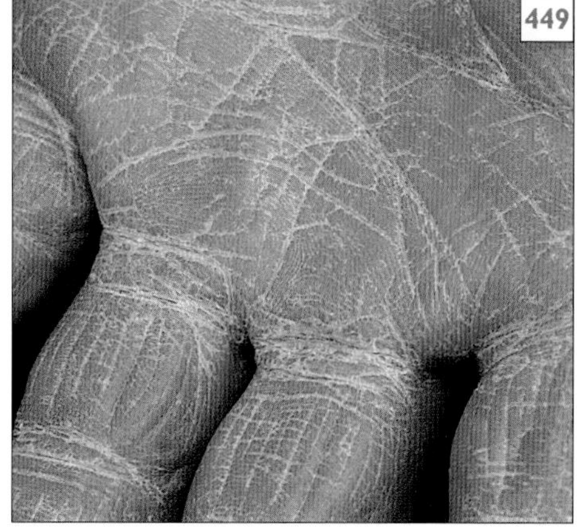

449 Tinea manuum.

Nail infection, tinea unguium, is very common and often an incidental finding. It is frequently associated with tinea pedis. A white or yellow discolouration first affects the free edge of the nail and spreads down towards the cuticle (**450**). The nail becomes thickened and crumbly. Toenails are most commonly affected.

DIFFERENTIAL DIAGNOSIS

Tinea corporis should be distinguished from psoriasis and discoid eczema. Candidal infection is less clearly demarcated than tinea cruris. Non-inflammatory scalp ringworm shows scaling and broken hairs, in contrast to alopecia areata. Tinea pedis may resemble bacterial infection of the toe webs, and eczema or psoriasis when affecting the soles. Unilateral involvement helps differentiate tinea manuum from psoriasis, eczema, and keratoderma.

INVESTIGATIONS

Direct microscopy and culture of skin scrapings and nail or hair clippings. Hair infected by *M. audounii* and *M. canis* shows bright green fluorescence under Wood's light (UV 365 nm). This is of particular use in tracing affected individuals in epidemics.

TREATMENT

Localized infection of glabrous skin can be treated with topical antifungals. Infection of hair, nails, and palms requires systemic therapy.

Pityriasis versicolor

DEFINITION AND CLINICAL FEATURES

A superficial, chronic cutaneous infection with the lipophilic yeast, *Malassezia furfur*. It presents as slightly scaly or pale brown patches and macules that fail to tan on sun exposure. It is usually asymptomatic and mainly affects young adults. The rash mainly affects the upper trunk, but may spread to the proximal limbs and neck (**451**). Different species of *Malassezia* exist as part of the normal skin flora and densely colonize the scalp, upper trunk, and flexures. Sweating and application of oils to the skin may increase susceptibility to this complaint.

DIFFERENTIAL DIAGNOSIS

Erythrasma, seborrhoeic eczema, vitiligo.

INVESTIGATIONS

Microscopy of skin scrapings shows characteristic mycelium together with spherical thick walled yeasts – likened in appearance to 'spaghetti with meatballs'.

TREATMENT

Topical antifungal preparations work well but relapse is common. Oral itraconazole may be used. Patients should be warned that repigmentation may take several months.

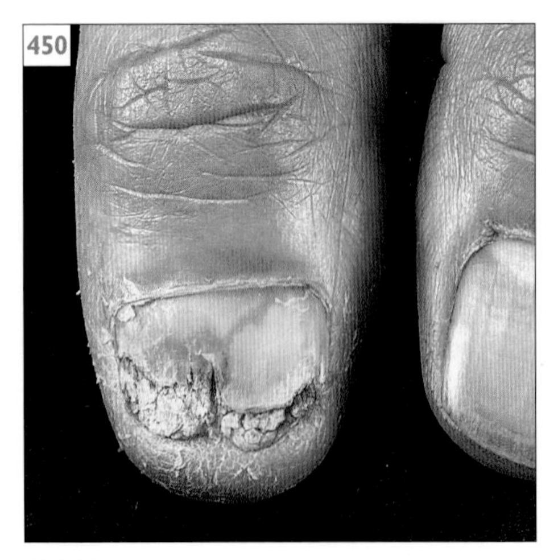

450 Tinea unguium.

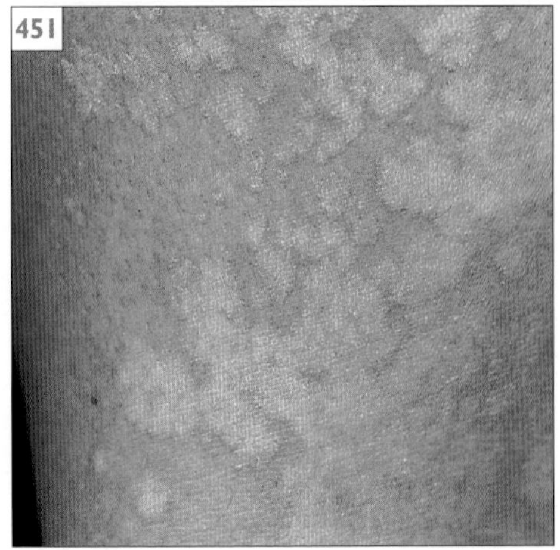

451 Pityriasis (tinea) versicolor.

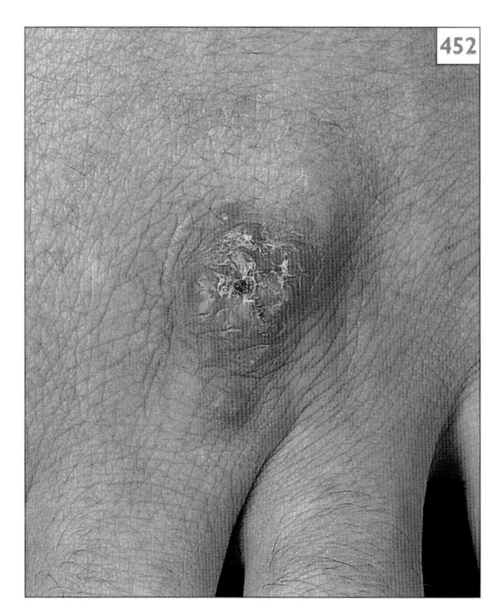

452 Sporotrichosis nodule.

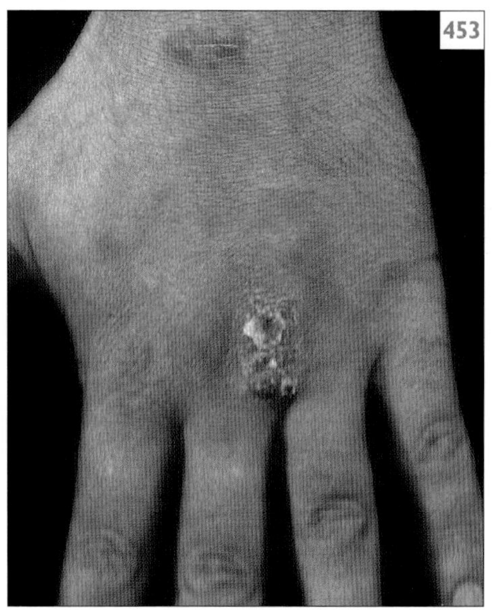

453 Nodules along local lymphatics in sporotrichosis.

Sporotrichosis

DEFINITION AND CLINICAL FEATURES

An uncommon deep fungal infection caused by *Sporothrix schenckii*. This fungus is widely distributed on decaying vegetation and infection is usually acquired following a minor injury. A nodule or warty plaque forms at the site of injury (**452**) and then, characteristically, nodules appear along local lymphatics (**453**).

DIFFERENTIAL DIAGNOSIS

Individual lesions can be mimicked by leishmaniasis and foreign body granulomas. The spread of lesions along lymphatics may also occur with fish tank granuloma (see p.220) and is known as sporotrichoid spread.

INVESTIGATIONS

Mycological culture. Histological examination is often non-specific.

TREATMENT

Treatment is with systemic antifungals. Oral potassium iodide is a cheap, effective alternative.

Candidal infection

DEFINITION AND CLINICAL FEATURES

Candidiasis is an infection caused by the yeast *Candida albicans* or occasionally other candidal species. This yeast may be a normal commensal in the oral and vaginal mucosa. It commonly causes superficial infections of the mucous membranes, intertriginous areas, and nail folds in susceptible individuals. Host susceptibility may be increased following antibiotic therapy, in Cushing's syndrome, diabetes, pregnancy, and with HIV infection. Systemic infection is rare and life-threatening and mainly occurs in immunosuppressed, debilitiated individuals.

The mucosal surfaces show white plaques that detach and leave erythematous areas (**454**). Submammary and groin flexures become sore and itchy with glazed erythema, often with satellite lesions (**455**). Chronic paronychia caused by candidal infection results in a painful swelling of the nail folds and usually of the fingers (**456**). Candidal paronychia often occurs in nail folds that are already damaged by trauma, irritants, and eczema and affects people with occupations involving repeated wet work. Chronic mucocutaneous candidiasis is a hereditary immunodeficiency resulting in the destruction of the nails (**457**) and in a chronic mucosal infection with spread to the oesophagus.

DIFFERENTIAL DIAGNOSIS

Flexural candidiasis must be distinguished from erythrasma, tinea cruris, and flexural psoriasis. Oral lesions may be confused with lichen planus, dysplasia, and hairy leukoplakia.

INVESTIGATIONS

Culture of swabs. Blood cultures in candidal septicaemia.

TREATMENT

Treatment with either topical or systemic anticandidal agents depending on the site and severity of infection. Further management includes the exclusion of underlying factors.

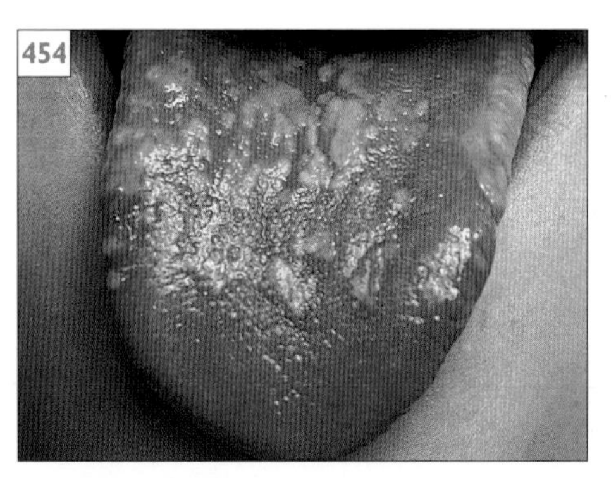

454 Oral candidiasis.

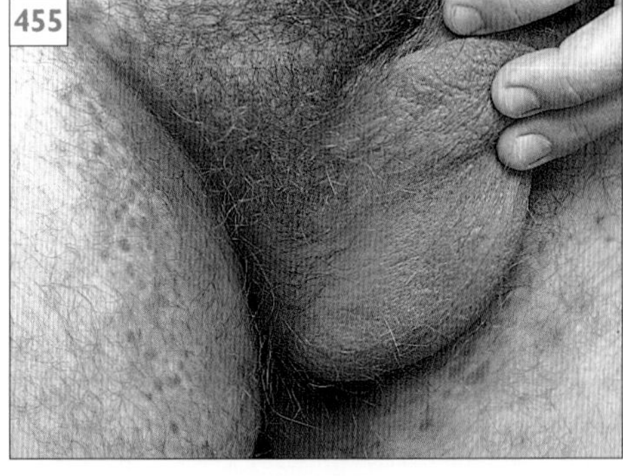

455 Flexural candidiasis with satellite lesions.

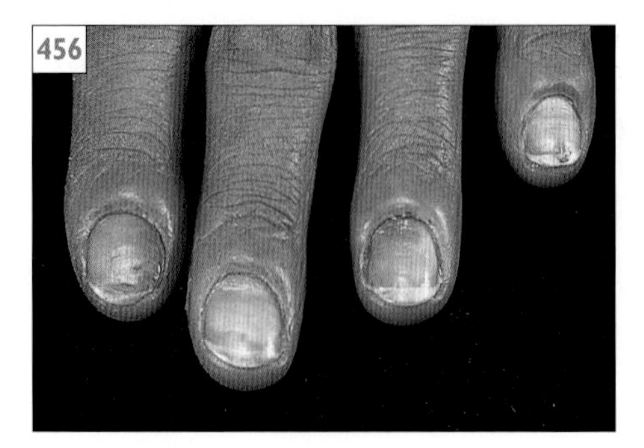

456 Candidal paronychia.

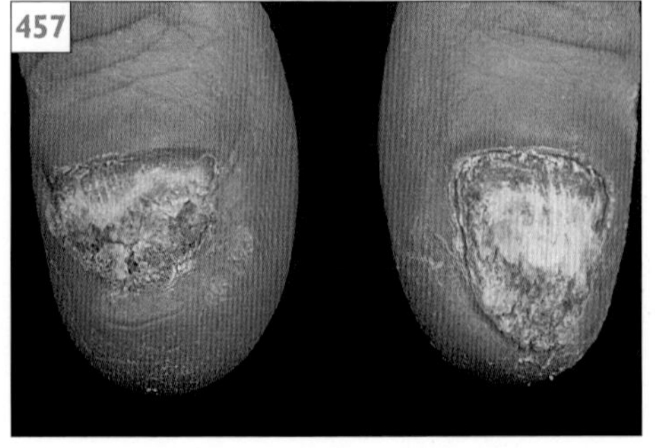

457 Chronic mucocutaneous candidiasis.

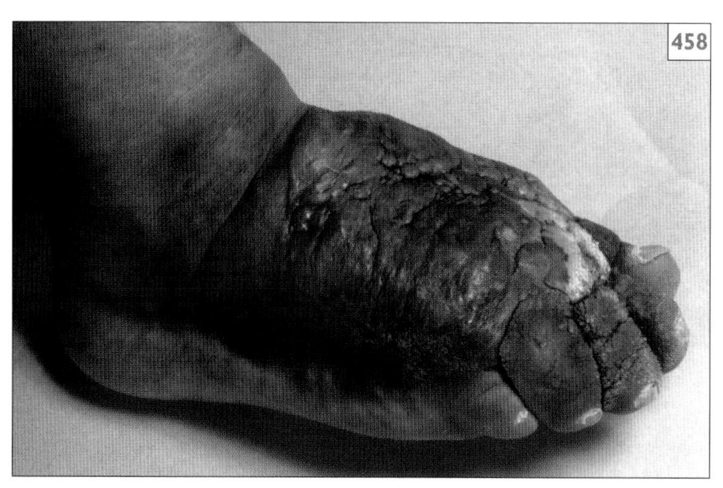

458 Mycetoma.

Mycetoma

DEFINITION AND CLINICAL FEATURES

A chronic localized infection caused by various species of fungi or actinomycetes (filamentous bacteria) and characterized by the formation of clusters of organisms ('grains') within abscesses. Causative organisms vary in different parts of the world and include *Madurella mycetomatis*, *Streptomyces somaliensis*, and *Nocardia*. These occur as saprophytes in soil or vegetation and are often implanted subcutaneously by a penetrating injury such as a thorn. Most lesions are on the lower leg and present as nodules and pustules, hard, swollen skin with discharging sinuses (**458**). This may result in serious deformity and gross swelling of the limb.

DIFFERENTIAL DIAGNOSIS

Chronic bacterial osteomyelitis, elephantiasis.

INVESTIGATIONS

Grain colour and microscopy may give a tentative diagnosis, but for accurate identification of the causative organism, culture is required. Referral to a reference laboratory is recommended.

TREATMENT

Systemic antifungals or antibiotics such as rifampicin, dapsone, streptomycin, and cotrimoxazole may be of benefit, but therapy may not be curative and ultimately amputation of the affected limb may be needed to prevent the infection from spreading.

VIRAL INFECTIONS

Measles

DEFINITION AND CLINICAL FEATURES

This is an infection with an RNA myxovirus, giving rise to upper respiratory symptoms, rash, and fever. Measles is usually contracted in childhood. It became less common with effective immunization. The incubation period is about 10 days. Clinical features are fever, catarrh, and conjunctivitis, followed after 3 or 4 days by the appearance of Koplik's spots (pale spots on a red base) on the buccal mucosa. The rash usually develops a day or two later. It first shows behind the ears but rapidly becomes generalized as a maculopapular rash (**459**). After 7–10 days the rash fades with fine peeling. In immunosuppressed or malnourished patients the rash can either be more severe with purpura or may be minimal with rapid spread of the virus to the lungs and brain.

DIFFERENTIAL DIAGNOSIS

Kawasaki disease, scarlet fever, drug eruptions.

INVESTIGATIONS

Clinical appearance is usually sufficient. Serology may confirm diagnosis retrospectively.

TREATMENT

Antibiotics may be required to control secondary bacterial complications. Passive immunization with normal human globulin reduces the risk of infection in those at special risk following exposure to the virus.

Rubella

DEFINITION AND CLINICAL FEATURES

This is an infection with an RNA togavirus, giving rise to a macular exanthem, with mild constitutional symptoms. Epidemics were a regular occurrence before the introduction of immunization. Rubella presents as a fever, sore throat, conjunctivitis, and sometimes arthritis which precede the rash by a few days, particularly in older children and adults. Younger children often present with the exanthem which is a red macular eruption starting on the face and spreading downwards. As it progresses a confluent, blotchy erythema develops (**460**). Lymphadenopathy, characteristically affecting the occipital nodes, may be a presenting feature and often occurs before the rash. The eruption disappears in about 4 or 5 days, clearing from the face downwards.

DIFFERENTIAL DIAGNOSIS

Other viral exanthems.

INVESTIGATIONS

Paired serology or raised IgM against rubella.

TREATMENT

There is no specific treatment.

SPECIAL POINTS

The incubation period is 2–3 weeks. Congenital rubella produces multisystem abnormalities.

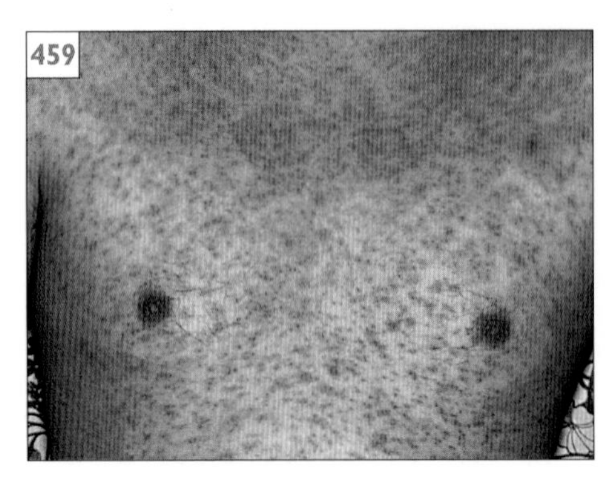

459 Generalized maculopapular measles rash.

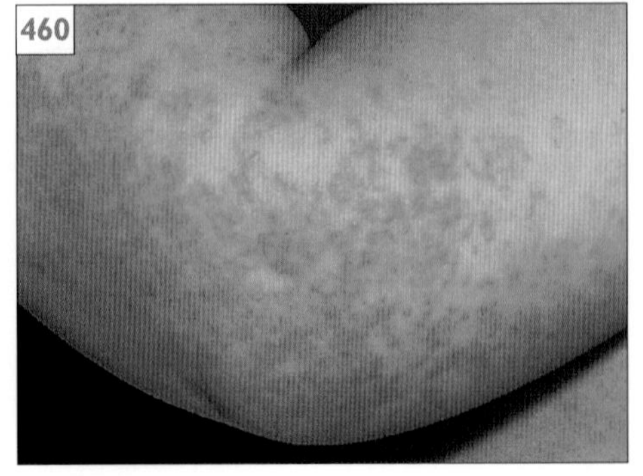

460 Rubella.

Erythema infectiosum

DEFINITION AND CLINICAL FEATURES

Erythema infectiosum is caused by infection with parvovirus B19. The first sign of infection is a rash on the cheeks. Initially there are red papules that later coalesce to give a raised, red, slapped cheeks appearance (**461**). A reticulate rash may also affect the buttocks and upper arms, and spread proximally and distally (**462**). The palms and soles may be involved, with the rash lasting 7 days. Mucous membranes may show red spots. - Low-grade fever is common. Older children and adults may develop arthralgia, often with minimal or absent rash. Sickle cell crisis may occur in susceptible children. An acute acral dermatosis, papular-purpuric 'gloves and socks' syndrome, has been reported in association with parvovirus B19 infection.

DIFFERENTIAL DIAGNOSIS

Other exanthems. Rash may suggest Kawasaki disease but systemic upset is less marked.

INVESTIGATIONS

In the acute phase, virus can be detected in the serum. Specific IgM to parvovirus B19 remains raised for up to 3 months.

Hand, foot, and mouth disease

DEFINITION AND CLINICAL FEATURES

A viral infection with Coxsackie A strains giving rise to stomatitis and blisters on the hands and feet. Oral lesions are rapidly ulcerating vesicles which break to form painful ulcers. The hands and feet show oval grey blisters with surrounding erythema (**463**). The sides and backs of the digits, and the palms and soles can be affected. Fever is mild. The condition lasts up to a week. Oral lesions are most marked in adults.

DIFFERENTIAL DIAGNOSIS

The fully developed condition is characteristic.

TREATMENT

No specific treatment.

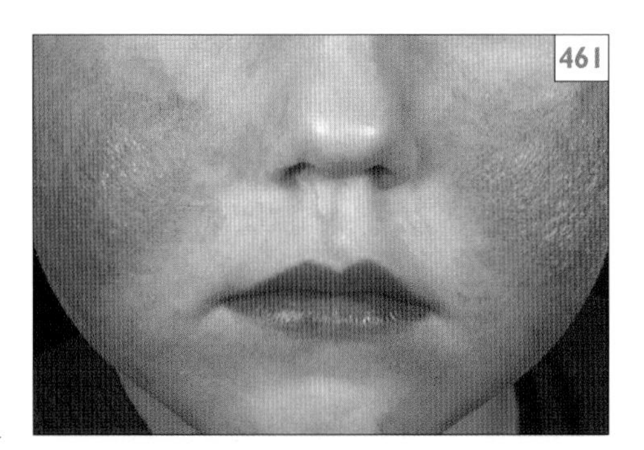

461 Erythema infectiosum (fifth disease or 'slapped cheek' disease).

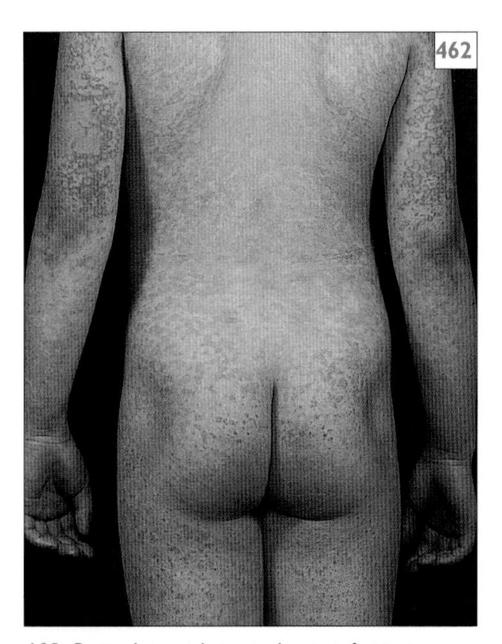

462 Reticulate rash in erythema infectiosum.

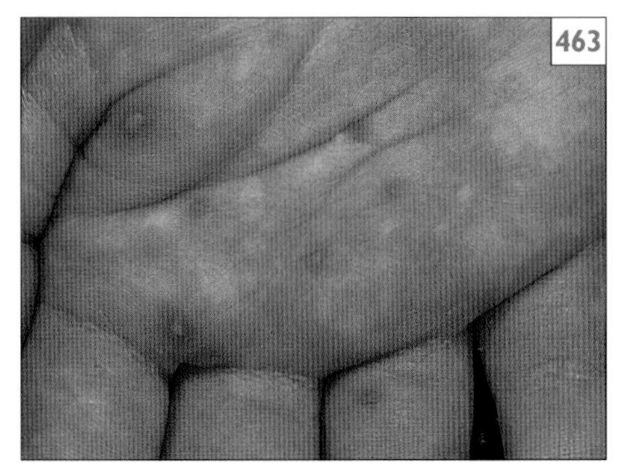

463 Hand, foot, and mouth disease.

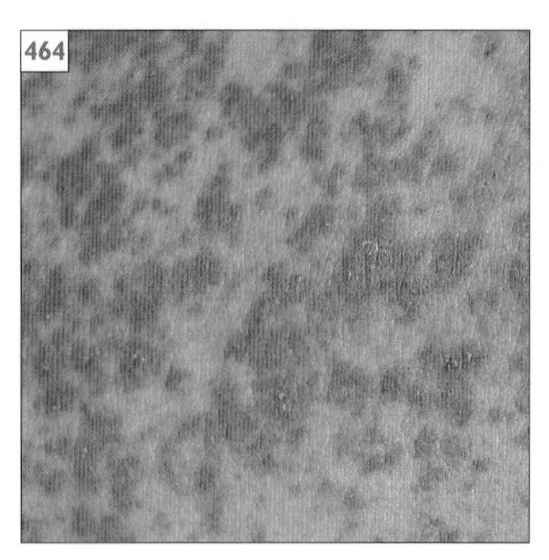

464 Glandular fever rash.

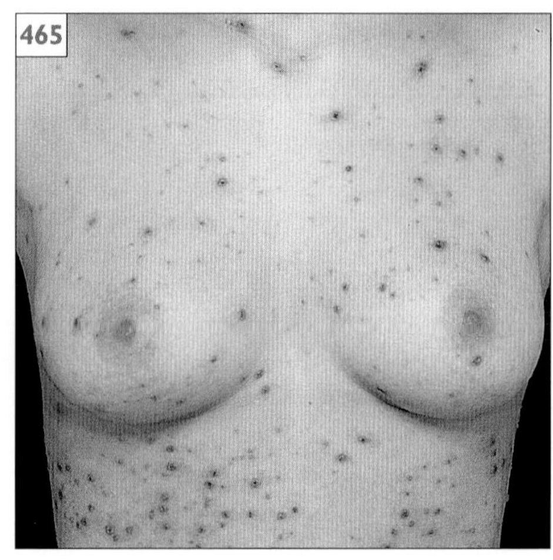

465 Chickenpox (varicella).

Glandular fever
(infectious mononucleosis)

DEFINITION AND CLINICAL FEATURES
This is an infection with the Epstein–Barr virus causing fever, sore throat, and lymphadenopathy. Spread is by droplet infection or direct contact (the kissing disease). Malaise and fever are followed within a few days by a sore throat which is associated with purpura on the junction between the hard and soft palate. Lymphadenopathy may be marked and splenomegaly is common. A rash occurs after 4–6 days in about 10% of cases and is usually macular or maculopapular, affecting the trunk and face (**464**). Acute urticaria may also occur. If ampicillin is taken, a widespread maculopapular or morbilliform rash is almost inevitable.

DIFFERENTIAL DIAGNOSIS
Scarlet fever, other viral exanthems.

INVESTIGATIONS
Atypical lymphocytes are seen on a blood film. The Paul–Bunnell test is positive in most patients after 1–2 weeks.

TREATMENT
No specific treatment.

Chickenpox (varicella)

DEFINITION AND CLINICAL FEATURES
This is an infection with the varicella zoster virus (VZV), giving rise to an acute vesicular eruption with fever. The fever and malaise, often mild, are followed by the development of a pruritic papular eruption that rapidly becomes vesicular, then turbid pustules. The eruption is most severe centrally and lesions appear in crops, resulting in a mixture of papules, vesicles, and crusts (**465**). Spread is thought to occur by droplet infection rather than skin contact. Scars are usually shallow unless the lesions become secondarily infected or deeply excoriated.

DIFFERENTIAL DIAGNOSIS
Widespread herpes simplex, as is seen in eczema herpeticum, does not have the typical centripetal distribution.

INVESTIGATIONS
Not routinely necessary. Electron microscopy and viral culture of vesicle fluid.

SPECIAL POINTS
The incubation period is 2–3 weeks.

TREATMENT
Oral antiviral therapy is indicated in adults with varicella and in the immunosuppressed or those of any age with severe disease.

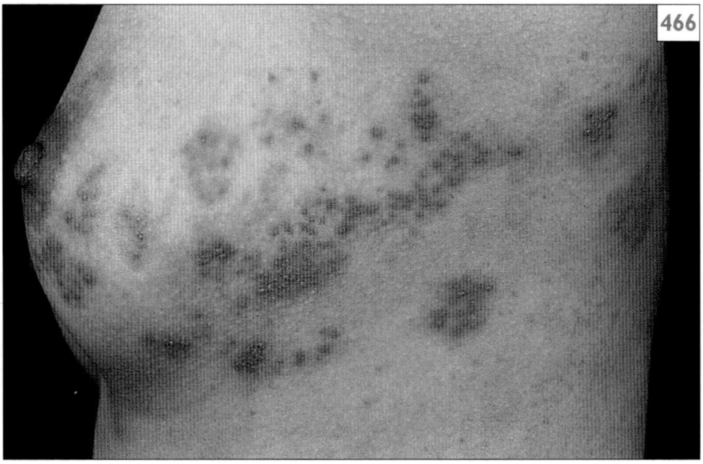

466 Herpes zoster.

Shingles (herpes zoster)

DEFINITION AND CLINICAL FEATURES

Reactivation of latent varicella zoster virus (VZV) from within sensory ganglia, giving rise to a vesicular eruption, in a dermatomal distribution. The eruption is often preceded by pain or paraesthesia within the affected dermatome. After 3 or 4 days, grouped, red papules appear in one or more dermatomes, becoming vesicular and then pustular (**466**). Pain, fever, and local lymphadenopathy are frequent, especially in the older patient. Thoracic and facial dermatomes are most frequently affected. Involvement of the ophthalmic region is complicated by keratitis. Motor nerve palsies can occur. Dissemination of lesions is seen in immunosuppressed patients. Lesions usually clear within a few weeks, though pain and dysaesthesia can be persistent and disabling.

Incidence of shingles increases with age. Immunosuppression from malignancy, medication, and AIDS increases both the incidence and severity. There is no evidence that contact with chickenpox provokes shingles but shingles is infectious and can give rise to chickenpox.

DIFFERENTIAL DIAGNOSIS

The pain prior to the development of the eruption is a frequent diagnostic catch and can mimic cardiac and pleural pain. Early shingles can be confused with herpes simplex.

INVESTIGATIONS

Not routinely necessary. Electron microscopy and viral culture.

TREATMENT

Prompt treatment with oral antiviral therapy such as aciclovir can prevent progression of the eruption, lessen pain, and reduce the risk of post-herpetic neuralgia.

Herpes simplex

DEFINITION AND CLINICAL FEATURES

An infection with herpes simplex virus (HSV) 1 and 2 causing a vesicular eruption. Primary infection with HSV1 usually causes stomatitis, whereas HSV2 affects the genital mucosa (see p. 94). Subsequent attacks can occur without re-exposure to the virus as it is carried in the sensory ganglia.

Initial exposure to HSV1 usually occurs in children who develop herpes stomatitis, a febrile illness with painful vesicles and ulcers on the hard and soft palate. Herpes can also develop following direct contact. On the fingers this results in deep, painful, grouped vesicles on the finger tip (herpetic whitlow) (**467**). Facial lesions, which may be multiple, can spread through rugby packs ('scrum pox') (**468**) and among wrestlers.

Recrudescence of the latent virus, usually in the trigeminal ganglia, produces grouped vesicles on the face (**469**), usually on the lips (i.e. cold sores). It is not known why some individuals have recurrent attacks and others do not. Attacks may be precipitated by sun exposure and concurrent illness; they are heralded by a tingling of the affected skin. The vesicles crust over and, in the absence of any secondary infection, clear in a week. When the skin is damaged, as in eczema and some other skin conditions, herpes can spread widely and become life threatening (eczema herpeticum (**470**), Kaposi's varicelliform eruption). Immunosuppression can result in atypical widespread lesions with the risk of systemic spread. Chronic ulcerative lesions are sometimes seen in AIDS patients.

DIFFERENTIAL DIAGNOSIS

Severe aphthous ulcers and some strains of Coxsackie virus can resemble primary herpes stomatitis. Herpetic whitlow must be distinguished from bacterial infection. Herpetic cold sores can resemble impetigo; severe infections should be distinguished from herpes zoster and chickenpox.

INVESTIGATIONS

Electron microscopy and/or culture or immunological examination of vesicle fluid.

TREATMENT

Severe infection, particularly in the context of eczema or immunosuppression, requires treatment with systemic antiviral agents such as aciclovir. Spread of infection into the eye can result in potentially blinding keratoconjunctivitis.

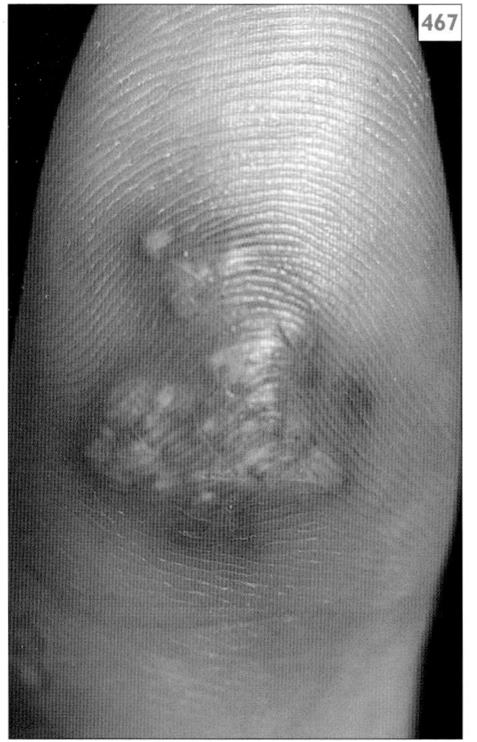

467 Herpetic whitlow.

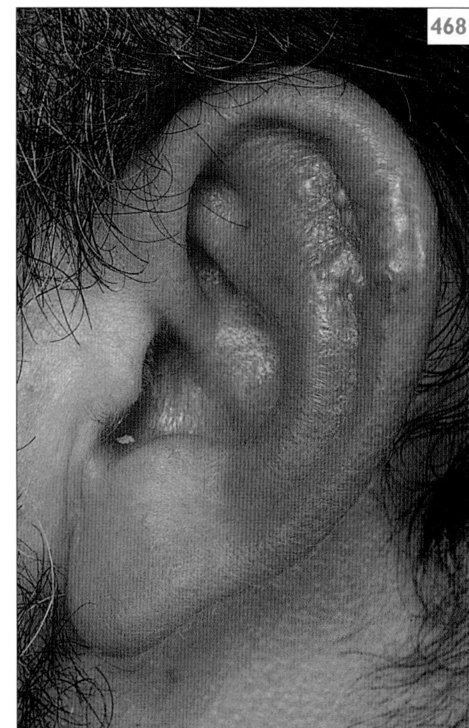

468 'Scrum pox'.

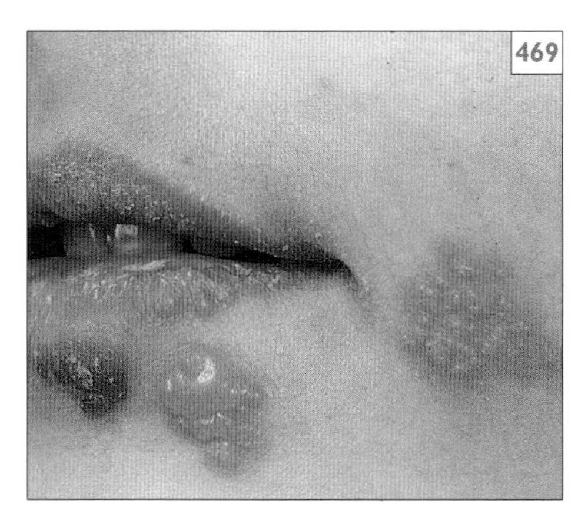

469 Herpes simplex labialis.

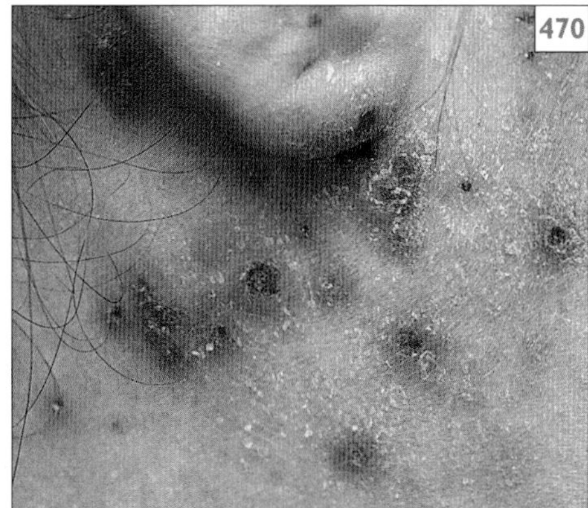

470 Eczema herpeticum.

Viral warts, verruca

DEFINITION AND CLINICAL FEATURES

Infection of the skin and mucous membranes with human papilloma virus, resulting in skin-coloured papules. Appearance and site is determined by the subtype of virus. Viral warts are extremely common, most often in children but no age group is exempt. Immunosuppression results in more widespread and numerous lesions. Hand warts are more common on the hands of raw meat and fish handlers. The main types of wart are as follows:

- Common warts are usually found on the hands but may develop on any area. Their spread is by direct contact, especially to abraded or damaged skin. Lesions are spread from the hands to the elbows, knees, and face. Lesions are hard, rough, skin-coloured lumps that range from a few millimetres to large confluent masses (**471**).
- Filiform or digitate warts are commonly found on the face and are finer and more thread-like than common warts (**472**). If they spread into the shaving area then eradication can be difficult.
- Plantar warts (i.e. verrucas) are found on the soles of the feet and sometimes cause pain (**473**).
- Mosaic warts, found on the soles of the feet, are numerous individual warts grouped together to form a plaque (**474**).
- Plane warts are smaller and flatter than the other types and may spread widely, usually on the face and dorsal surfaces of the hands (**475**).
- Genital warts.

DIFFERENTIAL DIAGNOSIS

Non-viral papilloma, solar and seborrhoeic keratoses can resemble warts.

TREATMENT

Most warts, particularly in children, clear spontaneously in 2–3 years. Treatment for recalcitrant lesions includes keratolytic paints and destructive measures such as cryotherapy.

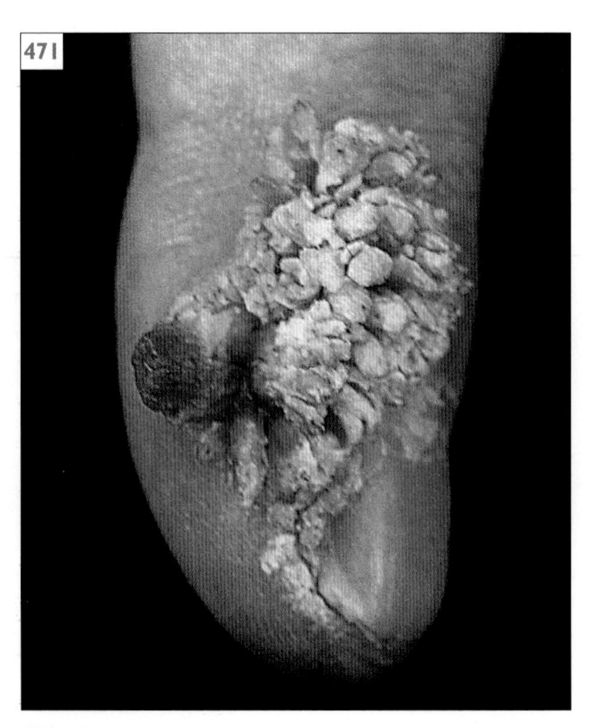

471 Common warts.

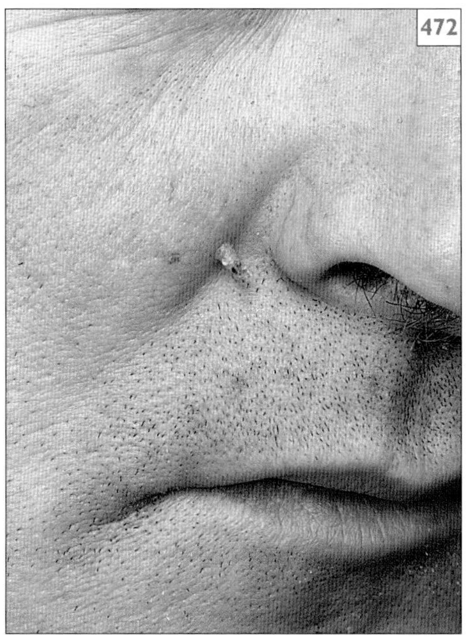

472 Filiform or digitate wart.

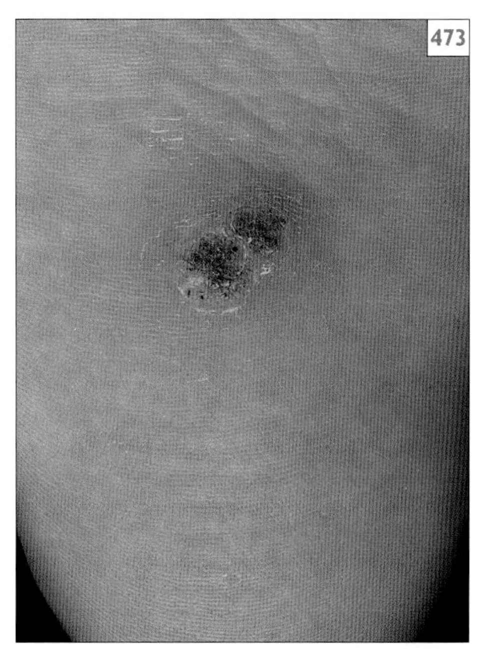

473 Plantar warts (verrucas).

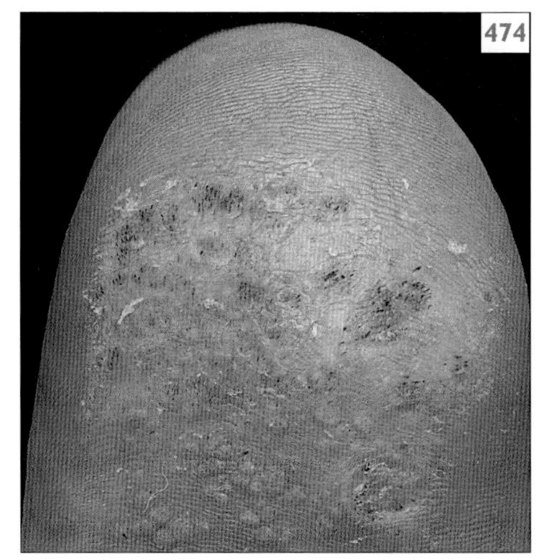

474 Mosaic warts.

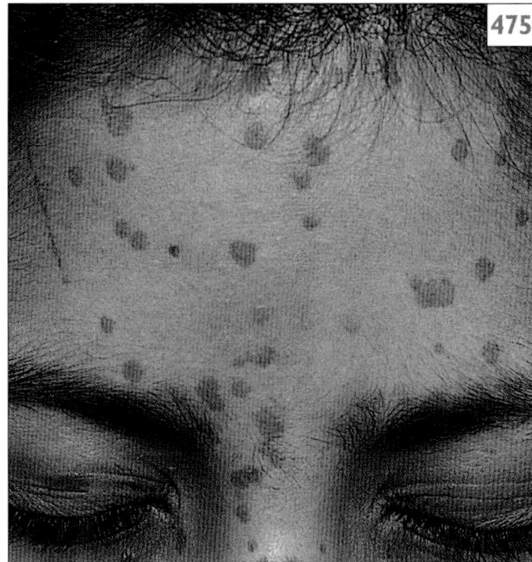

475 Plane warts.

Epidermodysplasia verruciformis

DEFINITION AND CLINICAL FEATURES

An inherited disorder in which there is widespread persistent infection with human papilloma virus and a predisposition to squamous cell carcinoma. Lesions on the face are typical of plane warts, but on the body, they are larger and may be hyper- or hypopigmented resembling pityriasis versicolor (**476**). Seborrhoeic keratosis-like lesions also occur. Warts usually develop rapidly in childhood but may appear at any age.

DIFFERENTIAL DIAGNOSIS

Pityriasis versicolor, generalized lichen planus, acrokeratosis verruciformis.

INVESTIGATION

Histology shows wart virus changes with extensive vacuolation of keratinocytes.

TREATMENT

Patients should avoid excessive sun exposure and be followed up for development of carcinomas and pre-malignant lesions. Oral retinoids may improve the clinical appearance, but do not clear the virus.

Molluscum contagiosum

DEFINITION AND CLINICAL FEATURES

Benign papules caused by a poxvirus that present as shiny, umbilicated, slightly translucent, pink or skin-coloured papules. They grow slowly, usually being less than 1 cm in diameter (**477**, **478**). Lesions can occur at any site, usually on the head, neck, and flexures; they are more widespread and larger in immunosuppressed patients and those with HIV infection. Rarely, grouped lesions can form large plaques. The infection mainly occurs in childhood, but may be sexually transmitted in adults.

DIFFERENTIAL DIAGNOSIS

Solitary giant lesions can be confused with a wide variety of lesions including keratoacanthoma, basal cell carcinoma, and viral warts.

INVESTIGATIONS

None routinely necessary. Histology of lesions shows diagnostic changes. Consider HIV testing in adults with widespread infection.

TREATMENT

Treatment is usually not necessary as the infection is usually self limiting. Troublesome lesions can be treated by curettage, cryotherapy, or by gently expressing or disrupting the contents.

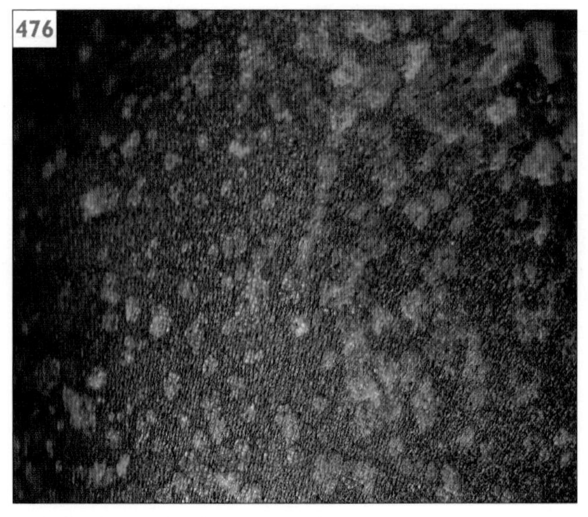

476 Epidermodysplasia verucciformis.

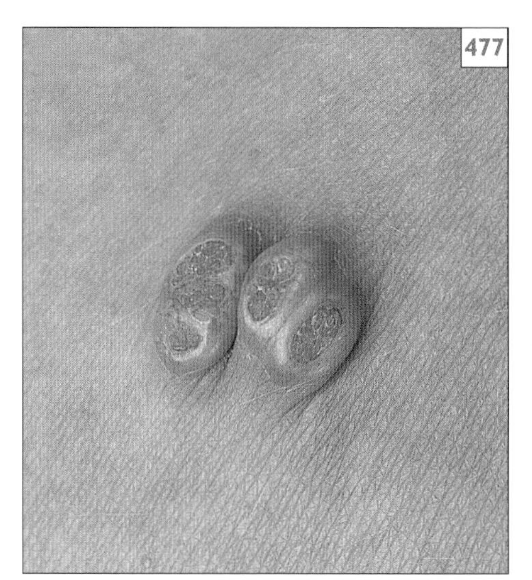

477 Molluscum contagiosum.

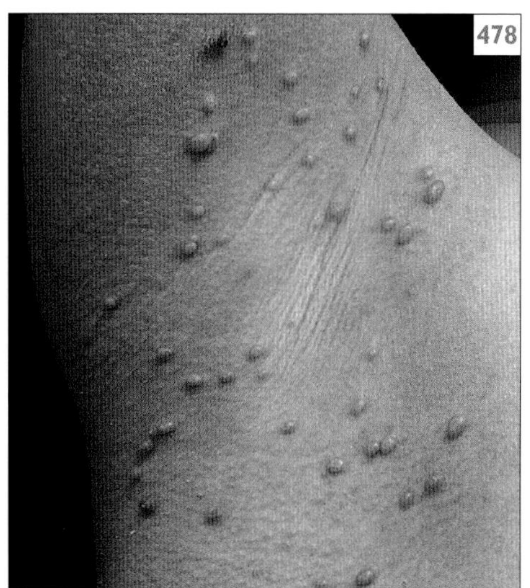

478 Molluscum contagiosum.

Orf

DEFINITION AND CLINICAL FEATURES

Infection caused by a parapoxvirus. The disease is widespread in sheep and goats and mainly affects young lambs which infect humans by direct contact, causing vesicopustular nodules. Early lesions are purplish papules. Over a few days these become umbilicated, haemorrhagic vesicopustules with central crusting, surrounded by a grey halo on an erythematous base (**479**). The lesions are usually solitary, on the hands and may reach 2–3 cm in diameter. They heal spontaneously in 3–5 weeks.

DIFFERENTIAL DIAGNOSIS

Herpetic whitlow, bacterial infection.

INVESTIGATIONS

Not usually necessary. The virus can be identified on electron microscopy.

SPECIAL POINTS

Erythema multiforme may occur after orf infection.

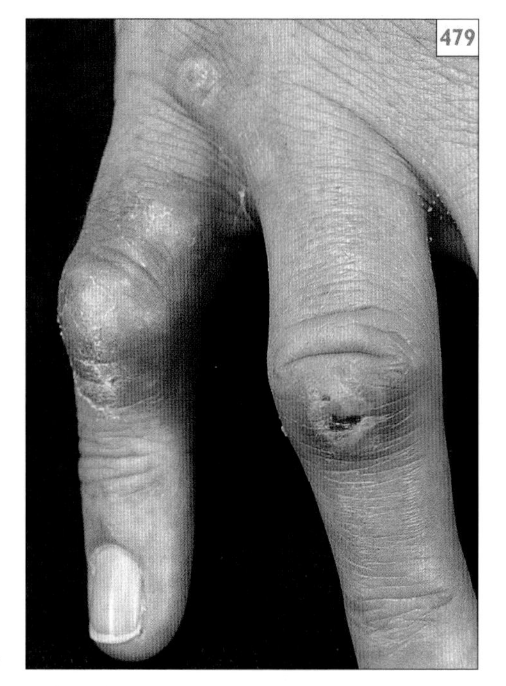

479 Orf.

HUMAN IMMUNODEFICIENCY VIRUS (HIV) INFECTION

HIV-associated dermatoses

DEFINITION AND CLINICAL FEATURES

HIV is the viral agent responsible for the acquired immunodeficiency syndrome (AIDS) which was first recognized in the early 1980s. Through its infection of immunocompetent cells, namely CD4 T- lymphocytes and macrophages, it causes a range of diseases due to evolving immune dysfunction which affect many systems of the body. Dermatological manifestations are wide-ranging and have been recognized as an important diagnostic and prognostic feature of HIV infection. The proportion of patients affected and range of skin complaints increases with the advancement of disease and progressive immunosuppression. Many of these dermatoses are seen less frequently since the advent of highly active antiretroviral therapy (HAART) which has had a dramatic impact on the survival and wellbeing of patients with HIV. However, therapy may trigger dermatological changes as part of the 'immune reconstitution syndrome' as well as novel drug side-effects.

The main routes of transmission are via sexual intercourse, transplacentally to the foetus, and through intravenous drug abuse. HIV is a RNA virus which gains access to cells by binding to the CD4 receptor and, by a process of reverse transciption, viral DNA is integrated into the host DNA. Viral proteins and RNA are synthesized and continually released into the plasma in HIV-infected untreated patients ($>10^8$ viral particles/day).

Acute primary infection causes a non-specific symptomatic illness with malaise and fever in nearly all individuals within 6 weeks of exposure to HIV. A seroconversion rash affects 75% of people and appears as a symmetrical, maculopapular exanthem involving the torso, palms, soles, and face (**480**). Other dermatological features include oro-genital ulceration, erosive genital intertrigo, and Stevens–Johnson syndrome.

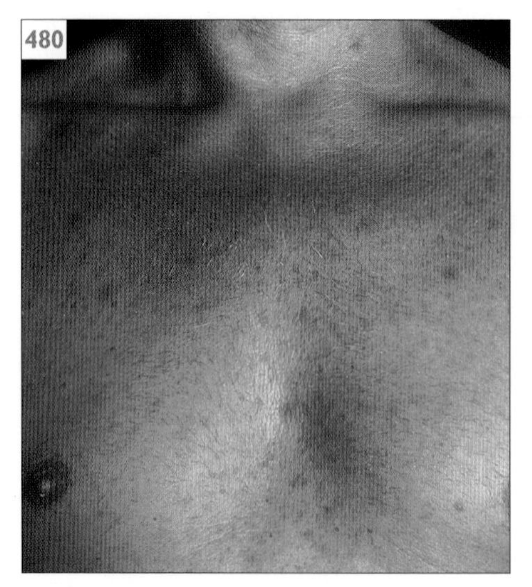

480 Seroconversion rash in HIV.

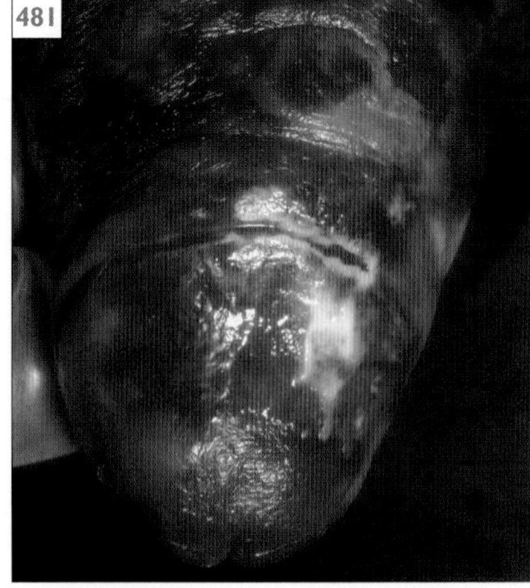

481 Chronic ulcerative herpes simplex virus infection in AIDS.

Several infectious dermatoses occur in severe, recalcitrant forms in people with established HIV infection. Molluscum contagiosum (see pp. 236–237) may present with widespread cutaneous lesions, and an underlying diagnosis of HIV infection should be considered in any adult presenting with multiple papular or nodular lesions on the face and neck. Severe chronic ulcerative herpes simplex virus infection of the anogenital area is a well recognized feature of AIDS (**481**). Reactivation of cytomegalovirus infection occurs in the context of advanced immunosuppression, and may occasionally present with ulcerated nodules and plaques. Viral warts (see pp. 234–235) may be more extensive and atypical in patients with HIV. Oral hairy leukoplakia, is thought to be caused by Epstein–Barr virus infection and is an early specific sign of HIV infection. It appears as a rough white patch on the lateral borders of the tongue (**482**) and is usually asymptomatic. Atypical, chronic, widespread, verrucous forms of varicella can occur.

Oral candidiasis (p. 226) is classically associated with immunosuppression from varied causes including HIV infection, and oesophageal candidiasis is an AIDS-defining diagnosis. Tinea infections are common, especially onychomycosis with *Trichophyton rubrum* (p. 223, 224). *Cryptococcus neoformans* infection may cause disseminated disease in AIDS, and skin involvement is characterized by necrotizing papulonodular lesions (**483**).

Bacterial infections may also occur in association with HIV infection. They include syphilis, which may present atypically and should be considered in any patient with a papulosquamous eruption, and orogenital ulceration. Bacilliary angiomatosis is an uncommon HIV-associated infection caused by the Gram-negative cat-scratch disease organism, *Bartonella*. The latter presents with purple-red nodules and papules, resembling Kaposi's sarcoma (**484**).

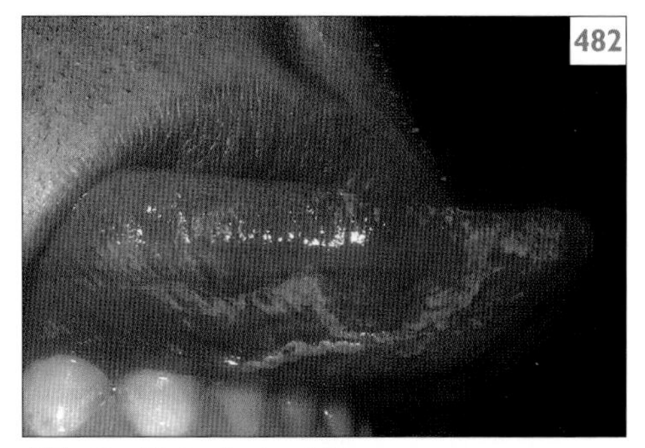

482 Oral hairy leukoplakia.

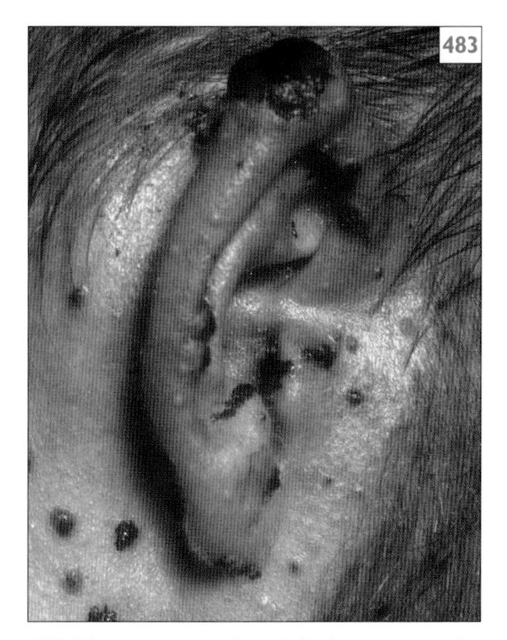

483 Necrotizing papulonodular lesions caused by *Cryptococcus neoformans*.

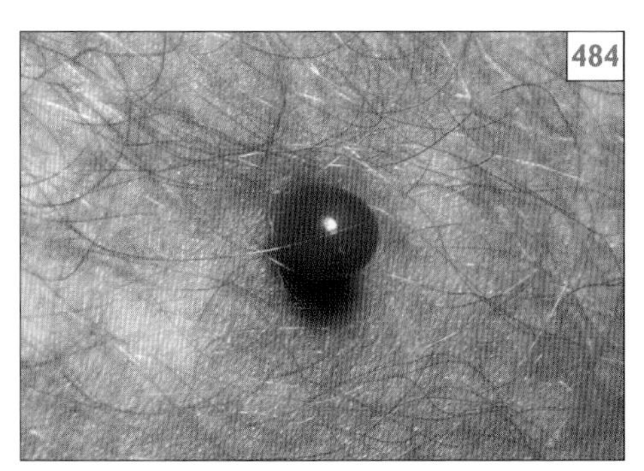

484 Purple-red nodules and papules caused by *Bartonella*.

A range of inflammatory dermatoses have been reported more commonly in HIV infection. Seborrhoeic dermatitis is characteristically more widespread and florid, and psoriasis may be more severe and atypical. Pruritis, xerosis, and ichthyosis are also common problems. Eosinophilic folliculitis is an HIV-specific disorder which appears as intensely pruritic, perifollicular papules and sterile pustules (**485**). Histology is characteristic with perifollicular degranulating eosinophils and mast cells. Scabies occurs frequently in HIV infection, and is often atypical with involvement of the head and neck. Norwegian (crusted) scabies may occur (see p. 245) and is highly contagious. Its occurrence should raise suspicion of underlying HIV infection.

Kaposi's sarcoma is well recognized as an AIDS defining diagnosis. AIDS-related KS is caused by HHV-8 and is multicentric, frequently involving the face, oral mucosal (**486**, **487**), palate, and genitalia. Lymphoedema may follow (**488**). There are also well documented case reports of intraepithelial neoplasia and invasive carcinomas of the anogenital region in patients with HIV infection.

Generalized drug eruptions are also a problem. In particular, fixed drug eruptions characteristically occur in the anogenital area. This has been well documented with penile erosions in patients receiving pentamidine. Other adverse effects of antiretroviral medication (see below) include nail darkening with AZT (**489**), lipodystrophy with protease inhibitors (**490**), and Stevens–Johnson syndrome with zidovudine.

DIAGNOSIS

HIV infection is most commonly diagnosed by detecteding antibodies to the virus. IgG antibodies appear 6–12 weeks following infection in the majority of patients. The gap between the time of intial exposure with HIV and the time antibodies are detectable is called the window period, or seroconversion. Throughout this period, the infected person may have high levels of virus in their body and may be highly infectious. Antibody tests are usually ELISA (enzyme-linked immunosorbent assay) and positive results are then confirmed with a second test, for example a Western blot. A rapid HIV antibody test which takes about 30 minutes also exists.

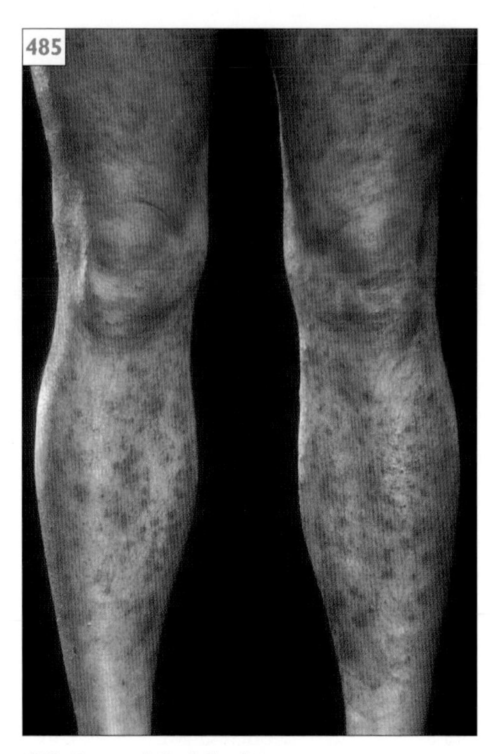

485 Eosinophilic folliculitis.

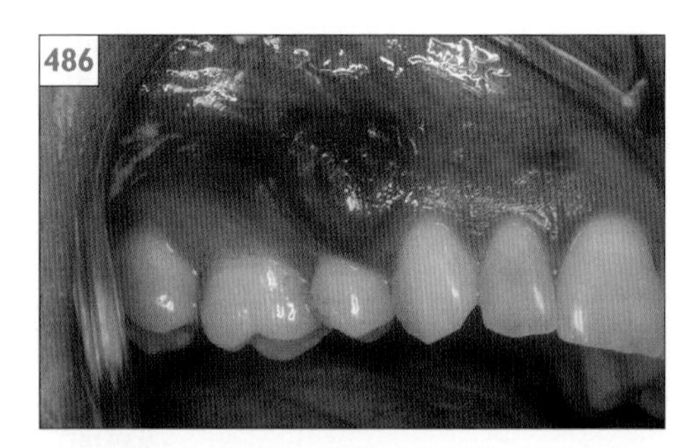

486 Oral Kaposi's sarcoma.

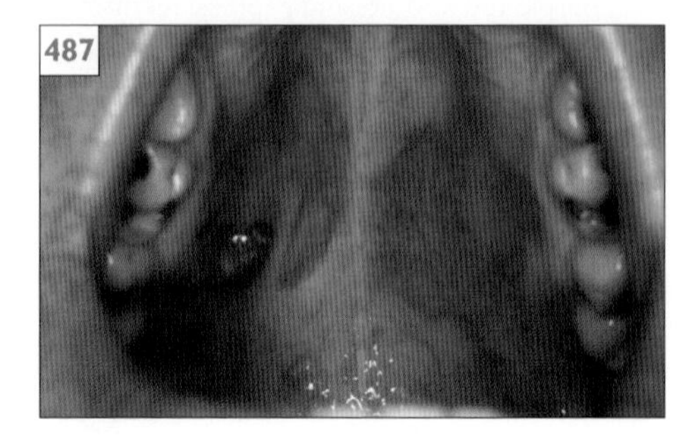

487 Oral Kaposi's sarcoma.

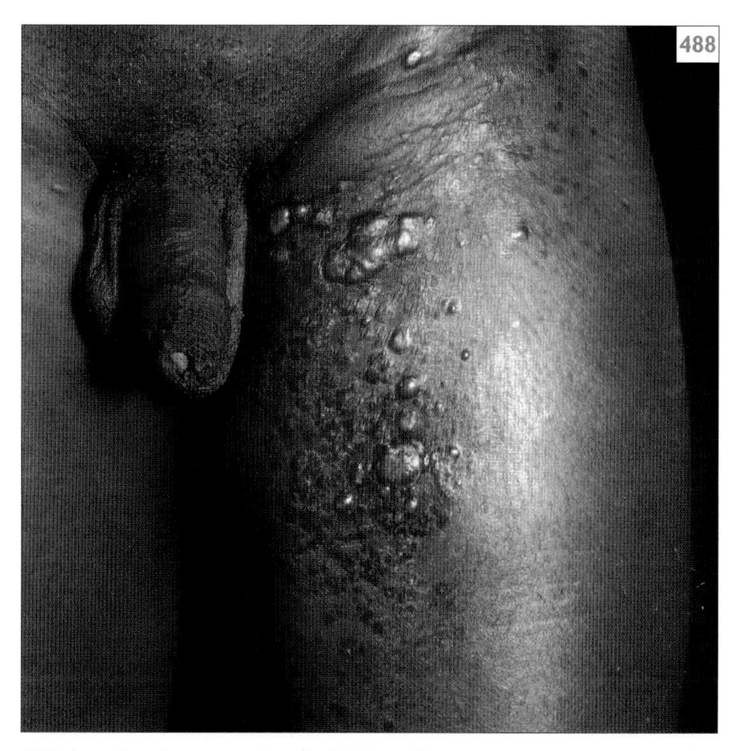

488 Lymphoedema associated with Kaposi's sarcoma.

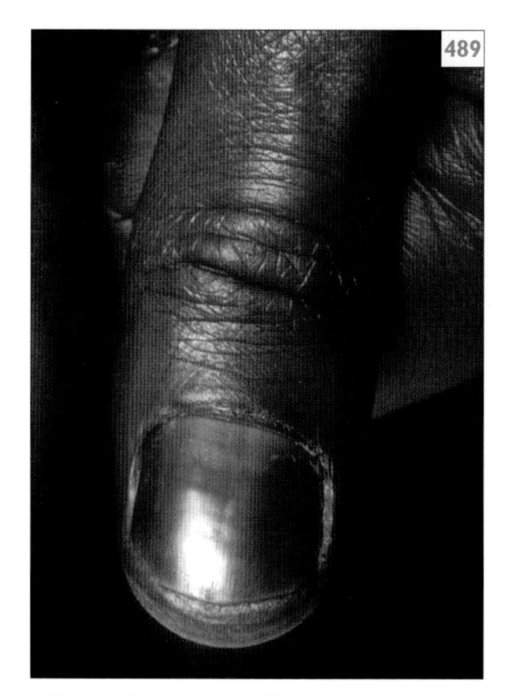

489 Nail darkening with AZT.

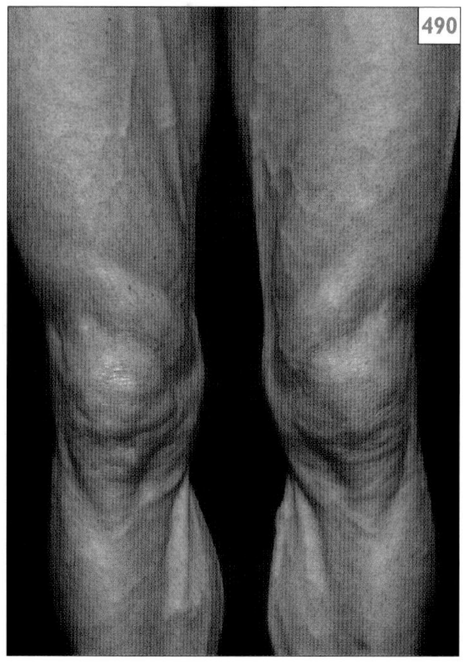

490 Lipodystrophy with protease inhibitors.

Another type of testing is based on detection of viral antigens, usually the protein P24, which is present early in infection and before seroconversion. P24 antigen tests are sometimes used to screen donated blood. A third type of test is based on detecting viral DNA or RNA. These tests can identify HIV in the blood within a week of infection. Babies born to HIV-positive mothers may be tested by amplifying viral DNA using polymerase chain reaction based techniques. Blood supplies in developed countries are screened for HIV using a RNA test known as NAT (nucleic acid amplification testing). In patients known to be infected with HIV, a viral load test to detect HIV genetic material can be used to monitor disease and response to treatment. DNA/RNA tests are rarely used to diagnose HIV in adults as they are very expensive and more complicated than a standard antibody or P24 test.

INVESTIGATIONS

In patients with HIV who present with rashes, investigations are frequently necessary and depending on the disease may include skin scrapings for mycology, viral and bacterial swabs, and histology of skin biopsies. Samples should be collected with due care so that no infectious hazard is created for the operator or other members of staff.

TREATMENT

Highly active antiretroviral therapy (HAART) consists of a combination of three or more anti-HIV drugs. Appropriate HAART therapy has contributed to a great improvement in survival of patients with HIV infection. There are four groups of anti-HIV drugs. Nucleoside/nucleotide reverse transcriptase inhibitors (NRTIs) also known as nucleoside analogues or 'nukes', were the first type of drug available to treat HIV infection in 1987. NRTIs interfere with the action of viral reverse transcriptase and thereby decrease viral replication. NRTIs are considered the 'backbone' of combination therapy because most regimens contain at least two of these drugs. The second group of antiretroviral drugs are the non-nucleoside reverse transcriptase inhibitors (NNRTIs), also known as non-nucleosides or 'non-nukes'. These also stop viral replication by inhibition of reverse transcriptase. The third type of antiretroviral drugs are protease inhibitors. They inhibit proteins involved in the process of viral replication. The fourth and newest category of drugs are entry inhibitors (EIs) which prevent HIV from entering human immune cells. These are not used as first-line therapy.

The most common combination HAART given at the onset of HIV treatment consists of two NRTIs (e.g. zidovudine and lamivudine) combined with either a NNRTI (e.g. efavirenz) or a 'boosted' protease inhibitor. A low dose of the drug ritonavir is most commonly used as a protease booster.

Resistance to antiviral therapy can occur with the emergence of mutant strains of HIV, and adverse effects and non-adherence to therapy are also common problems. Response to treatment may be monitored by measuring viral load and lymphocyte CD4 counts. There is ongoing research into when HAART treatment is best started. As this is a rapidly changing field the most up to date information should be consulted before instituting therapy.

INFESTATIONS

Insect and mite bites
(papular urticaria)

DEFINITION AND CLINICAL FEATURES
Multiple weals, papules, excoriations, and sometimes bullae as a reaction to insect or mite bites.

Fleas, gnats and mosquitoes are the most common biting insects, with geographical and seasonal variation. Reaction depends on individual response, from none, through innocuous itchy papules, to blisters. Season and circumstance are usually sufficient to identify bites from gnats and mosquitoes. Flea and mite bites, when numerous and recurrent, can cause diagnostic difficulty and the term papular urticaria is used. Lesions are most numerous on the legs and lower trunk (**491**) but any area can be affected. Pruritic papules and weals may be grouped, sometimes linearly. A punctum may be seen at the centre of a lesion but this is usually obliterated by scratching because of intense itching. Bullae may occur, particularly on the legs (**492**). The condition is more common in children, though adults may also be affected. Cat and dog fleas are the most common pests. Bird fleas and mites can also cause problems. Secondary bacterial infection is a common complication.

DIFFERENTIAL DIAGNOSIS
Follicular eczema, dermatitis herpetiformis.

INVESTIGATIONS
Inspection of brushings from the cat or dog, and its bedding. Examination of the animal itself rarely shows infestation.

TREATMENT
Tracking down the causative agent is often difficult. Symptomatic treatment with topical antipruritics, oral antihistamines, and insect repellants may help.

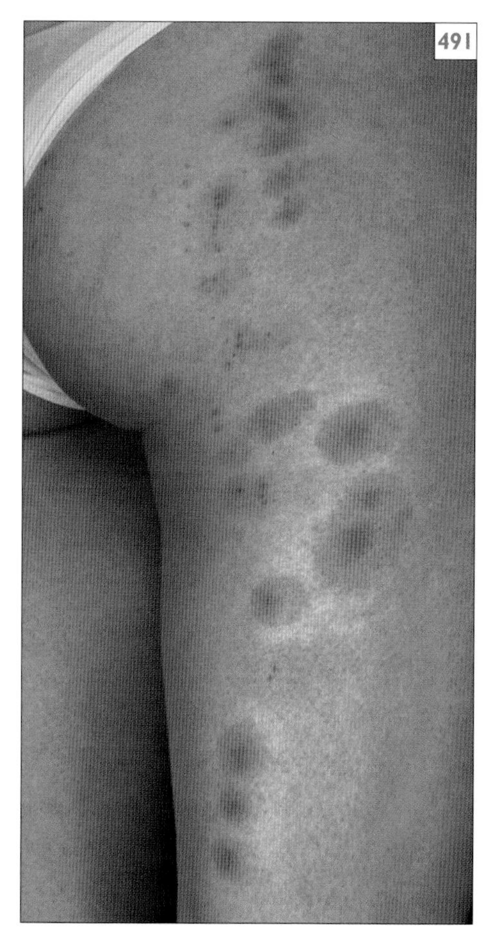

491 Papular urticaria.

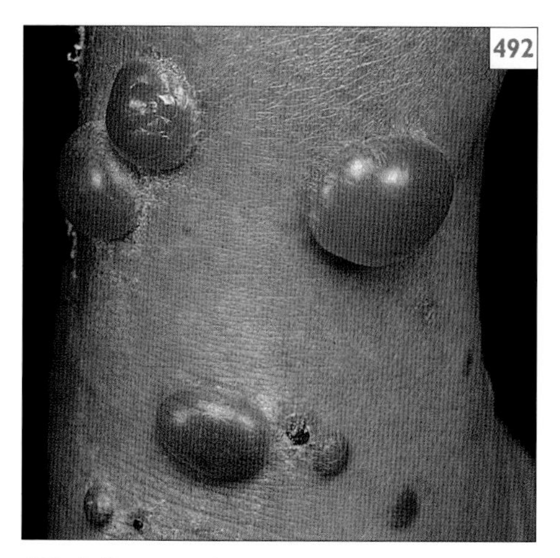

492 Bullous papular urticaria.

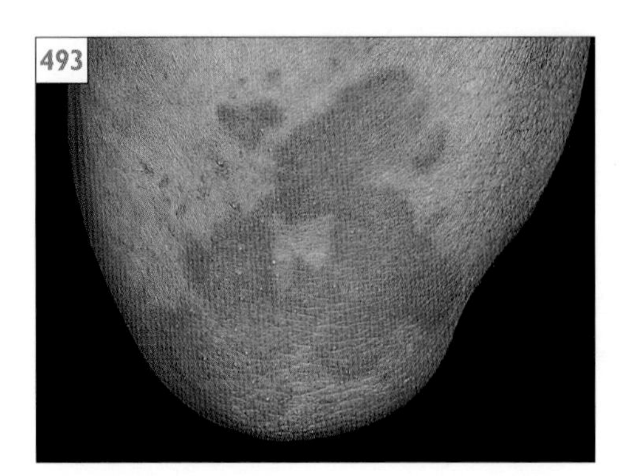

493 Insect sting reaction.

Insect stings

DEFINITION AND CLINICAL FEATURES

A local and sometimes systemic reaction to stings from insects, including wasps, bees, and ants. The injection of venom causes immediate pain, with gradually increasing swelling and erythema. Systemic reactions, such as wheeze, hypotension, and anaphylaxis, as well as florid local reactions (**493**) are usually caused by hypersensitivity to insect antigens.

INVESTIGATIONS

Radioallergosorbent tests (RASTs) can identify raised IgE levels to wasp or bee venom.

TREATMENT

Systemic allergic reactions need rapid treatment with adrenaline and supportive care; systemic antihistamines are sufficient for local reactions. Hyposensitization may be undertaken by skilled medical personnel in those with a history of life-threatening reactions, and only if resuscitation equipment is available.

Scabies

DEFINITION AND CLINICAL FEATURES

Infestation with *Sarcoptes scabiei*, a mite that burrows within the skin, giving rise to an intensely pruritic eruption. Mites are spread from person to person by close physical contact such as prolonged hand holding. Spread is facilitated by a latent period during which the scabies mite is carried asymptomatically. Itching starts 3–4 weeks after the infestation is acquired, and is so severe that sleep is frequently disturbed. The pathognomonic lesions of scabies are small linear burrows containing the mite (**494**). These can often be found on the hands, wrists, and feet or genitals, but may be sparse. The pruritus, urticated papules and occasional vesicles are thought to be a hypersensitivity reaction (**495**) and a widespread eczematous eruption usually occurs. Inflammatory papules on the penis are highly characteristic of scabies (**4968**) and are a helpful diagnostic clue when burrows cannot be identified. Scabietic nodules are intensely itchy and may persist for months after effective treatment (**497**).

Norwegian or crusted scabies is an uncommon subtype in which a deficient immune response allows huge numbers of scabies mites to multiply. The crusts and psoriasiform scale, loaded with scabies mites, affect the hands, scalp, face, and trunk (**500**). Itching may be minimal. Susceptible individuals are often only marginally immunosuppressed and may simply be elderly, pregnant, or have learning difficulties. It is not uncommon in patients with AIDS. Norwegian scabies is highly contagious and may give rise to outbreaks within hospitals and institutions.

DIFFERENTIAL DIAGNOSIS

Diagnosis is not difficult in the presence of typical burrows. Papular urticaria, eczema, pemphigoid, and many other itchy dermatoses have all been misdiagnosed. Animal scabies and mites can cause similar urticated erythematous papules without burrows.

INVESTIGATIONS

Microscopy of a mite or scrapings from a burrow confirms the diagnosis.

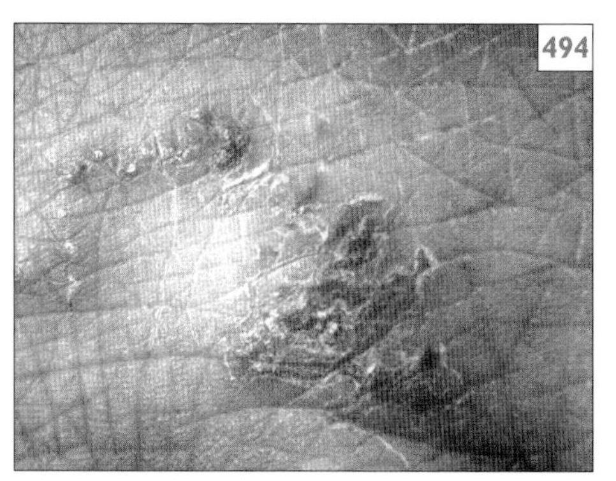

494 Scabies burrows.

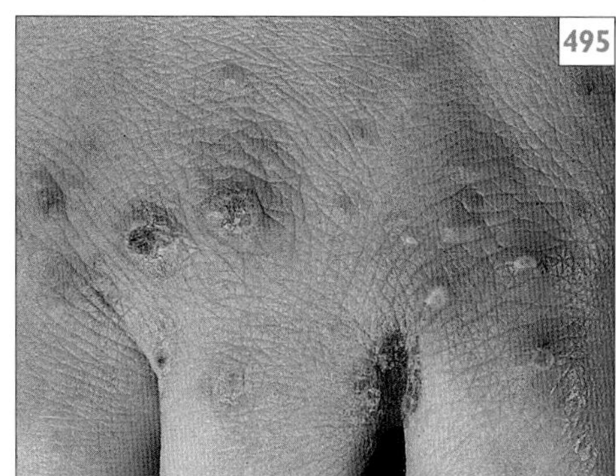

495 Scabies papules.

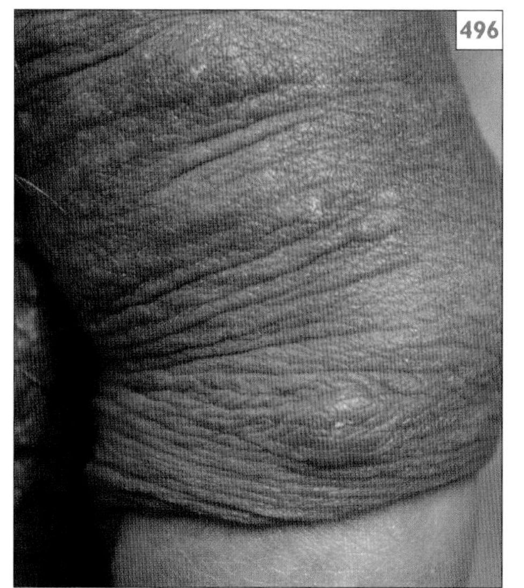

496 Scabies penile inflammatory papules.

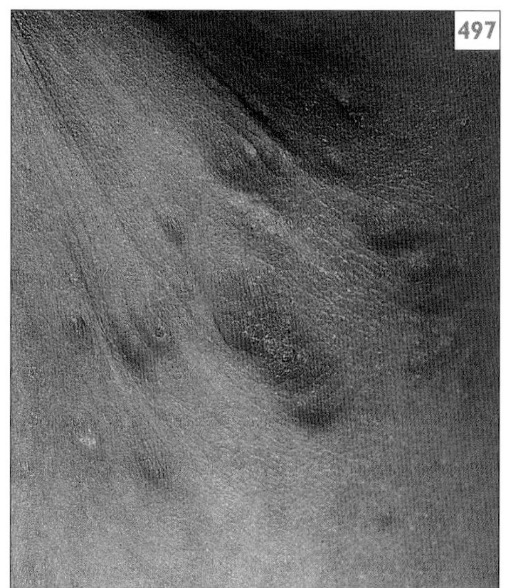

497 Scabietic nodules.

TREATMENT

A range of topical agents with scabicidal activity are available including permethrim and malathion. These should be applied for 12–24 hours and treatment repeated after a week. All close contacts must be treated simultaneously whether symptomatic or not in order to prevent reinfestation. Oral ivermectin appears safe and effective and is useful in management of outbreaks of scabies in institutions but is unlicensed. Ordinary laundering of clothing and bedding is adequate to clear infestation.

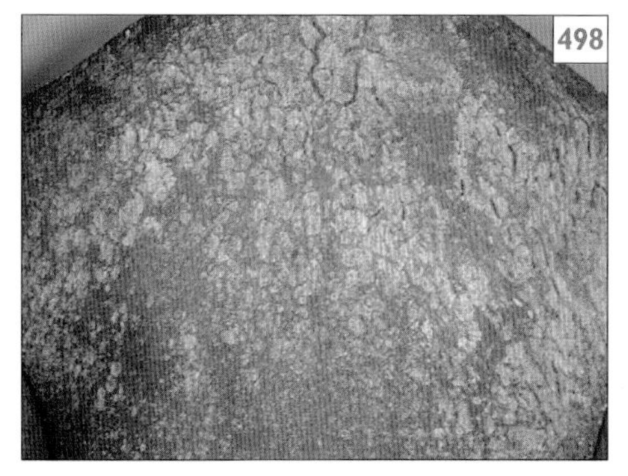

498 Crusted scabies.

Bed bugs

DEFINITION AND CLINICAL FEATURES

Bites from the blood sucking insect *Cimex lectularius*. Bed bugs live in cracks in walls and furnishings and under loose wallpaper and usually feed at night. They can survive long periods of starvation. Bites usually affect the face, neck, and arms. They appear as itchy papules, with a central punctum, are often grouped or linear (**499**). Bed bugs are visible to the naked eye – they are brown, oval, wingless bugs with flattened bodies (**500**). Similar bugs, normally affecting birds, can also bite humans.

DIFFERENTIAL DIAGNOSIS

Bites from flying insects.

TREATMENT

Bites may be treated symptomatically with topical antipruritics and antihistamines. Furniture and bedding must be thoroughly treated to eradicate bed bugs.

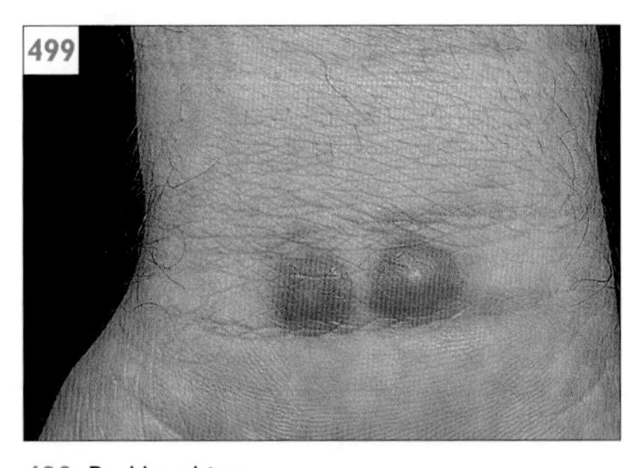

499 Bed bug bites.

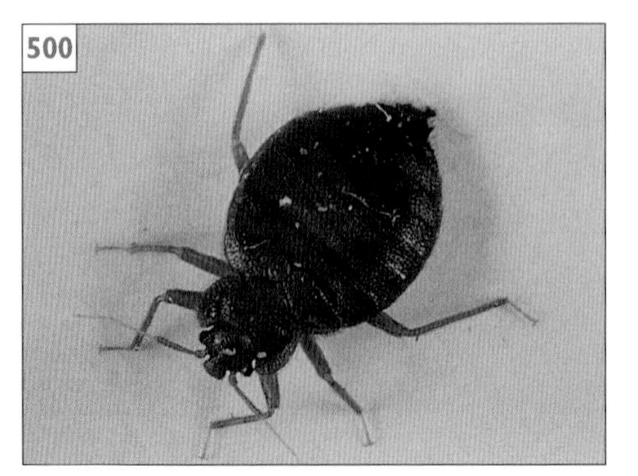

500 Bed bug.

Lice

Humans may be parasitized by three species of louse, *Pediculus capitis*, the head louse, *Pediculus humanus*, the body louse, and *Pthirus pubis*, the pubic or crab louse.

Head lice
(pediculosis capitis)

DEFINITION AND CLINICAL FEATURES

This is an infestation of the scalp with the head louse. It is endemic among primary school children and is commoner in girls. Pruritus may lead to excoriations, secondary infection, and lymphadenopathy. Adult lice are usually scanty but their nits (the white oval eggs) can be found adhering to hair shafts (**501**), particularly around the nape of the neck and ears.

TREATMENT

Topical insecticides such as malathion, carbaryl, and permethrin are effective pediculocides. However, widespread resistance is emerging and non-chemical alternatives include repeated removal of lice with a fine tooth comb after shampooing and conditioning.

SPECIAL POINT

Head lice are difficult to eradicate and may affect adults.

Pubic lice (pediculosis pubis)

DEFINITION AND CLINICAL FEATURES

An infestation of the pubic area by the crab louse, which presents with an itching in the pubic area. Crab lice are transmitted by close contact, and are usually sexually transmitted. Lice and nits can be seen. In children, crab lice may colonize the eyelashes and scalp (**502**).

TREATMENT

Topical pediculocides. All sexual contacts should also be treated and patients should be screened for other sexually transmitted infections.

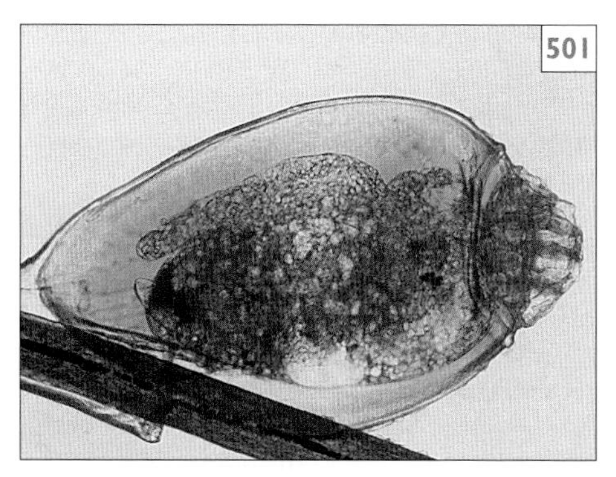
501 Head lice nit (egg).

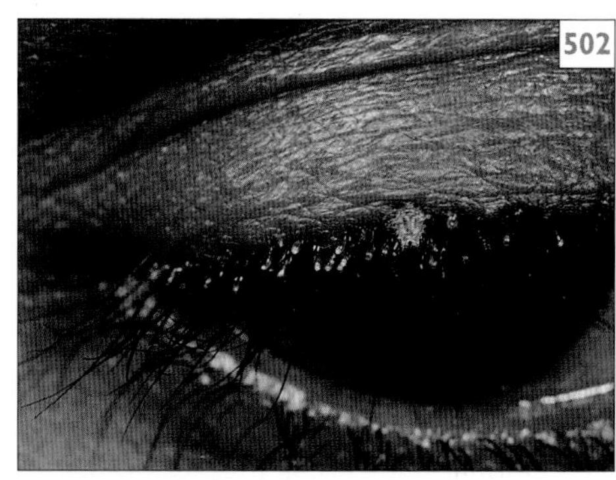
502 Crab louse in the eyelashes.

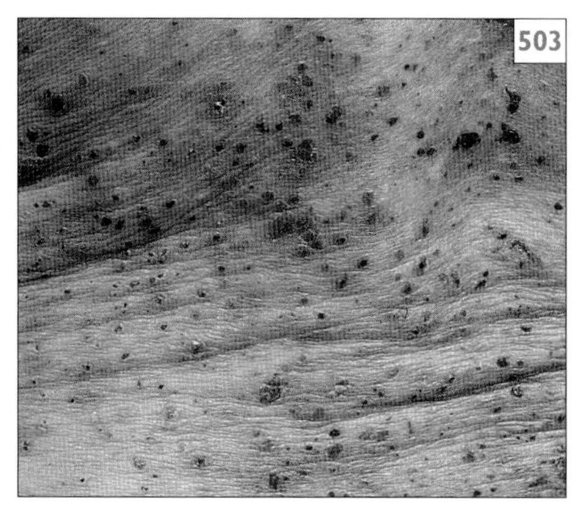
503 Body lice lesions.

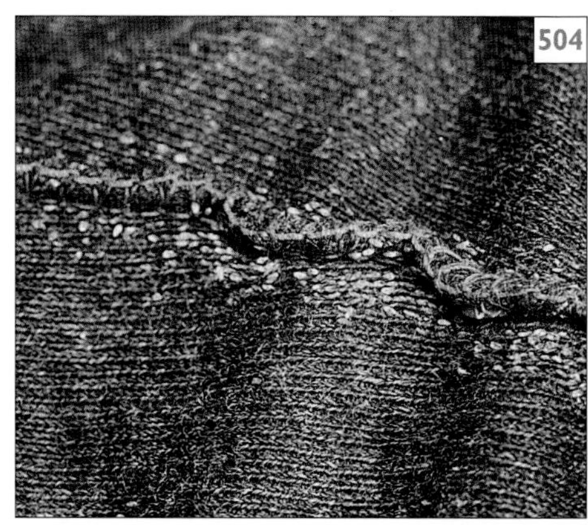
504 Body lice in a seam.

Body lice (pediculosis corporis)

DEFINITION AND CLINICAL FEATURES

Infestation of the body and clothing by the body louse. This infestation occurs in situations of poverty and neglect, and in developed countries, mainly affects vagrants. Itching results from sensitization to louse saliva. The body may be covered in excoriations with secondary infection and pigmentation (**503**). Red macules and papules can sometimes be seen. Inspection of clothing reveals lice and their eggs in the seams (**504**).

DIFFERENTIAL DIAGNOSIS

Pruritus of systemic disease may be confused, particularly in a hospitalized patient in clean pyjamas.

TREATMENT

Clothing needs to be destroyed or treated with topical insecticides or hot laundered in order to prevent reinfestation.

TROPICAL INFECTIONS

Cutaneous leishmaniasis
(oriental sore)

DEFINITION AND CLINICAL FEATURES

This is a localized cutaneous reaction to infection by the protozoon *Leishmania* which is transmitted by sandfly bites. It may cause cutaneous, mucosal, or visceral disease. Many species of *Leishmania* exist but most cases seen in travellers returning from tropical areas are due to *L. tropica*, *L. major*, and *L. aethiopica*. It is a disease of warm countries, occurring around the Mediterranean coast, North Africa, South America, central Asia, and China.

In the dry urban form, a small, brownish-purple nodule forms after an incubation period of around 2 months. This slowly enlarges to around 1–2 cm, at which time a shallow central ulcer covered by an adherent crust forms (**505**, **506**) which eventually heals by scarring after 8–12 months.

In the wet rural form, the lesions begin earlier after inoculation, and ulceration also occurs earlier (**507**). Secondary nodules may occur around lymphatics (**508**) and healing usually takes place in 2–6 months.

DIFFERENTIAL DIAGNOSIS

Boils due to *Staphylococcus aureus*, or secondarily infected insect bites heal within a few weeks.

INVESTIGATIONS

Skin biopsy or smear for identification of organisms and specialized culture. A cutaneous test (the leishmanin test) is positive in about 90% of cases.

TREATMENT

Small lesions may heal spontaneously but leave scars. Pentavalent antimonials are the drugs of choice and may be used intralesionally or systemically. Small lesions may respond to cryotherapy, heat therapy, or excision. Other drug options include azoles and terbinafine.

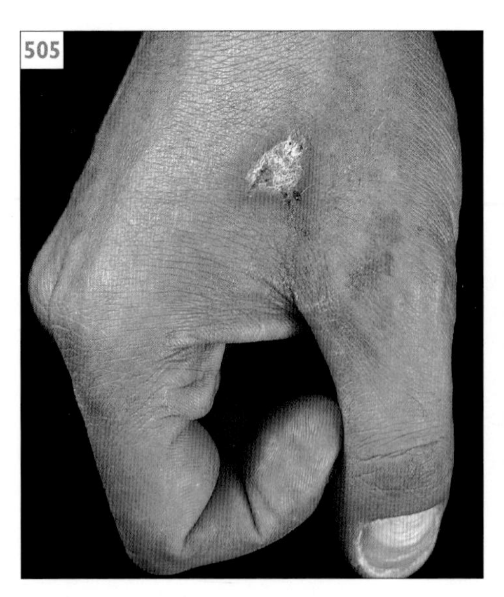

505 Cutaneous leishmaniasis.

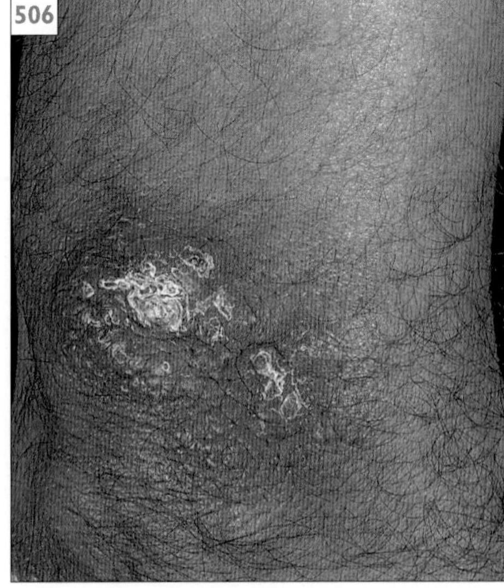

506 Cutaneous leishmaniasis.

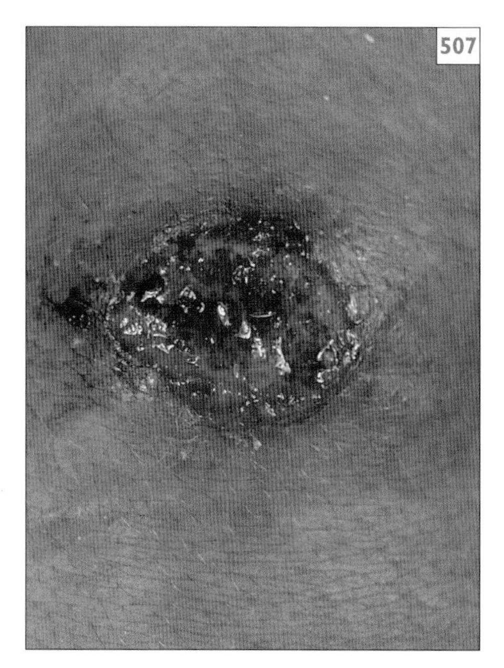

507 Ulcerated cutaneous leishmaniasis.

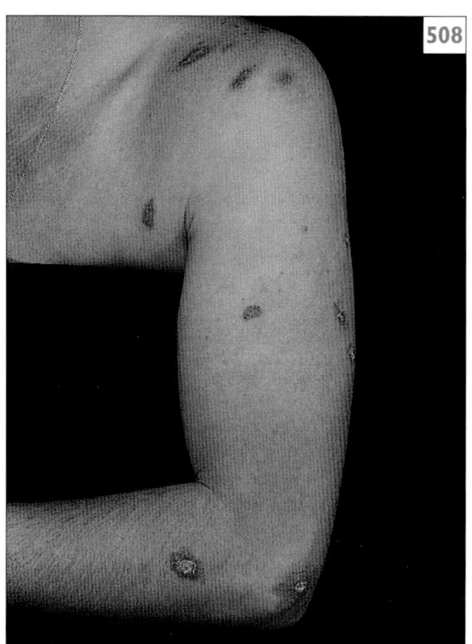

508 Secondary nodules of cutaneous leishmaniasis.

Cutaneous myiasis

DEFINITION AND CLINICAL FEATURES

Myiasis is the infestation of skin of humans and animals by the larvae of flies (Diptera). Infestation may be obligate, where a parasitic phase is essential to the life cycle, or facultative where larvae usually develop on decaying matter but may infest wounds. Larvae (maggots) may be capable of penetrating intact skin (e.g. botfly, blow fly, tumbu fly) to produce furuncle-like lesions (**509**) especially on exposed sites such as the face, scalp, or limbs. Lesions are extremely painful and discharge serosanguinous fluid. Other larvae are secondary invaders of neglected wounds and ulcers (e.g. blue bottles and houseflies).

DIFFERENTIAL DIAGNOSIS

Furunculosis.

INVESTIGATIONS

None usually necessary.

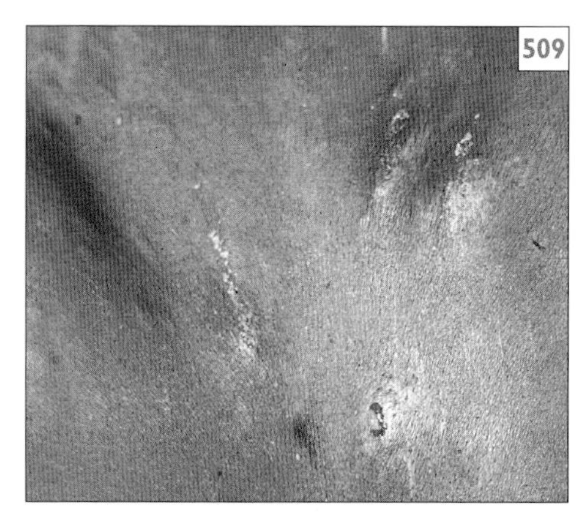

509 Cutaneous myiasis.

TREATMENT

Larvae may be expressed from furuncular lesions by firm pressure after surgical enlargement of the punctum and injection of local anaesthetic.

Onchocerciasis

DEFINITION AND CLINICAL FEATURES

A filarial disease caused by *Onchocerca volvulus*. The disease usually presents with pruritus erythema and urticated papules followed by a non-specific papular rash. The buttocks and shoulders are commonly affected (**510**). Gross lichenification and small scars eventually develop (**511**) followed by atrophy and loss of skin elasticity.

Onchocercomata are painless swellings, sited close to bony prominences, where mature worms may be found. Onchocerciasis is found throughout tropical Africa, Arabia, Central America, and Mexico. Transmission of larvae occurs through the bites of tiny black flies. All ages are affected. Without treatment, symptoms increase in severity until atrophic changes are complete. Microfilaria also invade the eye and can lead to blindness.

DIFFERENTIAL DIAGNOSIS

General pruritus from other causes such as iron deficiency anaemia should be excluded. Scabies and body lice commonly cause a generalized pruritus but the presence of burrows or lice in clothing seams will help to separate these.

INVESTIGATIONS

Skin snips taken from the legs or buttocks at night are examined in saline for the presence of microfilariae. Nodules can be excised and submitted for histology. A filarial skin test is usually positive. A full blood count may reveal eosinophilia, and a filarial complement fixation test is positive in over 60% of cases.

TREATMENT

The antihelminth drug ivermectin is effective in a single oral dose and patients living in endemic areas may be retreated after 6–12 months.

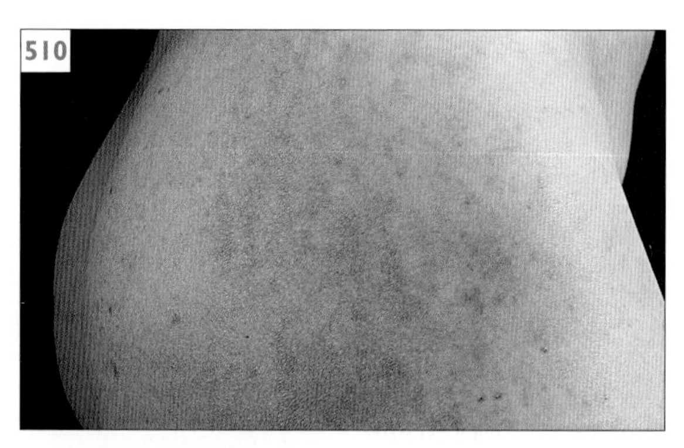

510 Onchocerciasis.

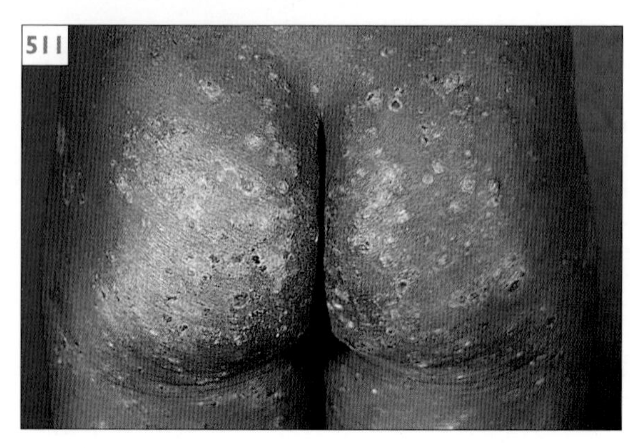

511 Onchocerciasis.

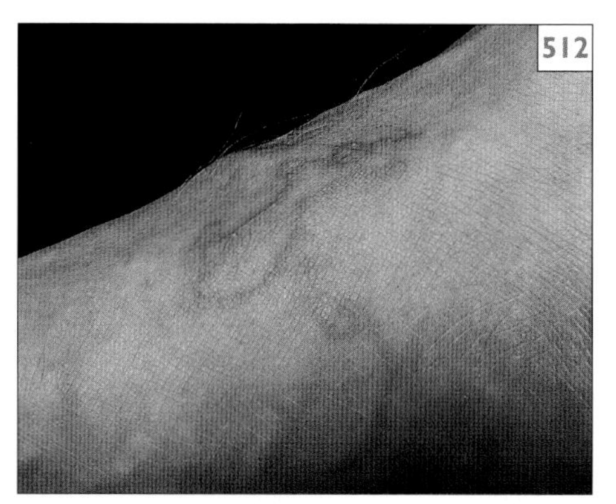

512 Creeping eruption.

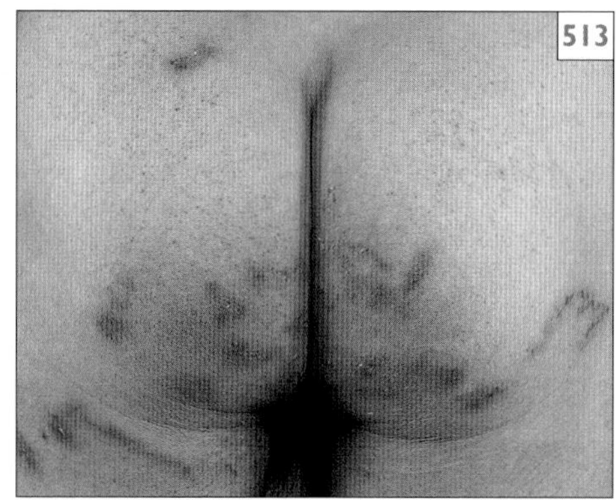

513 Creeping eruption.

Creeping eruption
(cutaneous larva migrans)

DEFINITION AND CLINICAL FEATURES

A self-limiting cutaneous eruption caused by the migration of animal hookworm larvae for whom man is a dead-end host. Most cases are caused by dog and cat hookworm larvae which penetrate the skin in moist, shaded, sandy areas such as tropical beaches. The eruption is composed of intensely itchy, serpiginous, pink tracks which advance about a centimetre per day (**512**). Large numbers of larvae produce a disorganized collection of tortuous tracks (**513**). Sites exposed to sand, such as the feet and buttocks, are the commonest areas to be affected in travellers returning from tropical countries. The larvae wander through the epidermis until they eventually die after around 4 weeks.

DIFFERENTIAL DIAGNOSIS

Lesions of *Strongyloides stercoralis* advance faster, are frequently perianal, and are associated with intestinal involvement. Migratory myiasis produces shorter tracks with a terminal vesicle which often breaks down.

INVESTIGATIONS

None usually required.

TREATMENT

The lesions respond quickly to treatment with a single dose of ivermectin or a 3-day course of albendazole.

Strongyloidiasis
(larva currens)

DEFINITION AND CLINICAL FEATURES

A parasitic infection with the roundworm *Strongyloides stercoralis*. It is most prevalent in warm damp climates, especially southeast Asia. Infective larvae penetrate the skin and may cause dermatitis. Larvae mature in the gut and may reinfect the patient by penetrating the perianal mucosal. Migrating larvae in the skin give rise to a wheal and flare response which follows the path of the larva. Generalized urticaria may also occur. Heavy worm infestation may cause enteritis and malabsorption.

DIFFERENTIAL DIAGNOSIS

Hookworm infestation also causes pruritis, but the clinical course is different with prominent pneumonitis and iron deficiency anaemia.

INVESTIGATIONS

Total IgE levels are raised and a full blood count usually shows eosinophilia. Larvae of *Strongyloides* spp. are demonstrated in the faeces and jejunal samples. Serological testing may also be performed for *Strongyloides* antibodies.

TREATMENT

Albendazole or ivermectin given orally. Patients should be followed up after 3 and 6 months with stool samples to ensure eradication.

INDEX